A HANDBOOK FOR INTERPROFESSIONAL PRACTICE IN THE HUMAN SERVICES

A HANDBOOK FOR INTERPROFESSIONAL PRACTICE IN THE HUMAN SERVICES

Learning to work together

Edited by Brian Littlechild and Roger Smith

PEARSON

Harlow, England • London • New York • Boston • San Francisco • Toronto • Sydney
Auckland • Singapore • Hong Kong • Tokyo • Seoul • Taipei • New Delhi
Cape Town • São Paulo • Mexico City • Madrid • Amsterdam • Munich • Paris • Milan

Pearson Education Limited

Edinburgh Gate
Harlow
Essex CM20 2JE
England

and Associated Companies throughout the world

Visit us on the World Wide Web at:
www.pearson.com/uk

First published 2013

© Pearson Education Limited 2013

ISBN 978-1-4082-2440-3

British Library Cataloguing-in-Publication Data
A catalogue record for this book is available from the British Library

Library of Congress Cataloguing-in-Publication Data
A catalog record for this book is available from the Library of Congress

10 9 8 7 6 5 4 3 2 1
16 15 14 13 12

Typeset in 10/13 pt Minionpro by 32
Printed and bound by Ashford Colour Press Ltd, Gosport, Hampshire

Brief contents

Contents

Contents

Chapter 9
Safeguarding children and child protection 117

Mary McColgan, Anne Campbell and James Marshall

Chapter 10
Children in need, looked-after children and interprofessional working 131

Nick Frost

Chapter 11
Older people 143

Michelle Cornes

Chapter 12
End-of-life care 159

Suzy Croft

Contents

Contents

Contributors

Professor Brian Littlechild is Associate Head of School of Nursing, Midwifery and Social Work at the University of Hertfordshire. As a social worker/manager, he specialised in work with children, young people and their families, and mental health. He continues to practise with young offenders.

Brian has researched and published widely on violence against staff, youth offending, child protection, mental health, and risk in social work and mental health. He has acted as a consultant to the Council of Europe on young people held in custody, and also on social exclusion, education and youth offending.

Professor Roger Smith is Professor in Social Work in the School of Applied Social Sciences at Durham University. As a practitioner, he worked in multi-agency settings with young offenders. Since becoming a social work academic, he has worked extensively in developing, delivering and evaluating interprofessional education as part of a wide-ranging multidisciplinary partnership in Leicester, which is recognised as a leader in the field. He has also researched and published widely in youth justice, research methodology and social work theory and methods.

Hugh Barr is Emeritus Professor of Interprofessional Education and an Honorary Fellow at the University of Westminster. He holds visiting chairs in that field in several other universities. He is President of the UK Centre for the Advancement of Interprofessional Education.

Hugh McLaughlin is Professor of Social Work at Manchester Metropolitan University. His research and teaching interests include the possibilities and limits of participatory research, critical professional practice and research informed practice. His recent books include *Understanding Social Work Research* (2nd edn.) (2012, Sage) and *Service-User Research in Health and Social Care* (2009, Sage).

John Hughes works as Director of Interventions in Hertfordshire Probation Trust where he has been employed as a senior manager for nine years. Prior to this he was the lead Criminal Justice Inspector in Northern Ireland, a senior probation officer in Somerset and a probation officer in Birmingham. He has masters degrees in social work and public sector management and an MBA.

Sue Urwin is a social sciences graduate from Birmingham University and qualified as a probation officer in 1977. She has worked in various generic and specialist probation posts and latterly has been seconded to Hertfordshire Criminal Justice Board to develop Diversion Panels and practice and policy for Mentally Disordered Offenders in furtherance of the recommendations of the Bradley Report. Sue was awarded the MBE in 2012 for services to Probation and Mentally Disordered Offenders work.

Dr Stephanie Sadler is Consultant Psychiatrist in Adult Mental Health with Hertfordshire Partnership NHS Foundation Trust; in her early career she worked as a general practitioner. Her research and teaching interests include bipolar disorder, schizophrenia, psychiatry and the law, and the management of mental disorder in pregnant women. Stephanie sits on the Hertfordshire Diversion Panel and was an adviser in the formulation of the Independent Safeguarding Authority.

Professor Di Bailey is the Head of Division for Social Work, Health and Social Care and Counselling at Nottingham Trent University. Di is a psychologist by background and a registered social worker. She has a special interest in the field of mental health, in particular interdisciplinary working and service-user involvement. Di is the author of *Interdisciplinary Working in Mental Health* (2012, Palgrave Macmillan) and editor of *At the Core of Mental Health Practice: Key Issues for Practitioners, Managers and Mental Health Trainers* (2000, Pavilion Publishing).

Michelle Culwick is Academic Subject Leader for Interprofessional Practice at the University of Wales, Newport. Her research and teaching interests include social work with children and families, interprofessional working and learning and evidence-based practice. Her current PhD research explores the experiences of social workers working with abused disabled children. She is co-author of *Sharing Assessment in Health and Social Care: A Practical Handbook for Interprofessional Working* (2009, Sage).

Carolyn Wallace is Principal Lecturer in Continuing Healthcare at the University of Glamorgan. Her research interests include the different ways in which professionals work together, public sector integration and frailty. Carolyn is the only nurse member of Welsh Crucible 2011. Among a number of other publications, Carolyn is the co-author of the new guidance for Multidisciplinary Working which was published by NHS Wales Continuing Healthcare programme board in September 2011.

Professor Mary McColgan has been a social worker and manager, and is now Head of School of Sociology and Applied Social Studies at the University of Ulster. Professor McColgan has published widely on a variety of childcare issues. Her recent contributions include book chapters in *Social Work Interventions* (2009), edited by Trevor Lindsay, and *Working with Aggression and Resistance in Social Work* (2010) edited by Brian Taylor.

Anne Campbell is a Senior Lecturer in Social Work at the University of Ulster. Her research and teaching interests include youth offending, substance misuse, women's mental health and research methods. She is a contributor to *Social Work Interventions* (2009), edited by Trevor Lindsay.

James Marshall is an Associate Lecturer in Social work at the University of Ulster, and also works as an independent social worker. His main teaching and research interests are child protection and the investigative interviewing of children for court. His recent publications include *Family and Child Care: Social Work Practice Guide* (2010, Belfast Health and Social Care Board).

Nick Frost is Professor of Social Work (Childhood, children and families) at the Faculty of Health and Social Sciences, Leeds Metropolitan University. Nick has published widely including most recently *Understanding Children's Social Care* (with Nigel Parton, 2009, Sage), as co-editor of *Beyond Reflective Practice* (with Bradbury *et al.*, 2010) and *Understanding Childhood and Families* (2011, Continuum). Nick worked in local authority social work for 15 years before commencing his academic career. He is Independent Chairperson of Bradford Safeguarding Children Board.

Michelle Cornes is a Research Fellow at the Social Care Workforce Research Unit at King's College London. Her main areas of interest are the social care workforce, interprofessional working and integrated care. She has completed evaluations on behalf of the Department of Health and the Scottish Government and has most recently completed an ESRC-funded study exploring multiple exclusion homelessness.

Suzy Croft is Senior Social Worker and Team Leader at St. John's Hospice and Research Fellow at the Centre for Citizen Participation at Brunel University. She has worked in palliative care social work for over 20 years and is an active member of the Association of Palliative Care Social Workers including as Chair. She has a background of work on participation and empowerment. She is a co-author of *Palliative Care, Social Work and Service Users*, published by Jessica Kingsley Publishers in 2007. She is currently a member of the Transition Board of the new College of Social Work.

Glenis Donaldson is a Senior Lecturer at Manchester Metropolitan University where she teaches on the physiotherapy degree programmes. She was a senior clinician specialising in paediatrics for 16 years and became interested in disability issues when working as a research assistant in Lancaster in 2003.

Bob Sapey is a Senior Lecturer at Lancaster University where he teaches mental health on the social work degrees. He was a practitioner with disabled people for 19 years before moving into higher education in 1993. He is co-author of *Social Work with Disabled People* which is now in its 4th edition.

Peter Beresford OBE is Professor of Social Policy and Director of the Centre for Citizen Participation at Brunel University. He has experience as a long-term user of mental health services and is Chair of Shaping

Our Lives, the independent national user controlled organisation and network. He has a long-standing involvement in issues of participation as educator, researcher, writer, commentator and activist. His most recent books include *Being a Mental Health Service User* (2010, PCCS Books) and *Supporting People* (2011, The Policy Press). He is a member of many government bodies and committees, including the Social Work Reform Board and the National Institute for Health Research Advisory Board.

Carmel Byers is a Senior Lecturer at the University of Hertfordshire. Her main teaching is in the area of social work theories, methods and interventions. She has a strong interest in service-user and carer involvement in planning, delivery and provision of services and social work education, and has been involved in writing, and research in this area, as well as presenting at conferences jointly with the 'Creating Links' – People Using Services and Carers group at the University of Hertfordshire.

'Creating Links'–People Using Services and Carers group at the University of Hertfordshire is involved in all aspects of the curriculum for the social work programmes delivered by the university, including teaching and assessment, new student selection, course development, writing, research and conference presentations. The highlight of the work of the group each year is the planning, designing and delivery of a week's block module on the BSc Social Work entitled, Working in Collaboration with People Using Services.'

Mary Rees taught in primary, secondary and special schools before moving to the School of Education, University of Hertfordshire, where she is currently Head of Regional Partnership Development. Her current research interest is in the impact of inquiry on practitioners.

Elizabeth Anderson is a Senior Lecturer in shared learning within the Medical School at the University of Leicester. She has led innovations for community education for medical students and for interprofessional education and is a National Teaching Fellow. She is joint author of the *Leicester Model of Interprofessional Education*, published by the Higher Education Academy in 2007, and has published widely on innovations in IPE. She was a contributor

to *Interprofessional Education. Making it Happen* in 2009 and *Listening to Children and Young People in Healthcare Consultations* in 2010.

Angela Lennox is a Senior Lecturer and Head of the Professional Development Unit at the Medical School in the University of Leicester. She is a general medical practitioner and advisor to the Department of Health. She is a joint author of the '*Leicester Model of Interprofessional Education*', published by the Higher Education Academy Subject Centre for Medicine, Dentistry and Veterinary Medicine, Special Report 2007. Her interests include inequalities in health and inner city regeneration.

Chris McKenna is a Senior Lecturer in Occupational Therapy at Teesside University. He developed his clinical expertise in learning disabilities services. In 1995 Chris began teaching occupational therapists, focusing on occupational therapy theory and the guiding framework for applying theory into practice. Current areas of interest are the issues impacting on individuals' motivation and OT perspectives on interprofessional working.

Cath Wright is a Senior Lecturer in Occupational Therapy at Teesside University. She has had experience in a wide variety of practice areas and had responsibility for a range of interprofessional teams. Her interests lie within leadership and service development and her current research is in the area of co-dependence. Cath has served as Council Member for the British Association of Occupational Therapists/College of Occupational Therapists.

Steve J Hothersall is a Senior Lecturer in Social Work at the Robert Gordon University, Aberdeen. He has worked as practitioner and manager in children's services and taught across the UK and Europe. He is the author, co-author and editor of several books and has a particular interest in work with children, young people and their families and applied philosophy, particularly pragmatism. Steve also practises as a children's safeguarder and a curator ad litem.

Patricia White is Senior Physiotherapy Lecturer in the School of Allied Health Professions, Faculty of Health and Social Care, University of The West of England, Bristol, and has contributed to the develpement of interprofessional education within the School.

Paul Illingworth is Head of School – Nursing and Midwifery at Birmingham City University. Paul has had over 35 years clinical, operational, project and strategic management experience in a variety of education, healthcare settings and additionally the civil service in the UK. His teaching/research interests are interprofessional/agency and partnership working; interprofessional education; mental health service-user/carer involvement; qualitative research methods; evidence-based practice and quality assurance. He co-edited and contributed to *Mental Health Nursing: Carving a Path to Practice* (2010, Pearson Education) and contributed a chapter on partnership working in mental health to *Caring for Adults with Mental Health Problems* (2007, Wiley).

Neena Lakhani is a Senior Lecturer in Clinical Pharmacy and Pharmacy Practice at the Leicester School of Pharmacy, Faculty of Health and Life Sciences, DeMontfort University. She is also a practicing pharmacist, with experience in hospital, community and primary care pharmacy. Her research interests include development and evaluation of interprofessional education programmes and practice research in the use of community pharmacy services by the South Asian Minority Ethnic population.

Brian Simon is a hospital pharmacist and a pharmacy lecturer at De Montfort University. He is a registered practitioner with the General Pharmaceutical Council.

Pamela Ward, BDS, MFGDP(UK), FHEA, has a background as a dentist in general dental practice spanning many years where the emphasis was on community dentistry. Her practice was selected as a Field Site by the Modernisation Agency to develop an approach based on the concept of dental teamwork. For several years she has been an examiner with the Faculty of General Dental Practitioners. In 2007 she joined, in its first year, the Peninsula Dental School as an Enquiry-based Learning Facilitator. In her various roles she has developed an interest in interprofessional practice.

Acknowledgements

Author's acknowledgements

To my parents, Charles and Violet, for setting me along the way. To Carole, my friend and wife for 30 years, for your support and unstinting commitment to our family. To our son Tom, who has been, and is, a constant source of joy and pride. Thank you both.

—Brian Littlechild

Roger Smith would like to acknowledge the contribution of colleagues from Corby JLB from whom he learnt the practicalities and value of collaborative practice, the many academic colleagues and students who have made interprofessional learning such a productive experience, and once again, Maggie, Emma, Claire and Daniel.

—Roger Smith

We would like to thank all the contributors to this book for their inspiration, hard work and commitment to this book.

Publisher's acknowledgements

The publishers would like to thank the anonymous panel of reviewers for their helpful comments on the initial proposal and the draft manuscript.

The publishers would further like to thank both Editors for the dedication, effort and skill they've demonstrated in producing this book, and also to thank the contributing authors for their chapters.

We are grateful to the following for permission to reproduce copyright material:

Figures

Figure 13.2 from *International Classifications of Functioning Disability and Health,* World Health Organization (WHO) (World Health Organization (WHO) 1980) p. 18; Figure 20.1 from *Changing Lives: Summary Report of the 21st Century Social Work Review,* Scottish Executive (Scottish Executive 2006) p. 16, Available at: http://www.scotland.gov.uk/Resource/Doc/91949/0021950.pdf; ISBN: 0755949382, Crown Copyright material is reproduced with permission under the terms of the Click-Use license.

Tables

Table on page 145 from *Comprehensive Assessment for the Older Frail Patient – Best Practice Guide,* 3.5, January, British Geriatrics Society (British Geriatrics Society 2010) p.1, http://www.bgs.org.uk/index.php?option=com_content&view=article&id=195:gpgcgassessment&catid=12:goodpractice&itemid=39 (Accessed 15th March 2010).

In some instances we have been unable to trace the owners of copyright material, and we would appreciate any information that would enable us to do so.

Introduction

Brian Littlechild and Roger Smith

Recent years have seen substantial changes in organisational and operational requirements and arrangements in respect of collaborative working between health and social care agencies and professionals. Consequently, there have been significant impacts on the education and training arrangements needed to prepare different professionals in light of the greatly increased emphasis on interprofessional and interagency working. There are more and more explicit expectations from UK and national governments in public statements, and in policy and regulatory documents, such as *Working together to safeguard children* (Department for Children Schools and Families, 2010), demanding effective interagency and interprofessional working arrangements in the planning and delivery of services.

Structural arrangements now encompass a number of professional groupings under one service heading, or under one roof, such as in some Community Learning Disabilities teams and Community Mental Health teams. To reflect these changes, there has been at the same time a distinct shift in expectations about the need for professionals to understand each other's roles and agencies, mirrored by more frequent opportunities for shared learning at qualifying and post-qualifying levels for different professionals.

This book provides a comprehensive account and analysis of key issues for those who are or will be working with different service user and professional groups, addressing for students, practitioners and managers the different levels and areas of knowledge – including, crucially, those from service users and carers – necessary to carry out fit for purpose interprofessional and interagency service delivery. It does this by marshalling and applying the knowledge base presented in the different chapters' key issues for the professional and service-user groups involved, thereby enabling professionals to understand the complexity of issues involved, and to work in interprofessional settings and contexts in a confident and effective manner.

There are relatively few texts that have addressed the needs of a wide range of professional groups to 'learn with, from and about each other' (Centre for the Advancement of Interprofessional Education, 2002), located within the different settings in which health and social care agencies and professionals operate. It is difficult not to favour one perspective or another, or to offer a sufficiently eclectic mix of expertise, experience and viewpoints. This book starts to fill that gap, in that it provides a wide-ranging resource for initial training and post-qualifying stages which can provide insights into both the generic challenges of collaborative working, and key contexts where these challenges need to be met, such as health and social care services, education and school services, offender services, children's services and continuing care.

The book provides an integrated and cross-cutting professional, cross-agency set of materials, giving a 360-degree view of interprofessional working. In particular, the book provides for the perspectives of service users and carers on shared working and its impact on service delivery, as well as those of the different professional groups concerned. The contribution of service users and carers has rarely been fully explored in the literature, although the main purpose of collaborative practice should be to improve services for these groups; to be best prepared to do that, we need to actively consider the issues from these groups' viewpoints, as this book does.

In doing so, we examine these areas in both theoretical and practical ways, not only examining research and policy areas which we need to understand in relation to the framing of such services, but also describing what each profession or agency covered in the book does. The book's contents identify key agencies and professionals within different professional and service-user group settings, their responsibilities and duties, locating these considerations within discussion and analysis of case studies, based on how the work is actually undertaken.

Our intention has been to offer insights from which different professionals will be able to have an understanding of the roles of the other professions in their area of work, and what the ways of working of those other professionals are; how best to understand those roles; and therefore how best to approach such working from this knowledge, focused on the needs and expectations of all involved, including service users and carers. In safeguarding children work for example, it is clear from a number of serious case reviews (see e.g. Brandon *et al.*, 2009; Ofsted, 2008) that professionals and agencies often do not understand well enough the roles or drivers of others, thereby increasing risks to children.

The book thus incorporates distinct thematic components, such as teamworking, boundary issues and power and status issues between professionals, set within policy/legal and theoretical and practice-oriented perspectives. In so doing it provides materials introducing and discussing 'live' examples from a number of distinct service areas, such as safeguarding children, work with young people, people with mental health problems, work with older people, and people with learning disabilities in Part Two. In Part Three we look at discipline-specific viewpoints, enabling the reader to gain insights into the challenges of collaborative working from the discipline-based perspectives of a number of professional groupings. By looking at that professional group's own internal workings and background, we can see how these relate to how interprofessional working can be best operationalised.

We believe this book is distinctive in that we have looked at the issues of how best to provide services from not only the core questions about interprofessional working from the different perspectives of all those involved, and worked through for particular service-user groups and the different professional groups, but also, crucially, reflecting recent developments and growing emphasis on the involvement of service-users and carers, and the place of these interest groups in the delivery and planning of services. The book features a number of contributions illustrating the challenges of delivering good practice from the service-user/carer perspective, which will help us to address issues such as collusion, dissonance and perceived power and influence differentials between professional interests, for instance. The inclusion of chapters by Peter Beresford on the effective inclusion of service users in interprofessional working, and Carmel Byers and the *Creating Links* group on the inclusion of carers, add important perspectives to ideas and approaches around interprofessional working.

We have attempted to provide the broadest spread of chapters with different emphases, providing a variety of perspectives on interprofessional working. For those reading the book in its totality, or selectively, the editors hope that the chapters will aid them in exploring what they need to know for their own areas of learning or work – and about assessments, interventions, and review of services while improving each agency and group's mutual understanding – an essential prequel to effective working practices.

A number of the chapters provide information about groups of service users or professionals, and also provide more general lessons for other areas and groups in the discussion about key issues for interprofessional working and interprofessional education. We have endeavoured to use examples of areas of practice which can give the widest lessons for all types of interprofessional working, professionals, agencies and service-user groups, so for example, we use an exemplar of Hertfordshire Mentally Disordered Offenders Interagency Panels, where the chapter draws on the actual experiences of the professionals and agencies involved to set out the general lessons for all involved in interagency working.

Part One provides the foundation for the rest of the book, examining the key areas that are necessary to take into account in any discussion of interprofessional working issues in qualifying and post-qualifying education and training programmes.

Part Two then follows these areas through into how we can apply our analysis to the different service-user groups across health and social care – child protection, mental health, learning difficulties, continuing care and work with older people, child protection/safeguarding of children, children in need/looked-after children, people with physical disabilities and end-of-life care.

Part Three then examines interprofessional working from the different perspectives of those who provide services, who they work with and issues for them in relating to other groups in their work settings. These chapters demonstrate the variety of professions involved in interprofessional working, and the great range of professions for whom this is an integral part of their everyday work, including some which are not always covered in detail in a book such as this, for example, teachers, dentists, pharmacists, occupational therapists, and physiotherapists.

Features of chapters

Features of chapters in Parts Two and Three in particular are included to aid readers in picking up on the key learning points in the chapter, and include exercises to allow the application of the chapters' key themes and ideas to readers' own learning within their areas of interest, service-user groups, and/or work settings. Different chapters address, where appropriate, considerations of the following:

- sharing information
- teamworking issues
- dealing with conflicting demands
- ethical and legal issues
- organisational and policy issues
- responsibilities and duties of professionals and agencies involved in the area of provision, and for each professional group
- roles/issues for each professional group/agency in that particular area.

At the start of each chapter, there is a *Chapter summary*, followed by a list of *Learning objectives* for the chapter.

Chapters will include where relevant *Case studies* that may be accompanied by exercises/guidance from the author(s), for the same purpose. These are developed as appropriate within each chapter, presenting main issues for readers to consider from that area of activity for the development of effective interprofessional working and the different relevant professionals/agencies. Case studies are used more in Parts Two and Three due to their particular focus.

Exercises are utilised in the chapters of Parts Two and Three in particular, designed to aid readers to consider the most important points they need to think about in applying the learning in that section to the development of their own understanding of the relevant interprofessional working issues, and how they might incorporate this to best effect in their own approaches to knowledge development and practice.

Summaries of *Key learning points* at several points within the text highlight key points from within it.

Closer look sections provide more detail about central themes, issues or policies in the chapter.

Further reading lists are given at the end of each chapter for readers who wish to follow up on the areas considered within that chapter.

Part One

In Part One the chapters cover key generic issues that we need to be aware of in order to understand the context and implications of trying to implement effective interagency and interprofessional working.

Roger Smith's chapters provide an overview of the subject of interprofessional working from two perspectives. First, he examines the conceptual and practical aspects of collaborative practice, in particular focusing on the purported advantages as well as the challenges likely to be encountered for those who are expected to work together, irrespective of the specific setting. He concludes with the observation that there are no guarantees and that for collaboration to be effective, we must work at it consistently.

In the second of these chapters, he considers the context, particularly the policy and professional drivers in support of increased levels of joint working, across virtually all aspects of health and social care provision, a trend likely to be further influenced by the current 'Big Society' agenda. Once again, the chapter considers both the positive aspects of greater encouragement to work jointly, and some of the persistent difficulties which may occur when necessary disciplinary and professional boundaries are not acknowledged by policy-makers. Learning how to combine skills remains a quite different exercise from learning how to do someone else's job, or supplant their areas of responsibility.

Hugh Barr provides an authoritative overview of the key areas which have influenced the development of interprofessional education from its inception up until the present day, with analysis of what can aid and hinder the effective working together of professions, including defensive practice and resistance to change. Barr argues that interprofessional education has a key part to play in enabling a profession to stand back and take stock of itself and its work with others, and can aid in promoting service, personal, professional and team development, giving examples of how this has happened in different settings and agencies. The place of interprofessional education in reducing risks to service users, and agencies, and aiding effective communication to achieve this is also covered.

Hugh McLaughlin provides a considered appraisal of the theory and workings of interprofessional practice, introducing a note of caution and realism, providing a critical reflection on why we need to avoid idealising its positive aspects, or overlooking the challenges of ensuring that collaborative working is effective and beneficial, and why the value of its outcomes are so highly valued.

John Hughes and Sue Urwin's chapter on working in partnership to provide a joined-up service for offenders with mental health needs provides a model for how an interagency service can be developed in this context. They take into account the lessons from government agency guidance, in this instance the National Audit Office, which can be applied to service development in a practical fashion, based on a review of the challenges presented to the different agencies involved. Using a case study from one

geographical area, instigated and followed through by the local probation service, this chapter looks at the possibilties and challenges for interprofessional working and the effects on local working practices, set out in a timeline analysis from the very start, including an evaluation of the process. In this way the chapter offers a template for development and resolution of issues arising in interprofessional working. These learning points are applicable to any form of systematic interagency planning and development.

In Sue Urwin and Stephanie Sadler's chapter on information sharing between agencies and professionals, they draw on the Hertforshire model set out in Chapter 5, and examine the issues involved in the subsequent development of an innovative protocol in 2010 in relation to the information sharing agreement (ISA) between the agencies involved. The scheme has been developed for use by all those who might work with the criminal justice system – police, probation officers, social and health workers, Crown Prosecution Service, magistrates, court officers, solicitors and the prison service. In exploring some of the professional, ethical and practice issues involved in information sharing between these groups and agencies, they set out lessons and areas of learning that have universal relevance and application across different service-user groups and agencies. The chapter again takes as an example a particular professional group, doctors, in examining in detail the issues that arise for different professions, based on their distinctive uniprofessional ethical and legal requirements, and using case examples to illustrate the application of such considerations in practice.

Part Two

This set of chapters brings into play how we can apply our analysis of generic knowledge of issues to the different service-user groups across health and social care, with the use of case studies and exercises to focus our thinking and learning.

In Chapter 7, on interprofessional working perspectives on mental health, Di Bailey covers the key policy changes that have framed the development of interprofessional working, and how community-based services in particular have had major changes including new specialist teams, new roles and new ways of working for existing professionals. It looks at how the latest Mental Health Act (2007) furthers this agenda, based as it is upon a greater degree of service integration that draws from a range of disciplines combining their different skills, theories and expertise. The important changes wrought by the growth of the survivor movement in mental health work based upon the recovery model are set out and analysed.

Michelle Culwick and Carolyn Wallace's contribution on learning disabilities explores how interprofessional working means knowing what to do, and having the right skills to do what needs to be done, in a competent and capable manner, with professionals conducting themselves with the appropriate attitudes, values and beliefs. Adopting a systems approach, Culwick and Wallace take the view that the demand for services originates from the service-user perspective of their need, and that those involved in the care system need to take into account social inclusion and person-focused approaches, and work together to meet and satisfy the holistic needs of the individual, developing the 'interprofessional willingness condition' – i.e. to do whatever is required to enable effective interprofessional working and service delivery for the service user.

Chapter 9, Safeguarding children and child protection by Mary McColgan, Anne Campbell and James Marshall examines the key issues for interprofessional and interagency working in one of the most high-profile and contested areas examined in this book. Nearly all public inquiries into child abuse deaths/serious harm have found that failings and deficits in the area of information sharing and interprofessional and interagency working have contributed to children not being sufficiently protected by the the professionals/agencies involved. This chapter addresses the dilemmas and the tensions experienced by the range of professionals involved in the complex arena of child protection, and explores the factors that facilitate effective practice in interdisciplinary working and good practice. Key findings relevant to interprofessional working are addressed, and are then applied to the Northern Ireland and wider UK situation, and to how procedures and processes to safeguard children are framed and at times constricted by interagency structures. The fundamental similarities and differences in the skills, theory and value bases across the agencies and identities of professional workers in health, social care, legal and educational settings in child protection work are discussed, how care versus control issues in child protection vary across the professions and agencies involved, and how this can affect interprofessional working.

The topics of 'children in need' and 'looked-after children' are then taken up by Nick Frost, who draws attention to the considerable enthusiasm in the policy world for sharing skills and resources to address children's needs, especially in light of a strengthening emphasis on holistic working and the interconnectedness of aspects of their lives. The result of this interest has been the development of a robust framework for shared working, supported by primary legislation and very substantial policy and practice guidance. As he concludes, the available research strongly supports collaboration in this area of practice, and emphasises the centrality of families themselves as part of the 'team around the child'.

Michelle Cornes' contribution on older people introduces the concept of personalisation which is at the forefront of the health and social care policy agenda, how this emphasises the importance of professionals working together to provide greater flexibility and choice for service users, and how at a strategic level, personalisation poses challenges for collaborative practice for local partnerships to work together to produce a broader range of services for people to choose from. Cornes points out how for front-line practice, personalisation should mean more power and resources being shared with people at the front line – service users, carers and front line workers – to 'co-produce' solutions to their difficulties and needs that they are best placed to know about.

In her chapter on palliative care settings, Suzy Croft provides an account of the types of issues that arise in understanding and dealing with the key matters which occur within such close teamworking in this area. The chapter provides a particular focus from the perspective of social workers as a means to examine key issues for good practice in interprofessional working, and how this relates to such issues for other professions. Croft examines how the role of this one profession, with its wide-ranging and holistic nature, does or does not easily fit with the other professions which have perhaps clearer and more closely focused boundaries. Arising from this perspective, general issues for all professions working in such settings – the effects of the status and power of each group, information sharing, roles of the different professions in relation to assessments, managing interventions and decision making in interprofessional working in this area – are considered. Grappling with this consideration then gives wider, more generalised lessons for other areas of interprofessional working, as explored at the end of the chapter.

Drawing on the example of the work of physiotherapists to illustrate the issues involved in interprofessional working in this area, Chapter 13 makes use of findings from studies of disabled peoples' experiences of wheelchair use and of physiotherapy, in their discussion of interprofessional working perspectives for people with physical disabilities. Glenis Donaldson and Bob Sapey examine the roles and functions of the different professionals working in this field. The chapter sets out how, between them, professionals can best provide an effective service to people in need of it from the use of a social model of disability and a rehabilitation model, which they argue should guide all interprofessionals working with people with disabilities.

Part Three

In Part Three we examine interprofessional working from the different perspectives of those groups of professionals who provide services, who they work with and what is important to know about them and their work with other groups in their various work settings. In accordance with our emphasis on the effects of all this on service users and carers, and their expectations of, and contribution to interprofessional working, we commence Part Three with chapters on these specific areas.

Peter Beresford in his chapter on service-users' rights, needs and expectations, looks at interprofessional working as perceived by service users, and the evidence of what this group needs and are entitled to expect from professionals who are providing services across organisational and professional boundaries. Too often, this key perspective is not placed sufficiently at centre stage in considerations of interprofessional working, and what its aims, outcomes and best ways to include service users as partners are and should be.

In pursuance of our aim to make the experiences of service users and carers a key feature of the book, Carmel Byers and the Creating Links group's two chapters focus on the areas professionals and agencies should be aware of in order to make carers' experiences, views and needs central to their delivery of services across interdisciplinary boundaries. The chapters are based not only on a review of the literature and research, but also on a process of discussion around key themes and the development of case studies between carers in the Creating Links group, and consultation with informal carers associated with carers organisations in Hertfordshire and foster carers in order to represent their views on the effectiveness of interprofessional working and how far they can be considered to be part of the care team. Until the present, there has perhaps been surprisingly little attention paid to carers' perspectives within interprofessional working and their part in interprofessional processes.

In Chapter 15, the carers identify practice issues that, in spite of policy statements and best practice initiatives, pose difficulties for them in their attempts to work in partnership with professionals and become valued as members of the interprofessional team. In the second chapter, they continue to explore the experiences of carers, building on the issues of communication, holistic approaches and values discussed in their first chapter, and the structural barriers that impede carers' participation are explored, the three most significant of which, as identified by the carers in the consultation, are issues of power, control and the impact of agency agendas. Practical pointers are also given in both chapters on how to assess and improve carers' partnership working with professionals and agencies in interprofessional arrangements.

In her chapter on teachers, Mary Rees focuses on interprofessional practice through the eyes and experiences of the one of the largest professional groups, with particular reference to their professional role and training, the organisation and accountability of the education system and teachers relationships with families and parents. The chapter draws on a number of research projects on interprofessional practice, including those on the impact on outcomes for children with additional needs, and professionals' perceptions of the nature and extent of sexual exploitation in one county, using case studies and fictionalised accounts from the research. It sets out the professional and policy basis upon which teachers have a role not only in the formal education of the child, but also in considering the child within the family, alongside other professional groups. The implications for schools having become more autonomous in their management of budgets and staffing, how the wider coordination of services by Local Authorities has declined and how this may affect interprofessional working for children and families who go to their schools are discussed. Rees introduces the conceptual framework of 'knotworking' as a way of helping agencies and professionals consider a sustainable model of interprofessional practice.

Doctors and interprofessional working is the theme of the chapter co-authored by Liz Anderson and Angela Lennox. Their account considers the history of doctors' involvement in joint practice, from its origins in a reaction against the dominant status ascribed to them at one time through a growing recognition of the importance of aligning mutual expectations with other professionals, to a point where their 'leadership' role is now tempered by a readiness to engage as partners with other professionals. This is recognised as a difficult journey for the profession, and one that requires reciprocal recognition of changing relationships.

Chris McKenna and Cath Wright consider occupational therapists and interprofessional working in Chapter 19. They draw specific attention to the value base of occupational therapists and how this, of itself, puts them in an important position to work with and

for people who use services, and to advocate with other professionals. In many ways, occupational therapists share a similar position to social workers in that they are required to take a holistic view of service-user's needs and aspirations, even though their area of distinctive professional expertise is clearly very different. Thus the centrality of their role as partners in service delivery is clearly emphasised.

Steve J. Hothershall then looks at how social work's concerns with looking at the holistic needs and sets of circumstances of the wide variety of service-user groups it works with fits with its relationships and working practices with other professionals. The chapter provides a clear account of what social work's main functions and approaches are as distinct from other professions. The key issues for current formulations of social work around its role in areas such as the protection and management of risks for vulnerable adults and children, its skills and values base, which emphasise respect for, and interpersonal skills used with, service users and carers, are examined in relation to how these affect social work's relationships with other professions and agencies involved in providing services to the groups social workers work with.

Patricia White's chapter examines the place of physiotherapists in arenas of interprofessional working, while also providing a particular focus on examining interprofessional learning within a university which provides a wide range of professional qualifying educational programmes, and how the planning and development of interprofessional education in order to learn with and about each other is a key prerequisite to effective collaboration following qualification. The chapter examines the work of physiotherapists, the profession's history and development, their roles and work settings, and then moves on to consider the need for physiotherapists and other professions to have joint education at this level, what has affected the planning and implementation of collaborative education at the University of the West of England, and how IPE has been integrated within its qualifying programmes.

In his chapter on nursing, Paul Illingworth examines the work of one of the largest professional groups in health care, their professional background and approaches, and relationships with other professional groupings in health and social care. Drawing on the Nursing & Midwifery Council's professional code, Illingworth sets out how nurses' association with other professions and agencies is framed. The parts played by nurses in interprofessional working are discussed, together with not only the potential benefits but also the tensions these associations can raise. Case scenarios are then provided which explore these issues in the context of the different fields of nursing: adult, child, mental health and learning disabilities. In the use of these case studies, the chapter provides illustrations of the types of situations that occur in different fields of nursing and the typical responses of nurses in what they can provide, with whom, and how they go about it.

In their chapter on pharmacists, Neena Lakhani and Brian Simon reflect on the challenges and opportunities for their profession in two distinct settings: the hospital and the community. In these situations, the requirements and relationships for joint working differ, but there are also common themes, such as the central role of the pharmacist in engaging with patients/service users, and their ability to understand and respond to possible 'gaps' which may arise between treatment plans and the lived reality. Utilising the common strand of a single case study, the authors illustrate both the role of pharmacists as a source of continuity and a channel of communication, and the different tasks, working relationships and mutual expectations which are likely to arise depending on the context.

Pam Ward in her contribution on dentists brings a previously rarely considered professional group under the spotlight. Using several very different case examples, she shows how dentistry can make a very significant contribution to shared working, whilst also challenging narrow conceptions of the dentist's role and tasks. This chapter illustrates that a 'readiness' to work interprofessionally and to consider the possible areas of collaboration in almost every practice setting is now an essential attribute of all health and social care professions.

Our aims and aspirations

Given the vast array of agencies and professions that are involved in the many different levels of interprofessional education and interprofessional working, we are aware that there will still be some unevenness even in a book of this length. Despite that, we hope that we have produced a book which will be of value to students, practitioners and policy-makers in gaining a better understanding of each profession's and agency's own internal areas of work and views of itself, and that students and qualified professionals might make use of the different sections of the book to gain a broad as well as deep knowledge of interprofessional working and interprofessional education. Within an account of the general debates and key areas for consideration, we hope that the book will show not only that we need to be able to work better across professional and agency boundaries for the benefit of service users and carers, but also that there are ways and means of putting in place mechanisms and skills and promoting values which will result in improved provision and outcomes in jointly provided social and health care services.

References

Brandon, M., Bailey, S., Belderson, P., Gardner, R., Sidebottom, P., Dodsworth, J., Warren, C. and Black, J. (2009) *Understanding Serious Case Reviews and Their Impact: A Biennial Analysis of Serious Case Reviews 2005–7*, London: Department for Children Schools and Families (DCSF).

Centre for the Advancement of Interprofessional Education (CAIPE) (2002) *Defining IPE*, accessed 13 July 2011 from: http://www.caipe.org.uk/about-us/defining-ipe.

Department for Children Schools and Families (2010) *Working Together to Safeguard Children (WT): A Guide to Inter-agency Working to Safeguard and Promote the Welfare of Children*, London: DCSF.

Ofsted (2008) *Learning Lessons, Taking Action: Ofsted's Evaluations of Serious Case Reviews 1 April 2007 to 31 March 2008*, London: Ofsted.

Part One

KEY ISSUES IN INTERPROFESSIONAL AND INTERAGENCY WORKING IN HEALTH AND SOCIAL CARE

1 Working together: why it's
   important and why it's
   difficult

2 The drivers and dynamics
   of interprofessional
   working in policy and
   practice

3 Change and challenge in
   interprofessional education

4 Keeping interprofessional
   practice honest: fads and
   critical reflections

5 Working in partnership to
   develop local arrangements
   for interagency and
   interprofessional services:
   a case study

6 Information-sharing
   agreements between
   agencies and professionals:
   making use of law, policy
   and professional codes

Chapter 1
Working together: why it's important and why it's difficult

Roger Smith

Chapter summary

This chapter aims to introduce a number of key aspects of interprofessional or collaborative working, in order to focus specifically on the opportunities and challenges presented. It first identifies some of the benefits as well as potential disadvantages associated with working together. Building on this framework, the chapter proceeds to discuss the underlying preconditions and the practice requirements necessary to ensure that collaboration is effective, and of fundamental importance, and actually works to the benefit of people who use health and social care services. In setting out these elements of good practice, however, there is no attempt to hide or minimise the kind of interpersonal, professional and structural obstacles which stand in the way of successful cooperation.

Learning objectives

This chapter will cover:

- the origins of interprofessional working
- the potential advantages of collaboration
- potential shortcomings in collaborative practice
- the challenges and opportunities of joint working
- key elements of effective collaboration
- the value base for working together.

A closer look

Why should we work together?

Victoria Climbié died as a result of extreme abuse and neglect on 25 February 2000, aged 8. One of the witnesses to the subsequent inquiry into her death described it as 'the worst [case] I have ever dealt with, and it is just about the worst I have ever heard of'.

(Laming, 2003, p. 2)

Writing about the lessons learnt from Victoria's history of abuse and the inadequate responses of a range of agencies and professionals, the president of the Royal College of Paediatrics and Child Health wrote: 'Prevention depends on collaboration . . . [I]t is not just organisations, committees and boards that must work together. Children like Victoria die when individual professionals do not work together.'

(Hall, 2003, p. 203)

Starting from the beginning

The impression is sometimes created that working in partnership has only become recognised as an important aspect of professional practice relatively recently. It is certainly the case that books such as this, and other publications on the subject, have only been produced in any quantity in the past decade or so. This does not mean, though, that the move towards better mutual understanding and cooperation in practice has no significant history. In fact, it is more likely that collaboration in some form or other has always been the norm as the modern welfare state has developed. This is certainly the view of some of those who have commented on the subject previously. Pietroni (1994, p. 77), for example, has suggested that 'The development of "groups of workers" coming together to look after a patient began with the emergence of the hospital'. As health and social care provision began to be developed as a systematic form of activity, so there also emerged an increasing number of specialised roles and tasks. While at first the interface between different specialised functions may have been highly structured and regulated, the 'militarisation' of medical services meant that tasks and relationships between practitioners also came to be differentiated and closely specified. This also ensured that services tended to be organised in a hierarchical fashion, with little scope for mutual negotiation or exchange of professional opinion. But what it did mean was that even from this early stage the need for specialist skills, systematic allocation of tasks and effective communication and 'transfer' arrangements was recognised quite clearly. Ironically, in fact, the gradual development of very specific functions in health and welfare also led to a parallel requirement for those carrying out these functions to share responsibilities and develop effective ways of combining their inputs in the interests of service users/patients.

The process of specialisation has sometimes been equated to the equivalent developments in industrial production and other commercial spheres. The pioneer of this kind of approach is believed to be Frederick Taylor (Rastegar, 2004, p. 79), who was driven by the perceived need to improve the quality, productivity and efficiency of manufacturing processes. Taylor believed that complicated activities could be broken down into a series of relatively straightforward tasks, which could then be streamlined and integrated to maximise overall performance. Whether or not it has been motivated by exactly the same logic or demands, the same kind of trends have been identified in the welfare sector, with a similar increase in the number and range of specialised activities. However, it is also acknowledged that a simple transfer of lessons from industry to health and welfare may be to underestimate the inevitable complexities of human services:

> While it is fairly straightforward to look at outcomes of a discrete condition or stage of care (situations where specialists tend to perform better), it is much harder to do so for patients with a variety of acute and chronic illnesses cared for in different settings for an extended period.
>
> (Rastegar, 2004, p. 80)

There have been other drivers, too, that have created an increasing variety of professional identities, with responsibilities which may only be effectively discharged if they are linked with the work of others. Of course, this trend has partly been about the search

Exercise 1.1

Can you identify and distinguish separate lists of 'old' and 'new' professions in health and social care? Looking at these two lists, what are the features which differentiate them? Do you think these differences might lead to tensions and conflict?

A closer look

Finding common ground

When I was asked to join a youth diversion team comprising a teacher, a police officer, a social worker, a youth worker and a probation officer, it quickly became clear that we had to find a balance between representing our own agency and its working principles and combining to deliver the specific collaborative task for which we were responsible. In order to do so, two essential preconditions had to be met. We all had to be prepared to give up some areas of practice for which we might previously have claimed exclusivity, and we all had to be ready to accept the validity of other disciplines' distinctive skills and expertise.

for a distinctive rationale, value base and identity which has occupied the thoughts of many practitioner groupings, especially those which have been established as distinctive occupational roles relatively recently (the 'new' professions).

This in turn itself sets up some interesting and challenging dynamics, given that becoming effective collaborators might mean giving up some aspects of your autonomous standing, which may have been hard won over a period of time.

At the same time, as Leathard (1994, p. 6) has wisely observed, difficulties 'can arise over the use of the word "professional"'. If other practitioners, or non-professional interests and viewpoints are marginalised by this use of terminology, purely because they do not see themselves as 'professionals', genuinely collaborative working may also be made more problematic. This issue becomes more significant still when we reflect on the importance of keeping 'carers' and those 'cared-for' at the centre of the process, and seeing them as key members of the 'team'.

So, two distinct trends of specialisation and professionalisation have been increasingly influential in shaping the working environment in health and social care. As tasks have become more discrete, and to some degree routinised, so have those responsible for carrying them out sought to articulate and maintain their own standing as professional experts with a degree of autonomy, authority and discretion. In light of this, it is perhaps not surprising that there has been an emerging recognition of the tensions and barriers inherent in these changes, and the need to address them. This has certainly been recognised as a significant challenge in the world of policy and practice guidance for some time (Pietroni, 1994), an awareness which has been compounded by the recurrent evidence from major inquiries that a failure to

collaborate effectively may amount to risky and, indeed, harmful practice (Stevenson, 1994).

Against this backdrop, then, there is a definite sense that the priority accorded to collaborative working has been enhanced in recent years, and that it has come to be seen as the starting point for effective practice in many areas across the service spectrum, rather than an optional extra. This impetus has been supported by many examples of 'good practice', such as the present author's own experience of multi-agency juvenile diversion (Smith, 2007), or the evidence from collaborative rehabilitative interventions for older people (Lymbery, 2003).

In parallel with these developments 'on the ground', we have also seen considerable behind-the-scenes activity on the part of government and other policy-making bodies (see Chapter 2). It has become almost a matter of faith that collaborative working is desirable and has the potential to resolve many of the difficulties encountered by people who feel that they are let down by health and social care agencies. But it is as well to begin with a cautionary note, as sounded by an earlier commentator:

What remains to be seen is whether the pressure on health and welfare professionals to work together will have a positive outcome . . . will clients, patients and users receive quality care and be enabled to make choices on a meaningful basis? Or will professional identities, under the cloak of rationalization and skill-mix realignment, become diluted and the standards of care undermined? Time will test the interprofessional resolve.

(Leathard, 1994, p. 9)

In light of this observation, it is worth stressing that in order to be able to work well with colleagues from other disciplines you will need to have and hold a clear and confident view of your own profession's purposes and principles.

Gains and losses 1: possibilities

As in almost any sphere of activity, collaboration in health and social care presents both opportunities and risks, and has always done so. It has been relatively easy to make a case for partnership in recent times based on the observable consequences of fragmented services and poor communication, but it may be that pressure to find easy solutions and 'quick fixes' has led to an underestimation of some of the endemic difficulties involved. As suggested elsewhere (Smith, 2009), a number of both advantages and disadvantages are attributed to working collaboratively. On the positive side of the coin, we might expect improvements in the following areas:

- **Improved efficiency.** There are a number of essentially practical ways in which sharing arrangements to work with service users should make provision more accessible and efficient. Thus, for instance, a number of discrete resources may be accessible to users from a single point of delivery. At the same time, practitioners may find that it is easier to communicate, and to share information and referrals with colleagues from different disciplines where they work from a shared working environment, or under the aegis of a common 'team' identity. It may be the case, for example, that recent trends towards offering combined mental health services have proved beneficial in this respect. Some of the challenges of working across different service boundaries, and negotiating competing policies on issues such as confidentiality

and sharing records, may be reduced under this sort of arrangement.

- **Better skills mix.** Similarly, the capacity to offer a broader range of skills may be a direct consequence of collaborative working strategies. In an increasingly specialised world, practitioners very often feel that they are being asked to undertake tasks at the limits of or beyond their own levels of competence, and which they have not been trained to undertake. In such instances, the scope to be able to draw on the expertise of colleagues and to integrate these into the overall service on offer may be very valuable. Police officers, for instance, have often been heard to complain that they have to act as social workers in crisis situations. Models of practice which facilitate closer working between the two might well go some way to alleviating this kind of frustration. Additionally, the availability and use of other sources of expertise may also contribute to a recognition of each other's specific knowledge and competences, reducing levels of suspicion or mistrust.

- **Greater levels of responsiveness.** People who use services are themselves often frustrated by the partial or inaccessible nature of the responses to their felt needs. Services which adopt a collaborative approach should be able to alleviate this concern in a number of ways. Firstly, it should be possible to 'signpost' someone to the relevant specialist service more easily. Secondly, practitioners themselves should have a better sense of what is on offer, and thus be empowered to make a greater range of options available. And it should be possible to tailor service mechanisms, such as assessment procedures, to address a variety of potential needs. This is clearly the intention of policy innovations such as the Common Assessment Framework for children; logically, common assessments also need to be linked to a suitable menu of interventions depending on the needs and aspirations identified.

- **More 'holistic' services.** Service users often find it irritating and confusing to be told that different providers will be responsible for different aspects of their 'problems'. At the same time, there is clearly a risk that atomised services will only address one aspect of need, while regarding anything else as 'someone else's job'. A holistic approach enables more facets of a complex situation to be addressed in tandem and in ways which complement each other. For instance, for disabled people this might mean that what they see and experience as arbitrary distinctions between medical and social needs can be eliminated and integrated services provided which bridge these divides. (See Figure 1.1.)

- **Innovation and creativity.** Not only does collaboration offer the possibility of a more rounded approach, it may also generate a creative environment for innovation. Where practitioners are able to share ideas and approaches, they may well gain fresh insights and feel enabled to exercise their imaginations. There is also the possibility that roadblocks arising from the constraints imposed by one organisation or procedure may be open to negotiation or circumnavigation when representatives of other agencies become involved. The involvement of other agencies in the juvenile diversion project in which I worked some time ago enabled the police to be much more confident about exercising their discretion and pursuing alternatives to prosecution.

- **Greater likelihood of user-centred practice.** It may be felt, too, that the experience of working together in the interests of service users can have an impact on organisational dynamics. Practitioners may indeed find the focus shifting because their interventions are organised around the service user, rather than along lines predetermined by the agency. By centring the service user in this way, collaborative practice may be seen as having the potential to empower user and practitioners alike, as they seek to reframe services so that they are tailored to individual needs and circumstances. The original intentions of person-centred planning seem to represent a manifestation of this principle in policy and best practice guidance (Department of Health, 2001).

There is thus considerable potential for collaborative practice developments to change some of the dynamics of intervention, by breaking down arbitrary distinctions between different aspects of service delivery and agency responsibilities. Such developments may also, by their nature, be more likely to place service users at the centre of processes of assessment, planning and intervention; and this, in turn, may lead to a greater sense of freedom and creativity for the practitioners concerned. These, then, are some of the positive aspects of interprofessional working.

Gains and losses 2: pitfalls

On the other hand, we might still expect a number of recurrent problems to arise. These may not be exclusive to interprofessional working, by any means, but they may become more acute in this context. Working towards collaboration may well be an uncomfortable experience for those involved, and they may feel at times that they are not fully supported in the pursuit of this aim by agencies which are also competing for resources and status:

- **Boundary disputes.** One of the issues likely to emerge in any attempt to establish effective interprofessional working arrangements is the nature and extent of each partner's role and responsibilities. This is especially the case because most professions, including those with long and established traditions, have a limited and unclear view of their own boundaries; what is or is not 'my job' may be a difficult question for many involved in partnership working (Hudson, 2007). As a result,

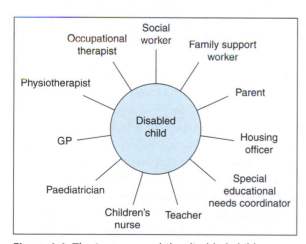

Figure 1.1 The team around the disabled child

two opposing problems may arise: some tasks, especially those which are seen as particularly problematic, may be shunned, for example. On the other hand, certain aspects of the combined function may be the subject of 'colonisation' attempts, whereby one professional group will lay claim to an exclusive role at the expense of others. These tensions illustrate another important consideration for collaborative practice: that is, to achieve a fully integrated approach, joint teams must go beyond simply sharing out tasks and begin to adopt principles of collective responsibility and accountability.

■ **Status issues.** Bringing diverse practitioner groups together with their different traditions and mutual expectations is almost bound to raise status issues. Unequal standing is probably manifested in a number of ways, some of them quite tangible. A simple look round the car park will probably bring this observation into sharp relief! The tension between the notion of an equal partnership and the traditional hierarchies sketched out by Pietroni (1994) is perhaps inevitable. It can materialise in a number of ways, including the assumption by some participants that they are able to instruct others, on grounds of professional expertise rather than organisational position, as opposed to working with them to agree collective solutions. Lymbery (2006, p. 1124), likewise, has suggested that 'the uncertain professional status of social work creates a particular problem in relation to the development of collaborative working' with older people.

■ **Language barriers.** As we have already observed, the difficulty of agreeing a common language is quite fundamental, starting with the long-running debate about how we should define the people with whom we work: are they 'patients', 'service users', 'clients', 'customers' or just 'citizens' (Billingsley and Lang, 2002, p. 32)? Beyond this, though, is a more extensive concern about the ways in which language structures professional identities, assumptions and practices. It is undoubtedly the case that the development of specialist terminology and shorthand (especially acronyms) is associated with the perceived need to establish professional identities and credibility. On the other

hand, however, it is also well documented that such use of language can be exclusive and divisive, both between practitioner groups and between providers and service users. This is not to suggest that no such terms or forms of use are appropriate, just that the impact of their applications must be borne in mind and moderated as far as possible.

■ **Competing practice models.** Lying behind differing language practices may be more substantive differences in the ways in which people who use services are defined, their problems identified and interventions constructed. One of the most obvious of these is the apparent opposition between 'social' and 'medical' models in work with people with disabilities (Baxter and Brumfitt, 2008), or those who have mental health needs. Similar, perhaps less clear-cut oppositions arise in the field of criminal justice where young people who offend can be defined first and foremost as 'criminals', or, on the other hand, as having welfare needs which should be prioritised. Such differences of perspective obviously have very substantial implications for the ways in which practice is organised.

■ **Complex accountabilities.** In the midst of the potential differences between professional groupings outlined previously, there are also likely to be complicating factors arising from structural and organisational tensions. Where collaborative services are organised, the question of accountabilities becomes a testing issue. For some, it may be quite disconcerting to think that they may be supervised, managed or evaluated by someone who does not share their background or training. The underlying concern may be framed in terms of the question: 'who will take the blame if this goes wrong?' (Smith, 2009, p. 136). Equally, though, practitioners may feel uncomfortable with the idea that their own performance may be judged by someone who does not really appreciate what their role involves in terms of skills and expert knowledge. It may seem inappropriate that career prospects could be affected by such 'uninformed' opinions.

■ **Disputed decision-making powers.** In the same vein, the issue of the legitimacy of judgements about one's professional performance are paralleled by concerns about who has the ultimate authority to make operational or strategic decisions. At what point does collective team responsibility have to be ceded in favour of the 'lead' organisation for a particular service function? This seems to have been a recurrent issue in areas of practice characterised by the risk of harm, or a sense of urgency, such as child protection, for instance. The decision over whether criminal inquiries by the police should supersede collective action to protect children from harm may impose considerable strains on underlying safeguarding arrangements. The issue raised here is whether collaborative practice is only sustainable in 'fair weather', and when things get difficult agencies revert to more individualised ways of working based on their unique priorities and operational rules.

- **Imported inequalities (of gender, ethnicity or culture, for example).** It is also important to not just concentrate on what might be seen as essentially *internal* tensions facing the collaborative practice agenda. There are likely to be other externally defined inequalities and imbalances at play, represented, for example, by established categories such as gender, ethnicity and culture. External social divisions may be imported into the interprofessional arena, and played out once again in terms which intensify differences of practice, orientation and values. It is well known, of course, that professional hierarchies tend to replicate gender divisions, with those at the 'top' of the tree being more likely to be male-dominated. As the world of health and welfare changes are increasingly rapidly, we may also see similar divides emerging on grounds of culture and ethnicity. It is, of course, crucially important that implicit professional hierarchies do not become another vehicle through which forms of social inequality and oppression are made manifest.

Towards effective partnerships: challenges and opportunities

Given that there are likely to be both positive attractions and inbuilt tensions in the project of establishing effective partnerships, it will help here to set out some of the ways in which challenges and opportunities may be approached in undertaking this task. First, it is clear that there are a number of endemic obstacles to better levels of cooperation, although each of them may be seen to represent an underlying test of commitment, running from the strategic and structural levels all the way through to the individual practitioner. Thus, for example, there is a fundamental question as to the level of resources which it is thought appropriate to invest, and what represents a comparable level of input, given that agencies have very different capabilities in terms of what is available to them. In fairly simplistic terms, of course, this may be reduced to a question of how much each partner is willing to invest; however, it is not just a question of making a cash contribution, especially given that some will find this easier than others. Also involved in this kind of calculation is the extent to which parent agencies will make key personnel available, and on what basis. Other contributions 'in kind' may be important; a commitment to share information, as far as legally permissible, may be seen as a significant symbolic contribution, too.

Of equal significance in symbolic terms is the readiness of agencies to demonstrate their support, by taking an active role in collective management, perhaps, or by showing a common readiness to respond to external pressure or adverse publicity. In my own past experience of interagency practice, I can recall how important it was to feel that senior managers were involving themselves in the project, simply by attending management committee meetings. It became distinctly awkward for those practitioners whose managers never seemed to be able to attend; this implied an underlying lack of interest, of course.

As well as the substantive and symbolic value of resource commitments of various kinds, it is important to develop a common sense of purpose and working practices, especially where the initiative in question is breaking new ground. It is at this point that the issue of 'multi' versus 'interagency' working emerges with some impetus.

As one commentator observes, in the 'health literature the terms "multiprofessional" and "interprofessional" are often used interchangeably' (Finch, 2000, p. 1138). This can give rise to considerable confusion, and we are reminded that this is an important distinction to make, representing the difference between, say, working alongside one another in a common location, but on separate tasks; and, on the other hand, working on a commonly agreed and integrated activity which necessitates a level of shared understanding and mutual investment. This is much more clearly an interactive process than simply working in ways which are complementary, but do not involve any significant degree of collaborative engagement. It is suggested, for example, that fully interprofessional working requires participants to be effectively prepared for this in a number of ways. They must '"know about" the roles of other professional groups'; they must 'be able to "work with" other professionals in the context of a team'; and they should be ready to '"substitute for" roles traditionally played by other professionals' when this would improve processes and outcomes for service users (Finch, 2000, pp. 1138–9). This suggests, in turn, that we cannot expect genuinely interprofessional practice to 'just happen': it must be prepared for, both strategically and also at the level of practice. Participants should be entitled to expect that they will be offered joint training and preparatory activities such as team building, for example, but they must also be prepared to engage in joint working with open minds. In this spirit, a crucial question for those getting involved in collaborative practice is: 'what are you prepared to give up?' This is a question for agencies as much as it is for practitioners, of course, but it is of major significance if working together is to move beyond a token aspiration. Thus, for example, agencies may have to be prepared to give up decision-making powers, in certain respects, as when the police agreed to negotiate over whether or not to prosecute in the juvenile diversion project in which I was involved. Equally, though, it may be important for medical practitioners to reconsider the way in which they view the diagnostic process in some contexts. Not only does this sort of adaptation contribute significantly in equalising implicit power imbalances between disciplines, it also importantly underpins approaches which seek to engage service users more actively as partners and as key decision makers in their own right. The question of 'giving up' some aspect of one's professional author-

ity or operational autonomy should not be underestimated, though. We know, for instance, that the question of who is authorised to take certain statutory measures in mental health is a matter which has tested the strength of collaborative relationships in the recent past, and there are always likely to be problems if certain participants feel that they are being required to give up hard-won status and authority under duress. Similarly, the emergence of new roles in the interests of better collaboration can also have a disruptive effect, as with the introduction of 'primary care mental health workers' (Harkness et al., 2005).

Despite the evident challenges to be met, an equivalent range of opportunities present themselves, which can be summarised briefly here. The exercise of developing collaborative activities is, in itself, likely to provide a source of mutual support. Where practitioners may be seeking to develop new and creative services, the availability of mutual support from across professional divides may be of significant value. This, in turn, may well help to underwrite a sense of cohesion and common purpose, organised around the sense of shared goals which are represented in terms that transcend relatively narrow professional interests. Similarly, the availability of external sources of support may well enable developments to establish and maintain a degree of credibility amongst colleagues and in wider domains, even where they appear to be working 'against the grain'. Finally, and most importantly, the implementation of this kind of strategy offers the possibility of added value; that is, it can legitimately aspire to offer more than the sum of its parts, and to deliver a form of intervention which treats the service user as an integral whole, rather than a collection of atomised and unconnected 'problems'.

Given these alternative perspectives, it is perhaps unsurprising that the idea of interprofessional working generates some quite polarised views about its value and potential. In reality, of course, it is equally capable of achieving positive benefits, and leading to problematic outcomes and conflict. What is necessary, though, is to have a common view of aims and purposes, and to develop appropriate strategies and problem-solving approaches to enable these to be realised.

Strategies and approaches: making collaboration work

It will be helpful to outline at this point some of the probable ingredients necessary for effective collaboration, as well as thinking about some of the ways of combining these.

First, it may be useful to begin by acknowledging that working in partnership across agency or disciplinary boundaries is a special form of teamworking. In other words, many of the same principles apply, such as the need to recognise both the formal roles assigned to members and the roles that derive from their individual qualities and character. In a sense, then, 'normal' teamwork considerations will apply, but will need adapting somewhat to account for professional differences, not just of role, but also of status, expertise and social context. When I first began teaching interprofessional groups of students, I did not take sufficient account of the need first to establish a team ethos and identity before focusing on the inevitable issues of negotiating the formal boundaries of agencies and disciplines. Just as in a learning environment, it may be useful to undertake introductory exercises when establishing an interprofessional team, such as setting mutually agreed ground rules. This task will almost certainly help to clarify the specific challenges arising from complex patterns of obligation and accountability. Where, for instance, do we need to set the limits to openness and sharing of information, in light of agency confidentiality policies? It is, indeed, in the nature of partnership working that the roles adopted by participants will incorporate ambiguities and tensions. Questions of loyalty and belongingness naturally arise, and it is perhaps unsurprising if it appears that for some, their commitment to collaboration is tentative and provisional. They may be unwilling to make a fuller commitment for fear that they will be marginalised by their parent discipline in direct proportion to their level of investment in an interagency enterprise, especially if this is something that is not fully understood, endorsed or valued by erstwhile colleagues. Such tensions are not easily resolved, and are likely to be experienced by most of those involved in partnership working. The accusation of 'going over to the other side' may be difficult to take, and it may also be associated with fears about damaging one's career prospects, too. Retaining explicit and consistent links with parent agencies may be necessary, then; this is not, ironically, because of a lack of commitment to joint working, but because sustaining good relationships back 'at home' may actually enhance the ability to play a full part. So managing multiple accountabilities and allegiances is a necessary part of the groundwork for good interprofessional practice. A further aspect of this ambiguous position which may be advantageous is the opportunity to act as a mediator between different interests, and to bring opposing viewpoints into discussion, if not agreement. The interprofessional practitioner represents the joint project within his or her own agency as well as the reverse. As a probation officer, I found it particularly helpful, for instance, to be able to call on my teacher colleague's assistance when seeking to negotiate an arrangement to maintain a student in school. Her credibility with other educationalists was naturally much greater than mine.

This, in turn, highlights another sense in which the recognised attributes of good teamworking also apply to collaborative practice. Respect for one another as individuals must be paralleled by respect for each other's professional identities and practices. This is highlighted by long-standing tensions such as the apparent hostility between proponents of social and medical models of disability. Where different practice strengths are to be combined, it seems inappropriate and probably impractical to hold on to extreme variants of such positions. Rather, the starting point must be one of recognition and exchange, building up a mutual picture of the reasons that underlie different priorities and working practices.

It is important, too, to build on this recognition and appreciation of different skills and responsibilities to develop an approach which is complementary. Joint working is not about everybody doing everything, just as preparing for it does not mean learning how to do each others' jobs. Instead, the important skills to develop are the ability to recognise when each other's contribution is appropriate, and to hand over work as and when it makes professional sense to do so. Underlying this, in personal terms, it is also necessary to build up mutual trust and confidence in the other's abilities.

None of this is to suggest that there is no room for disagreement or honest expression of differences of opinion. There are bound to be foggy areas of practice where it is unclear as to who should take responsibility; again, here, the important principle to acknowledge is that constructive criticism is helpful, so long as it does not amount to a devaluing of another practitioner's sense of professional competence. It may not always be necessary, but formal mechanisms can be utilised for the expression and resolution of disagreements in order to acknowledge that it is legitimate to disagree, but that working together also necessitates a commitment to trying to resolve differences.

Effective collaboration, then, requires a shared sense of purpose, tempered by a recognition of individual skills and responsibilities, and supported by working arrangements and mechanisms which enable differences to be resolved relatively straightforwardly. Mutual respect is important, too, and this incorporates both personal and professional dimensions.

As we have seen previously, these principles have wider resonances in a social context where professional hierarchies may tend to reflect broader inequalities. Ultimately, it is argued

> Effective *interprofessional* collaboration appears to require practitioners to learn, negotiate and apply understanding of what is *common* to the professions involved; their *distinctive contributions*, what is *complementary* between them; what may be *in conflict*; and *how to work together*.
>
> (Whittington, 2003, p. 58)

Whether collaborations take place through established teams with a specific remit, or ad hoc arrangements to meet needs in a particular case, they require

---

Exercise 1.2

Do you hold stereotyped views of any other professional groupings within social care or health? Do you think these stereotypes have any basis in fact? Is it better to share them with colleagues or to suppress such beliefs in the interests of good working relationships?

---

similar processes of negotiation, preparation and trust-building, in order to facilitate effective interventions on behalf of people who use services. These may be difficult to sustain in light of organisational demands and competing pressures, but the centrality of the service user helps to underpin common commitments and focuses practice accordingly; if this is the staring point, then it becomes easier to sustain joint working, even in the face of tensions and interdisciplinary strains.

Looking ahead: pitfalls and possibilities revisited

There are, as we have seen, a number of contemporary developments which seem to point towards increasing expectations that partnership working will become the norm. However, these trends are likely to incorporate both possibilities and threats, as we have also acknowledged. In particular, these issues cohere around the challenge of finding a balance between investing considerable time and energy in the necessary working arrangements, on the one hand, and the potential for more effective user-centred services on the other. It is important to recognise, for instance, that a number of commentators have been quite sceptical about the value of collaboration for its own sake, questioning whether there is sufficient evidence available of its potential to justify the apparent levels of enthusiasm which it generates. Some concern has been expressed, for example, that interprofessional working has become 'a new orthodoxy' (Christie and Menmuir, 2005, p. 62), with untested assumptions informing this, to the effect that it is bound to lead to more efficient and effective practice, almost by definition. This may not be the case, though, if it leads to a diminution in professional standards, or the establishment of monolithic coalitions which turn their faces against service users. Thus, for instance, a collectively agreed decision to intervene in a family against parents' wishes may be harder to challenge where there are no alternative viewpoints being expressed. Clearly, this is not necessarily wrong, but the possibilities of 'groupthink' and unwillingness to acknowledge alternative viewpoints should be recognised:

> Collaborative projects tend to reflect the aims and priorities of the key stakeholders *only* if those stakeholders are involved from the planning stage onwards. This means that while such projects often address the needs of the professionals involved they do not necessarily meet the needs of users and carers.
>
> (Rummery, 2003, p. 208)

It has also been observed that joint working may lead to an improvement in the processes of assessment and decision making, there is 'no evidence' (Rummery, 2003, p. 208) that these in turn lead to better outcomes for service users. A number of other studies (Zwarenstein *et al.*, 2000) have been unable to generate substantial evidence of the benefits of interprofessional practice, and so we must be wary of idealising the notion that working together is always going to lead to improvements.

On the other hand, there is some evidence of improved services and outcomes, especially in the area of work with children and families. Frost *et al.* (2005) have carried out a fairly extensive review of multi-agency teams to support children and families. In particular, good working relationships can be seen to offer the opportunity to utilise different perspectives productively: 'Joined-up working does not necessarily mean doing away with difference' (p. 190). Indeed, it seems to be beneficial to actively seek out the alternative options that this may provide.

In areas of practice such as early years' services, joint working is fairly well established, and is more or less accepted as the norm (Gardner, 2003). Early years' services, for instance, have an established tradition of collaborative working, where centres are established within communities to 'bring resources together and provide a range of non-stigmatising service provision for families' (Smith, 2009, p. 142). In this context, it is suggested that bringing together generalist and specialist professional interests offers a number of potential benefits, including more needs-responsive and less stigmatising services. This was one of the underlying aims of Sure Start, where the aim of providing accessible 'joined-up' services to marginalised communities was at the heart of the initiative. It must be acknowledged, though, that subsequent evidence has been equivocal as to the real achievements of Sure Start overall. In addition, disentangling the impact of multi-professional working from the direct effects of additional expenditure, or the benefits of providing more local services, is a difficult task. Nonetheless, successful examples of this kind of model are identifiable, featuring jointly agreed 'meta-strategies', recognition and respect for 'differences', effective 'dissemination' of common aims and objectives and a willingness to learn from each other, at both practitioner and agency level (Gardner, 2003, p. 151).

We should perhaps be somewhat cautious about overstating the benefits directly attributable to the breaking down of agency and professional divides. On the other hand, we can begin to identify some common features of 'successful' multi-agency working, and what approaches might help to underpin this. The starting point must be a genuine and active commitment from participating agencies. This provides the basis of support which practitioners will require in order to feel comfortable about sharing ideas, taking professional risks and sometimes admitting uncertainty and asking for help.

Sometimes, too, it is a matter of making sure that practical challenges do not intrude, or create divisions. Where interprofessional teams are established, there are very often issues of parity of status, pay and conditions and authority, which can lead to persistent feelings of unfairness and unequal treatment. Thus, the groundwork is important, both at agency level and at practitioner level.

Practitioners themselves have to become familiar with different ways of working, different systems and multiple lines of accountability. While there is much rhetorical encouragement to work across conventional boundaries at present, this still necessitates some detailed adjustment in the mindset of those directly involved in new ways of working. Stereotyped views must be kept in check and taboos challenged; I remember being told forcefully and somewhat indignantly by a medical student at an interprofessional learning event: 'we're not all slaves to the "medical model", you know'.

Beyond this, a degree of openness and acceptance of challenge is required, which is sometimes arguably absent from the uni-professional environment, and so becomes even more difficult to activate in a multi-agency setting. By the same token, though, exchanges of this kind can only be productive if they are grounded in a spirit of respect and recognition of professional difference, and the value of other points of view. These considerations suggest that it is not just a question of attitudes and values, but that these must be demonstrated in action, through particular styles of working, which cannot be routinised or individualistic, but necessitate sharing, reflection, debate and then a mutual acceptance of responsibility for the outcomes of practice. This requires a substantial degree of mutual trust and respect, of course, and there are many reasons that this may be difficult to achieve in the real world of collaborative practice; there must, however, be underlying goals if such ways of working are to have any hope of being consistently effective.

Conclusion

The aim of this chapter has been to set out some of the key benefits and obstacles to collaborative working. In essence, it is clear that there is considerable support for the idea of joint working both in terms of government and agency policy, and in terms of professional, service user and practitioner aspirations. However, historical differences in the ways in which professions have developed have often acted as an impediment to collaboration.

We have also observed that **working together** may **lead to improved services, although this is not a given**. Precisely because of this, **effective joint working needs to be 'worked at'** consistently and continually.

Further Reading

Pietroni, P. (1994) Interprofessional teamwork: its history and development in hospitals, general practice and community care (UK) in Leathard, A. (ed.) *Going Interprofessional*, London: Routledge. A useful and concise summary of the historical trends and dynamics in interprofessional care.

Lymbery, M. (2003) Collaborating for the social and health care of older people in **Weinstein, J.** *et al.* (eds) *Collaboration in Social Work Practice*, London: Jessica Kingsley Publishers. For a summary of the key challenges in joint working for older people.

Belbin, R. (2010) *Team Roles at Work, 2nd ed*, London: Butterworth-Heineman. A useful and very influential source on team roles and effective team working.

Useful websites

http://www.belbin.com

Another source on team roles which offers resources (at a price) to enable practitioners to assess their own preferred team roles, and consider what this might mean for practice.

http://www.improvementfoundation.org/theme/mental-health/national-primary-care-mental-health-collaborative.

A source of good practice guidance in mental health.

References

Baxter, S. and Brumfitt, S. (2008) Professional differences in interprofessional working, *Journal of Interprofessional Care* 22, 239–51.

Billingsley, R. and Lang, L. (2002) The case for interprofessional learning in health and social care, *Managing Community Care* 10, 31–4.

Christie, D. and Menmuir, J. (2005) Supporting interprofessional collaboration in Scotland through a Common Standards Framework, *Policy Futures in Education* 3, 62–74.

Department of Health (2003) *Valuing People*, London: The Stationery Office.

Finch J. (2000) Interprofessional education and teamworking: a view from the educational provider, *British Medical Journal* 321, 1138–40.

Frost, N., Robinson, M. and Anning, A. (2005) Social workers in multi-disciplinary teams – issues and dilemmas for professional practice, *Child and Family Social Work* 10, 187–96.

Gardner, R. (2003) Working together to improve children's life chances: the challenge of inter-agency collaboration, in J. Weinstein, C. Whittington and T. Leiba (eds) *Collaboration in Social Work Practice*, London: Jessica Kingsley Publishers.

Hall, D. (2003) Child protection–lessons from Victoria Climbié, *British Medical Journal* 326, 293–4.

Harkness, E., Bower, P., Gask, L. and Sibbald, B. (2005) Improving primary care mental health: survey evaluation of an innovative workforce development in England, *Primary Care Mental Health* 3, 253–60.

Hudson, B. (2007) Pessimism and optimism in interprofessional working: the Sedgefield Integrated Team, *Journal of Interprofessional Care* 21, 3–15.

Laming, H. (2003) *The Victoria Climbié Inquiry*, London: The Stationery Office.

Leathard, A. (1994) Interprofessional developments in Britain: an overview, in A. Leathard (ed.) *Going Interprofessional: Working Together for Health and Welfate*, London: Routledge.

Lymbery, M. (2003) Collaborating for the social and health care of older people, in J. Weinstein, C. Whittington and T. Leiba (eds) *Collaboration in Social Work Practice*, London: Jessica Kingsley Publishers.

Lymbery, M. (2006) United we stand? Partnership working in health and social care and the role of social work in services for older people, *British Journal of Social Work*, 36, 1119–34.

Pietroni, P. (1994) Interprofessional teamwork: its history and development in hospitals, general practice and community care (UK), in A. Leathard (ed.) *Going Interprofessional: Working Together for Health and Welfare*, London: Routledge.

Rastegar, D. (2004) Health care becomes an industry, *Annals of Family Medicine* 2(1), 79–83.

Rummery, K. (2003) Social work and multi-disciplinary collaboration in primary health care, in J. Weinstein, C. Whittington and T. Leiba (eds) *Collaboration in Social Work Practice*, London: Jessica Kingsley Publishers.

Smith, R. (2007) *Youth Justice: Ideas, Policy, Practice*, Cullompton: Willan.

Smith, R. (2009) Interprofessional learning and multi-professional practice for PQ, in P. Higham (ed.) *Post-Qualifying Social Work Practice*, London: Sage.

Stevenson, O. (1994) Child protection: where now for interprofessional work?, in A. Leathard (ed.) *Going Interprofessional: Working Together for Health and Welfare*, London: Routledge.

Whittington, C. (2003) A model of collaboration, in J. Weinstein C. Whittington and T. Leiba (eds) *Collaboration in Social Work Practice*, London: Jessica Kingsley Publishers.

Zwarenstein, M., Reeves, S., Barr, H., Hammick, M., Koppel, I. and Atkins, J. (2000) *Interprofessional Education: Effects on Professional Practice and Health Care Outcomes (Review)*, Wiley, 10.1002/14651858.CD002213.

Chapter 2
The drivers and dynamics of interprofessional working in policy and practice

Roger Smith

Chapter summary

In this chapter, the aim is to summarise the contemporary and historical influences which have brought interprofessional working to prominence. We will consider some of the landmark events which have supported these developments, and a number of key themes will be identified. In particular, certain drivers are identified, such as scandal and the search for efficiency savings which collectively seem to provide justification for joined-up working. The contemporary policy agenda is reviewed and the chapter concludes with a brief discussion of some of the potential shortcomings of an uncritical endorsement of collaborative practice as an unqualified good.

Learning objectives

This chapter will cover:

- the historical influences which have informed current views of collaborative working
- some of the key national and international policy instruments which promote joint working
- the main drivers of policy relating to shared intervention strategies
- some of the possible criticisms of a uniform approach to the promotion of interprofessional practice
- messages for the future of collaborative practice.

More than just a passing fad

In this chapter, we will widen the focus somewhat to consider the historical and contemporary influences which have put such emphasis on the importance of developing effective collaborative practice. Given its current popularity, it might seem to some that as a way of working, joined-up practice has become something of a totem, to which everyone must pay lip service without really knowing what it means or what their contribution should be. It is perhaps unsurprising that something as self-evidently worthwhile as effective cooperation should be so widely endorsed in principle. On the other hand, there remains a nagging sense that it is being driven by rather more questionable interests and influences. When the traffic all seems to be flowing in the same direction, there is probably some justification for asking the question 'why?', rather than just being taken along for the ride.

It may be felt, for instance, that there is too close an identification of collaborative practice with a government agenda informed by 'managerialist' (Clarke *et al.*, 2000) preoccupations with setting standards and 'getting the job done' in the most efficient way to meet prescribed targets. For those involved in professional practice this may feel uncomfortably like a call for uniformity of delivery rather than a recognition that cooperating across boundaries involves a process of negotiating complexity and taking account of uncertainty (see Figure 2.1). We must be prepared, therefore, to consider the range of motives which may lie behind policy initiatives and structural adaptations in the interest of working together better. Equally, it is important to remember that some of these initiatives have emerged as a result of acknowledged problems in the past, where failures of trust, communication or awareness have been held responsible for dramatic and sometimes tragic outcomes.

The lessons of history are important for several reasons then, and these include the need to incorporate them into our practice rather than let prior learning evaporate, pending the repetition of earlier mistakes. It is surely no accident that our concerns over the adequacy of collaborative working arrangements are by now long-standing, and have not diminished noticeably over time.

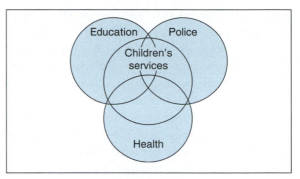

Figure 2.1 Children's services and child protection: individual and collective responsibilities.

Exercise 2.1

Child protection is an area of practice for which a number of agencies hold some responsibility, but it is not a core activity for many of them. What are the implication for leadership and coordination in situations where there are fears about children's safety?

Common agreement that joint working is a 'good thing' has not been sufficient to cement it in place at the centre of professional health and welfare services, or to ensure that when it is attempted collaboration has been effective and beneficial to the users of our services. So, we must combine a critical awareness of the origins and implications of particular 'drivers' and partial agendas, on the one hand, while on the other we must also ensure that messages from the past are carried forward, adapted and incorporated into our practice. This is the case for all those engaged in this task at present, irrespective of the differing lengths of time for which specific professional groupings have been recognised as significant players in interagency practice. Some may feel that they are coming relatively late to the party, but they are not necessarily disadvantaged in terms of their capacity to take advantage of past experience. Indeed, they may bring a welcome clarity of vision and purpose to issues which have confounded others for some while.

Historical lessons?

The policy drivers for interprofessional working are by no means a recent phenomenon. They have been well-established in welfare services for decades now. Thus, it has been pointed out that the 'establishment of children's coordinating committees' was recommended as long ago as 1950 by the Home Office (Hallett and Stevenson, 1980, p. 1). Such concerns have often been revealed in the aftermath of events which have given rise to serious doubts about the organisational arrangements for meeting welfare needs and safeguarding vulnerable people. While the focus of these concerns has often been harm to children, it has not been exclusively so, as several sources have indicated (Butler and Drakeford, 2005). Certainly, though, a central thread has been the sense of failure and the need to redress shortcomings in communication and coordination following evidence of poor and dangerous practice, whatever the setting. So it was that the inquiry into the death of Maria Colwell focused on the inadequacy of arrangements for cooperation at the time (the early 1970s). As a result, a number of recommendations were made which addressed both structural and procedural arrangements, making a case for umbrella bodies to oversee interventions in situations of serious concern, to be mirrored by formal collaborative procedures such as case conferences.

In fact, it may feel that many of the recommendations and reforms instituted in the subsequent period have had a very familiar feel to them, with the consistent themes of formalising collaborative arrangements at institutional level and supplementing these with changes in procedure and practice to guarantee better communication and shared working on the ground. However, even in the 1980s it was also possible to anticipate some problems in delivering idealised solutions of this nature. For example, different agencies might offer more or less commitment to working together, with their levels of involvement and active participation varying substantially. Indeed, this might be expected where there are no formal 'sanctions for non-participation' and differential limits are set on 'the extent to which autonomy' is ceded between organisations (Hallett and Stevenson, 1980, p. 6). Other problems associated with attempts to improve collaborative mechanisms could be the lack of common geographical boundaries, additional layers of bureaucracy, or the very different capacity or authority of participants to 'speak for or commit their colleagues' (p. 7). As this early review indicates, then, there is a long-established recognition that failures of coordination between agencies and professional groupings have been associated with serious and sometimes tragic outcomes, especially, but not only, for children. At the same time, many of the solutions proposed and implemented historically have had inherent shortcomings themselves, and there is certainly a risk that too much faith has been invested in these. The persistence of structural and procedural flaws has perhaps been underestimated, and this may be revealed in a distinct tendency for each new inquiry to identify many of the same failings; but then, also, to put forward again and again the same sort of solutions.

A closer look

Endemic problems?

In 1974, the official inquiry into the death of Maria Colwell, as a result of neglect and physical abuse, concluded: 'The overall impression created by Maria's sad history is that while individuals made mistakes it was the 'system', using the word in its widest sense, which failed her' (DHSS, 1974a, p. 86).

The failings of interprofessional collaboration have thus been a matter of repeated concern for many years, and yet they seem to be intractable. By the time of the Victoria Climbié inquiry, little seemed to have changed: 'The suffering and death of Victoria was a gross failure of the system. It is clear . . . that the agencies with responsibility for Victoria gave a low priority to the task of protecting children'.

(Laming, 2003, p. 3)

The bigger picture: the World Health Organization

Internationally, considerable impetus was given to the principle of collaborative practice by the World Health Organization (WHO) (1988), when it issued detailed guidance on the benefits of working interprofessionally, and the means by which shared education initiatives could support this. Building on an earlier WHO report noting 'a worldwide trend towards teamwork', and the 'Alma Ata Declaration' to this effect, this guidance took it as read that

> health workers could carry out their numerous tasks more efficiently if they were members of carefully composed teams of people with various types and degrees of skill and knowledge. A team as a whole had an impact greater than the sum of the contributions of its members.
> (WHO, 1988, p. 7).

These benefits could be achieved across the whole gamut of service delivery settings from prevention to rehabilitation.

The emphasis on combining skills to maximise outcomes has remained a theme for the WHO ever since. Returning to the subject in 2008's *World health report*, it stated that care that is person-centred, comprehensive, exhibits continuity and encourages participation of those concerned 'requires health services that are organized accordingly, with close-to-client multidisciplinary teams that are responsible for a defined population, collaborate with social services and other sectors, and coordinate' contributions from other services and agencies (WHO, 2008, p. xvii). Concrete examples are provided of the positive benefits of effective teamworking, internationally, for example in terms of improved outcomes in the Democratic Republic of the Congo (p. 31), and the report suggested that such arrangements foster trust amongst the communities served (p. 51).

Other international drivers of the trend towards closer cooperation at the level of practice are identified in social and political changes in the shape and dynamics of contemporary welfare states. Mixed economies of provision, including public, voluntary and private sectors, greater levels of demand and moves towards 'community-based services' (Rummery, 2006, p. 295) have been consistent developments across national and political divides. Thus, at a global and structural level, it appears that a number of influences are coming together to prompt change:

> This is due to the perception that the struggle to respond to rising demand for services (and the perceived failure of traditional welfare regimes to respond adequately to users' needs) is due, at least in part, to the failure of the

state to work properly 'in partnership' with the private and community sectors, and with welfare users
> (Rummery, 2006, p. 293)

In order to deal with this apparent inflexibility of state systems, whatever the regime, there has been a common push towards establishing and sustaining interorganisational partnerships, which can be more flexible and responsive to the expressed needs of service users. The international character of these developments may serve to create a sense of inevitability and 'naturalness' about them, which may, in turn, obscure some grounds for concern. Firstly, it may be that efforts directed towards establishing 'partnership working' actually divert energy from direct service delivery; secondly, the task of sustaining partnerships may then override the more important question of improving services; thirdly, this may lead to the establishment of 'success criteria' which are partnership-oriented rather than service-driven; and finally, there is very little concrete evidence to confirm that improved collaborative relationships are directly associated with better service outcomes (Rummery, 2006, p. 300). We should thus be cautious about overstating the presumed gains of better interprofessional mechanisms, while also recognising that the kind of questions to be asked about 'effectiveness' and service quality still need to be based directly on the concerns and priorities of people who use services themselves.

The drivers of collaborative practice: contemporary agendas

Scandal

In light of the above reflections, and especially concerns about the limited evidence base, it may be helpful to consider in a little more detail the current influences which seem to be driving the move towards greater collaboration in the specific organisational and practice contexts in which they operate. First, as we have already observed, there has been a persistent undercurrent of what might be termed 'defensiveness' which has been prompted by recurring evidence of system failure associated with damaging outcomes and personal tragedies. That is to say, the fear of scandal and attracting a bad press has definitely had an impact on strategic thinking in health and welfare services. Thus Parton (2006, p. 31), for example, states that it is impossible to 'overestimate the impact' of Maria Colwell's death and the subsequent inquiry on 'both policy and professional practice'. In accounting for the tragedy, a narrative emerged which put the blame as much, and perhaps more, on the 'system' as on a series of individual mistakes:

> It was recognised that there was no formalised inter-agency system for dealing with child abuse in most parts of the country [the UK] and that much was left to the initiative of individual workers.
>
> (Parton, 2006, p. 31)

This 'national' problem thus gained prominence at around the same time that the WHO was beginning to promote the benefits of collaboration, and the perhaps predictable outcome was the development of structures and procedures for seeking to avoid a recurrence of extreme forms of child abuse. It was this event which prompted the series of 'Working Together' documents initiated by the (then) Department of Health and Social Security in 1974 (DHSS, 1974b), and consistently revised and extended since then (for the latest version, see Department for Children Schools, and Families, 2010).

It has been shown elsewhere (Butler and Drakeford, 2005, for instance) that the 'scandal' surrounding harmful institutional practices extends well beyond the domain of children's services. Similar failings in the provision for adults have prompted parallel initiatives in the search for effective systemic responses. What is significant about the process of revelation and reaction is not the specific service setting, but the recognition that something serious has gone wrong which goes beyond essentially individual shortcomings and must be accounted for in a similarly 'systemic' fashion. This is a process whereby 'the specific comes to stand for the general' (p. 1), and this leads to the conclusion that problems cannot be solved just by changes of personnel, but necessitate a major overhaul of accepted practices. The consequences of this, however, may well be an unwillingness on the part of atomised public bodies to accept sole responsibility,

---

Exercise 2.2

Can you identify some key considerations which could be applied to help determine when collaboration is required and what it should be expected to deliver?

(e.g. 'The task involves sharing information which is not immediately accessible to everyone involved')

How should these be incorporated into policy and guidance?

---

and this may lead to responses which are framed in terms of collective obligations and the need for a shared response to the problem. In this sense, then, these essentially defensive adaptations themselves lead towards new manifestations of joint working and the acceptance of a range of interlocking responsibilities, as in Working Together and the equivalent policy frameworks for safeguarding vulnerable adults:

> In recent years several serious incidents have demonstrated the need for immediate action to ensure that vulnerable adults, who are at risk of abuse, receive protection and support.
>
> (Department of Health, 2000, p. 6)

The necessary framework for delivering an effective preventive and, where necessary, responsive service is one in which 'all responsible agencies come together to ensure a coherent policy' (p. 6).

We can see that certain aspects of collaborative practice are clearly prompted by prior system failure and represent reactive strategies which seek to put right collective shortcomings.

Complexity

The interprofessional education programme in which I am involved (Anderson and Lennox, 2009) incorporates no fewer than 13 professional groupings, and this is by no means all those with an interest in health and social welfare. It thus seems obvious that complexity is an aspect of contemporary service delivery which must be addressed in practice. For instance, it is recognised in the 'No Secrets' guidance that individuals' circumstances and needs may both be 'complex' (Department of Health, 2000, p. 12), and that services must be sufficiently flexible and comprehensive to be able to respond accordingly. Not only are needs recognised as multifaceted, but alongside this, social processes and organisational structures are also believed to be becoming ever more closely intertwined. Information and communication systems have proliferated with the digital age, and as a result we are faced with the task of processing and prioritising a continually increasing amount of data from a similarly expanding number of sources: 'In general, we found that the introduction of new technologies invariably creates turbulence within the work culture and within the organization' (Cullen, 2005, p. 167).

In one example reviewed in Cullen's study, the 'complexity and scale of a hospital-based information system was found to engender a form of "system dependency" and a propensity to a high level of disruption' (p. 169) in the event of technology failure. At the same time, the proliferation of information sources has been mirrored by an increasing specialisation of practitioner functions, so that communicative complexity finds its parallel in a diversification of roles, boundaries and relationships. Thus, not only is more information being generated and transmitted, but the number of routes and interfaces between professionals is also mushrooming.

One review of practice in community hospitals suggests, for instance, that

professional boundaries were flexible . . . with role diversification apparent, especially for nurses . . . This diversification of roles often challenged existing professional boundaries and, at its most extreme, could lead to breakdowns in communication with overall patient care suffering.

(Heaney *et al.*, 2006, p. 7)

The implications of greater specialisation and diversity of functions within health and social care have been recognised by government (Department of Health, 2004); the levels of care provided have been described as 'much more complex both technically and organisationally' than in the past (p. 66). It is also acknowledged that progressive functional specialisation means that responding to 'many conditions can

require a number of organisations and people to work together predictably, reliably and safely' (p. 67). The emerging recognition of complexity and its implications in policy documents suggests that this has clearly influenced thinking about the value of collaborative working (NHS Wales, 2009). It is also acknowledged that securing effective cooperative arrangements is itself far from straightforward: 'working in collaboration is a complex and challenging process which demands high quality leadership, management skills and interventions' (p. 1). The notion of 'partnership' is thus identified as a 'key element of the prevailing model of public service' (p. 3).

There appears, then, to be a complementary dynamic in play to the effect that changes in the social, professional and organisational environment are producing an array of new demands, expectations, skills and resources, all of which in turn prompt a greater emphasis on managing and coordinating this proliferation of factors impacting on the delivery of health and social welfare: 'Clearly, in this situation it is no surprise that people and organisations are motivated in different ways to seek collaborative ways to solving complex problems and delivering public services' (NLIAH, 2009, p. 3). This does not mean, of course, that there is anything like a consensus on the best ways to bring about shared working practices which are beneficial to the service user. There are in fact 'numerous interpretations and perspectives about the notion of integration' (p. 4).

Efficiency

Unsurprisingly, perhaps, a consistent policy driver for joint working has been the idea that it will lead to services which are more efficient, both from the point of view of those who access welfare services and that of the provider agencies. Thus, for example, the aim of ensuring that basic information about an individual and their circumstances is only collected once on behalf of all relevant professional interests seems self-evidently to be a sound objective. Not only is effective information sharing believed to be safer and more appropriate for those who use services, but it also seems to save time and money. The interlocking and pressing nature of welfare needs suggests that it is often the case that no one agency can possibly cater well for every aspect of the service required. It is simply not possible for any one professional to hold the full range of knowledge and skills required: 'The clients in question are frequently so vulnerable that their needs cannot be met by any single agency' (Tomlinson, 2003, p. 1).

In specific service areas such as child mental health, influential bodies such as the Audit Commission have for some time argued the case for improvements in shared working, suggesting that 'weaknesses' in the use of readily available information suggest a need for 'joint planning' and 'better collaboration' (1998, p. 62). This claim has gained further support more recently from the medical profession, which has often in the past been seen to be somewhat resistant to the idea of sharing patient data: 'For different agencies to work effectively together to achieve the best outcomes for patients, it is important that they are able to share information about each patient' (British Medical Association, 2006, p. 26). In the BMA's view, initiatives such as *Every Child Matters* (Department for Education and Skills, 2003) and the emergence of Children's Trusts have shifted the focus of activity and have prompted a greater need for 'professionals who are not specialists' (p. 27) in any given service area, but may be the first point of contact, to be familiar with the range of needs they are likely to encounter as well as the range of specialist services and skills available to address them. This, in turn, indicates the importance of training initiatives to improve awareness of others' roles and capabilities (2003, p. 28).

From the perspective of service users, children in this instance, it seems that collaborative arrangements offer a greater level of effectiveness because they better reflect the multifaceted nature of their own needs. From their point of view, 'seam free services' (Children First Children in Wales, 2002, p. 2) are much more likely to respond appropriately and quickly than those which require repeated referrals and assessments. The value of a 'single . . . point of contact', and a focus on the 'outcomes that are important' to children and families (p. 9) is recognised, and it is believed that multi-agency projects are best placed to offer this type of response, for instance in

A closer look

The five outcomes

The 'five outcomes' identified by *Every Child Matters* represent an attempt to describe the key features of a good life for children. These do not coincide neatly with individual service responsibilities, rather they imply that joint working will be essential to ensure that they are achieved, irrespective of individual children's needs or circumstances.

The five outcomes are:

1. Be healthy.
2. Stay safe.
3. Enjoy and achieve.
4. Make a positive contribution.
5. Achieve economic well-being.
          (Department for Education and Skills, 2003)

NB The change of UK government in 2010 led to a decline in the level of enthusiasm for the five outcomes amongst senior politicians, despite their relatively rapid acceptance as a common agenda amongst agencies and professional groups concerned with children's well-being.

the case of disabled children with a range of service requirements.

In any context where needs are likely to be complex and interlocking, there is clearly a contemporary consensus to the effect that good interagency arrangements can only work in the interests of more effective practice to the benefit of service users. Some tensions have to be acknowledged however, and it has already been noted that the expectation of more efficient use of resources is unlikely to compensate for cuts in individual service investment (Arblaster *et al.*, 1996). In fact, reductions in investment can actually reduce the capacity of agencies to work together effectively, it is argued.

'Joined-up services'

In the early years of the New Labour government, it became something of a mantra that we should aspire to the creation of an integrated service framework across the range of welfare provision, and that joined-up services at the point of delivery could and should be supported by organisational, strategic and structural arrangements which would facilitate this aim. Once again, the underlying impetus for this approach was provided by a number of concerns, such as those of service users meeting unhelpful responses from providers whose responsibilities did not match the service being requested, and simply being directed elsewhere. At the same time, the view became prevalent that failing to make connections could exacerbate problems, or at least fail to prevent things getting worse for some people. Thus, in areas of practice such as youth justice it seemed that failure to link the concerns of communities to the issues arising from the problematic behaviour attributed to young people would lead to partial and counterproductive outcomes, whereby nobody's concerns would be met.

Joining up services was not just a matter of efficiency, it was also about bringing together and reaching working agreements between agencies and others about what the central purposes and objectives of provision should be. Thus, the reforms in youth justice of 1998 were prompted largely by a belief that previously practice was characterised by 'confusion of purpose and a culture of making excuse for criminal behaviour' (Burnett and Appleton, 2004, p. 34). Not only were agencies and services hopelessly divided in structural and organisational terms, it was believed (Audit Commission, 1996), but they were also seen to be pulling in opposite directions, failing to convey clear messages about acceptable behaviour, and equally, having little impact on the levels and impacts of youth crime. Associated with this, it is perhaps predictable that agencies and practitioners will be less likely to demonstrate a spirit of mutual recognition and respect, and, indeed, it is more likely that suspicion and conflict would be the norm.

Creating a collaborative environment and facilitating joint working might seem an obvious way of establishing the basis for negotiation, mutual recognition and an emergent sense of common purpose, around the central objective specified by government of 'preventing offending by young people'. Of course, simply putting practitioners from different agencies together and asking them to cooperate may not be sufficient, as

Exercise 2.3

Think about youth justice, or any other service area with which you are familiar. Can you identify professional principles, ethics, targets or standards which might come into conflict depending on which agency you represent?

How would you go about trying to resolve potential conflicts of this kind?

seemed to be the case in the early days of the Youth Offending Teams, where some staff were believed to be 'frightened of change' or 'blocking and sabotaging' (Burnett and Appleton, 2004, p. 39), and important professional principles might even be under threat.

Similarly, a rather idealistic vision of 'joining up' services by establishing multi-agency teams might have the opposite effect; in reality, what might emerge is effectively yet another discrete service with its own boundaries to be agreed and negotiated by others:

Many of the YOT [Youth Offending Team] practitioners mentioned that they had lost contact with their parent agencies and explained that they consequently identified themselves more with the YOT than with their parent agency.

(Burnett and Appleton, 2004, p. 41)

Thus we should conclude this section with a note of caution about the drivers of the current inter-professional working agenda. Their very attractiveness as principles and goals ensures that they are likely to have a powerful impact on the service environment. On the other hand, this does increase the possibility that shortcomings and unrealistic aspirations will both be overlooked, and easy assumptions might come to prevail.

Working together: the policy agenda

The current popularity of 'partnerships' as the solution to problems of fragmentation and poor coordination between health and social services has been backed by a raft of measures.

(Glendinning, 2002, p. 116)

As the principle of collaborative practice has become accepted as conventional wisdom, so government policy has increasingly demonstrated a commitment to promoting and supporting joint working, notwithstanding some of the reservations we have already touched on. As indicated previously, the advent of the New Labour government gave a particular impetus to these developments, but it is also the case that earlier measures had pointed in the same direction. It is reported, for example, that in 'the UK, inter-agency approaches to complex social and economic problems have been encouraged since the 1980s' (Harris, 2003, p. 303).

Some specialist service areas may also have well-established traditions of collaboration such as provision for mentally disordered offenders (Home Office, 1995). Nonetheless, the trend towards greater emphasis on collaboration in policy has intensified in recent years. It is a theme which has become embedded in core documents and statements of aims rather than in supplementary guidance. Thus, the flagship White Paper *Our Healthier Nation* (HM Government, 1998) laid a great deal of emphasis on partnership working, for example. Subsequent legislation, in the form of the Health Act 1999, incorporated specific duties mandating service planning and delivery partnerships between health services and local authorities. It was this legislation which paved the way for joint service delivery arrangements, bringing practitioners from different disciplines under common management and organisational frameworks, using vehicles such as Care Trusts. Such arrangements now typically encompass service areas such as learning difficulties and mental health, with either health or local authorities taking the lead role. At around this time, a series of programmes and financial incentives were also put in place to promote collaborative arrangements, including Health Action Zones and Health Improvement Plans (Glendinning, 2002, p. 116).

As we have observed, structural and programme innovations of this kind have also been evident in other areas of practice, such as youth justice, where the choice over whether or not to get into partnership arrangements was removed by the Crime and Disorder Act 1998, which established interagency youth offending partnerships at the strategic level, and combined Youth Offending Team in the practice arena. Despite the superficial appearance of uniformity of purpose and activity, Glendinning (2002, p. 117) also points out that much is left unresolved by the 'absence of a single, standard blueprint' for the precise content and working arrangements of such joint initiatives. This may be felt in one sense to be appropriate, given the likely need for a degree of adaptation to local circumstances, diverse populations and varying needs and priorities. On the other hand, as she points out, this creates real difficulties for any attempt to analyse or evaluate the achievements of interagency working as a distinctive form of service organisation and delivery.

Strategic and structural initiatives such as those in the areas of health improvement and youth justice have sought to establish a culture and fertile breeding ground for enhanced cooperation at service level. These have been matched by substantive policy developments which have sought to map out the kind of changes in working methods and delivery goals which would reflect this more interconnected vision of the welfare arena. The language of documents such as *Every Child Matters* (Department for Education and Skills, 2003), for example, is highly instructive in this respect. The aim of *ECM* is to start from the child's perspective, and thus to construct a view of need and service provision which is determined not by pre-existing structures and divisions of labour, but as an integrated whole. Thus, the five outcomes that reflected agreed aspirations for children were identified: being healthy, staying safe, enjoying and achieving, making a positive contribution and economic well-being (Department for Education and Skills, 2003, p. 8). To achieve these, the mechanisms to deliver the range of services suited to children's diverse circumstances would need to change accordingly:

We want to put children at the heart of our policies, and to organise services around their needs. Radical reform is needed to break down organisational boundaries . . . Key services for children should be integrated within a single organisational focus.

(Department for Education and Skills, 2003, p. 9)

It is not just in relation to children's services that these ideas have taken hold. The advent of personalisation in relation to the care and support of adult service users bears many of the same features. The shift of emphasis towards user-defined assessments of need will require a parallel commitment to common frameworks and shared operating principles, it seems. The devolution of budgetary control to individual service users may well have similar consequences, to the extent that they will seek to 'mix and match' provision, according to their own preferences, perceptions and requirements. As for children, a common set of expected outcomes is identified. Service users should be enabled to: 'live independently', 'stay healthy and recover quickly from illness', 'exercise maximum control' over their lives, avoid children being required to act in inappropriate caring roles, 'participate as active and equal citizens', 'have the best possible quality of life, irrespective of illness or disability' and 'retain maximum dignity and respect' (HM Government, 2007, p. 3).

Not only will achieving these aims require integrated service delivery across specialisms, but it will also involve collaboration across sectoral boundaries, between statutory, private and voluntary organisations. The focus on securing real change at service level is made clear:

> This will not require structural changes, but organisations coming together to re-design local systems around the needs of citizens. The new local performance framework, which covers the delivery of all services by local government working alone or in partnership, will help to create an improved approach.
>
> (HM Government, 2007, p. 2)

As with children's services, concrete manifestations of this agenda are expected to include shared information systems, 'one-stop shops' and common assessment tools. These improvements in joint working seem self-evidently desirable, but it is worth sounding a brief note of caution; flexibility and common systems may also generate confusion and a loss of certainty about core professional identities and purposes.

The third aspect of the new policy agenda which can be identified is the establishment of common targets and performance measures; these can be seen as designed to secure common commitment to agreed service outcomes in a concrete way, creating incentives not just to collaborate, but to do so successfully. It is widely recognised that the welfare system has recently been subject to an ever-increasing array of mechanisms and measures to determine if and how it is achieving the goals set for it, and this has very quickly become a dominant feature of public service culture: 'The recent past has been dominated by words like targets, inspection and management' (Bichard, 2008, p. 5).

The kind of delivery frameworks established (such as Local Area Agreements and Public Service Agreements) have typically created expectations which include demonstrable evidence of coordination and partnership; 'The cross-cutting nature of government objectives is . . . explicitly built into the PSA architecture and, locally, professional bodies now have a statutory "duty to cooperate" in the creation of LAAs' (p. 8). As is clear from a brief history of recent approaches to public policy-making, the use of targets as drivers of 'cross-cutting' strategies has become commonplace (p. 19). In support of this, it is suggested that setting 'targets for health [has] broadly "worked", at least in the short term' (p. 25). It thus seems that 'performance management is here to stay'. Indeed, the progressive development of this sort of approach to service delivery is seen as having a positive role in promoting collaboration, and securing common commitment to shared goals and service standards.

The use of targets to drive change is not always welcomed, however. Concerns are expressed over the skewing effect of concentrating on those indicators which are relatively easily captured and subject to measurement, rather than less obvious or 'softer' evidence of positive achievement. These issues have gained a sympathetic hearing from the coalition government elected in 2010, which seemed determined to reduce such manifestations of bureaucracy and micro-control. It is clearly important not to become preoccupied with securing evidence of effective collaboration at the expense of fundamentally more important considerations such as the benefits of joint working for patients, service users or citizens themselves. We should always be prepared to recognise that joint working is not a prerequisite of good practice in all circumstances, and in some cases freestanding agencies and lone practitioners are able to meet people's needs or represent their interests perfectly well. It is sometimes felt that an overly prescriptive approach undermines local attempts to work out and organised suitable 'organic' arrangements (Institute for Government, 2008, p. 68). In this sense, ironically, we may find that overly intrusive attempts to ensure that partnership working takes place in the interests of local communities and individuals actually compromises their own attempts to take a genuinely user-centred approach to setting priorities and responding to need holistically. We can perhaps conclude that the policy environment is important in setting the tone in favour of collaboration and better integrated services; but at the same time, if this becomes too overbearing and specific, it may cut across the attempts by providers and practitioners to create real partnerships geared to better outcomes on the ground.

Before we move on to consider such criticisms briefly, it is important to take account of the final policy goal reflected in current exhortations to work together better, and this is 'troubleshooting'. As we have seen, critical and sometimes tragic failures in provision have frequently been explained in terms of poor or non-existent interagency communication, lack of clarity about mutual responsibilities, lack of mutual understanding and blurred accountabilities. In light of this, policy change has frequently been driven by the urge to resolve these shortcomings, as in the case of Victoria Climbié, for instance (Laming, 2003). This is not simply a matter of responding in reactive fashion to perceived failures or scandal, but is informed also by a more positive recognition that we can learn from mistakes, and even 'near misses'. Reviewing such cases, for example, illustrates some of the recurrent challenges facing those involved in collaborative working. Thus, where family circumstances change suddenly or unpredictably, the importance of maintaining pre-emptive information exchange becomes clear:

[T]he provision of a service to a child, including monitoring and protection, was complicated by the geographical mobility and frequent moves by the family. This was further compounded when several agencies . . . are involved with the family. Here good inter-agency communication becomes even more important.

(Sinclair and Bullock, 2002, p. 25)

It seems that policy is, in part, being driven by the lessons from experience. This suggests for instance that agencies need to incorporate routinely in their systems and procedures an expectation of openness and a readiness to share information and insights, even in the face of other policy imperatives which may create pressures in a different direction, such as expectations of confidentiality and data protection.

Policy frameworks of this 'anticipatory' nature are increasingly becoming the norm in health and social care, and seem to be related to the recognition that problematic issues need to be shared, rather than simply passed on. This notion of collective responsibility and accountability is reinforced by legislation, policy documents and implementation mechanisms, such as Local Safeguarding Boards and Partnership Trusts, which emphasise the common and interlocking commitments of all those concerned when it comes to dealing with problematic events or circumstances.

In this sense, the aim is to engender a fundamental culture change; the emphasis will shift from atomised responsibilities and functions to a practice culture which accepts and works across permeable boundaries, where working arrangements, responsibilities and interventions are guided by the need to respond to issues which cannot be neatly subdivided or parcelled out to free-standing sources of expertise. As a result, understanding these boundaries and the issues which arise becomes an integral part of the professional responsibilities held by each practitioner and the structural and organisational relationships of each agency which might be or become involved in the specific service context.

The collaborative policy agenda: some critical reflections

It will probably be important at this point to sound a note of caution. The policy agenda is overwhelmingly in favour of closer collaboration between professionals irrespective of their parent discipline, as we have seen. This weight of opinion can lead to a series of uncritical assumptions about the possible benefits. Poor communication, for example, cannot simply be attributed to institutional boundaries and lack of mutual understanding. This is to underestimate some of the factors which are common to all those in practice in health and welfare, such as heavy workloads, complex and bureaucratic procedures and competing organisational priorities. It is clearly the case, too, that service failures can be attributed to internal system failures at least to the same degree as they may be the result of deficiencies in interagency cooperation. To the extent that the push towards joint working may obscure some of these issues, it may compromise good practice rather than facilitating it.

It is also a matter of concern for many professionals that the value of their distinctive skills and functions should not be diminished to the extent that policy assumptions might imply that many aspects of their work are interchangeable. Some approaches to interprofessional education appear to incorporate such assumptions, and may have the consequence of leaving some practitioners feeling devalued rather than empowered by the collaborative policy agenda. Being encouraged to recognise and appreciate others' roles and responsibilities is not the same as learning to do someone else's job.

Other possible unintended consequences associated with a greater emphasis on partnership working include the loss of clarity about key roles and responsibilities; where responsibility is held jointly, this may lead to the diminution of individual initiative and accountability. Equally, the emergence of common operational agendas and assumptions may contribute to 'groupthink' and a parallel sense from the service-user's perspective that they are facing a seamless wall of vested interests which are not working conscientiously on their behalf.

If collaboration becomes an end in itself, it may indeed deflect attention from the fundamental importance of providing effective services which meet the needs of service users. In effect, the faultlines may be redrawn, so that statutory bodies and integrated provider organisations become more impermeable, and thus exclusive. Key members of the 'team' may find themselves left out, including, of course, service users, carers and other informal participants.

For practitioners this raises important questions about what the developing policy consensus around interagency working means to them. If it is driven by an administrative and procedural agenda, this may result in more elaborate and effective systems for exchanging information and making decisions, on the one hand while, on the other, and detrimentally, such improvements in efficiency may have unforeseen impacts, such as a loss of focus on those who should be at the centre of the process.

Conclusion

This chapter has sought to provide an overview of the historical and contemporary development of collaborative practice, and it has sought to outline some of the potential criticisms to be addressed if we are to achieve effective approaches to shared working in the interests of those who use our services.

Joint working has been progressively recognised over a period of time as **an integral component of high-quality service delivery, in principle, and in the right circumstances.** However, interagency collaboration has often been inspired as a response to high-profile failings in practice, and there is sometimes, therefore, a **tendency to take an idealised view of joint working as an unproblematic solution** to problems of poor interprofessional communication, under-resourcing, unsatisfactory practice or 'skills gaps'. **Collaboration is not an end in itself**, and should always be pursued only insofar as it can demonstrate its capacity to improve service outcomes.

Further reading

Butler, I. and Drakeford, M. (2005) *Scandal, Social Policy and Social Welfare*, Bristol: The Policy Press. An interesting account of the way in which critical events reflecting major system failures have influenced ideas and policy and encouraged greater commitment to the philosophy of joint working.

Glendinning, C., Powell, M. and Rummery, K. (2002) *Partnerships, New Labour and the Governance of Welfare*, Bristol: The Policy Press. An edited collection providing an overview of the influence of ideas of joined-up government on the forms of joint working undertaken in the early years of the twenty-first century.

Parton, N. (2006) *Safeguarding Childhood*, Basingstoke: Palgrave Macmillan. A critical account of recent developments in child protection, focusing on aspects of policy and systemic shortcomings and their possible explanations.

Useful websites

http://www.education.gov.uk
http://www.homeoffice.gov.uk
http://www.doh.gov.uk

Government websites all of which contain copious guidance on policies and procedures underpinning interdepartmental relationships and practice.

http://www.who.int

World Health Organization (WHO) site which provides examples of the international evidence and advice on multi-agency cooperation.

References

Anderson, E. and Lennox, A. (2009) The Leicester model of interprofessional education: developing, delivering and learning from student voices for 10 years, *Journal of Interprofessional Care* 23, 557–73.

Arblaster, L., Conway, J., Foreman, A. and Hawtin, M. (1996) *Inter-agency Working for Housing, Health and Social Care Needs of People in General Needs Housing*, York: Joseph Rowntree Foundation.

Audit Commission (1996) *Misspent Youth*, London: Audit Commission.

Audit Commission (1998) *A Fruitful Partnership: Effective Partnership Working*, London: Audit Commission.

Bichard, M. (2008) 'Foreword' in Gash, T., Hallsworth, M., Ismail, S. and Paun, A. *Performance Art: Enabling Better Management in Public Services*, London: Institute for Local Government, p. 5.

British Medical Association (2006) *Child and Adolescent Mental Health: A Guide for Health Care Professionals*, London: BMA.

Burnett, R. and Appleton, C. (2004) Joined-up services to tackle youth crime, *British Journal of Criminology* 44, 34–54.

Butler, I. and Drakeford, M. (2005) *Scandal, Social Work and Social Welfare*, Bristol: The Policy Press.

Children First/Children In Wales (2002) *Inter-agency Working with Disabled Children and Young People*, Conference Report, April 11.

Clarke, J., Gewirtz, S. and McLaughlin, E. (2000) *New Managerialism, New Welfare?*, London: Sage.

Cullen, R. (2005) *Health Information on the Internet: A Study of Providers, Quality, and Users*, Westport, CT: Praeger Publishers.

Department for Children, Schools and Families (2010) *Working Together to Safeguard Children: A Guide to Inter-agency Working to Safeguard and Promote the Welfare of Children*, Norwich: The Stationery Office.

Department for Education and Skills (2003) *Every Child Matters*, Norwich: The Stationery Office.

Department of Health (2000) *No Secrets: Guidance on Developing and Implementing Multi-agency Policies and Procedures to Protect Vulnerable Adults from Abuse*, London: Department of Health.

Department of Health (2004) *The NHS Improvement Plan*, Norwich: The Stationery Office.

Department of Health and Social Security (1974a) *Report of the Inquiry into the Death of Maria Colwell*, London: HMSO.

Department of Health and Social Security (1974b) *Non-Accidental Injury to Children*, LASSL 74, 13, London: DHSS.

Gash, T., Hallsworth, M., Ismail, s. and Paun, A. (2008) *Peformance Art: Enabling Better Management in Public Services*, London: Institute for Local Government.

Glendinning, C. (2002) Partnerships between health and social services: developing a framework for evaluation, *Policy and Politics* 30, 115–27.

Hallett, C. and Stevenson, O. (1980) *Child Abuse: Aspects of Interprofessional Cooperation*, London: Allen & Unwin.

Harris, S. (2003) Inter-agency practice and professional collaboration: the case of drug education and prevention, *Journal of Education Policy* 18, 303–14.

Heaney, D., Black, C., O'Donnell, C., Stark, C. and van Teijlingen, E. (2006) Community hospitals – the place of local service provision in a modernising NHS: an integrative thematic literature review, *BMC Public Health* 6, 309–20.

HM Government (1998) *Our Healthier Nation*, London: The Stationery Office.

HM Government (2007) *Putting People First: A Shared Vision and Commitment to the Transformation of Adult Social Care*, London: Department of Health.

Home Office (1995) *Mentally Disordered Offenders and Inter-Agency Working*, Home Officer Circular 12/95, London: Home Office.

Institute for Government Performance (2008) *Performance Art: Enabling Better Management of Public Services*, London: Institute for Government.

Laming, H. (2003) *The Victoria Climbié Inquiry*, London: The Stationery Office.

NHS Wales (2009) *Governing Effectively in Partnership: A Guide for Boards*, Cardiff: NHS Wales.

NLIAH (2009) *Getting Collaboration to Work in Wales: Lessons from the NHS and Partners*, Cardiff: NLIAH.

Parton, N. (2006) *Safeguarding Childhood*, Basingstoke: Palgrave MacMillan.

Rummery, K. (2006) Partnerships and collaborative governance in welfare: the citizenship challenge, *Social Policy and Society* 5, 293-303.

Sinclair, R. and Bullock, R. (2002) *Learning from Past Experience; A Review of Serious Case Reviews*, London: Department of Health.

Tomlinson, K. (2003) *Effective Interagency Working: A Review of the Literature and Examples from Practice*, Local Government Association Research Report 40, Slough: NFER.

World Health Organization (1988) *Learning Together to Work Together for Health. Report of a WHO Study Group on Multiprofessional Education for Health Personnel: The Team Approach*, Technical Report Series 769, Geneva: WHO.

World Health Organization (2008) *World Health Report*, Geneva: WHO.

Chapter 3
Change and challenge in interprofessional education

Hugh Barr

Chapter summary

Interprofessional education (IPE) took hold in health and social care in the United Kingdom (UK) during a period of unprecedented change 40 years ago when the shift of emphasis from institutionally based to community care demanded new models of teamwork and closer collaboration between the professions involved. Research into primary care teams exposed fraught relationships. Numerous work-based IPE 'initiatives' focused on the problems, but were succeeded by others which became more outward and forward-looking as its potential to further change was recognised. Post-qualifying IPE initiatives in universities and polytechnics reinforced that emphasis as they promoted progressive models of care.

Pre-qualifying IPE took off more slowly, but received a fillip when the post-1997 Labour government promoted 'common learning', not only to effect closer collaborative practice but also a more flexible workforce to further its strategies to modernise health and social care. These objectives, and established understanding of IPE were reconcilable, as this chapter explains, but with difficulty.

No less radical reforms for health and social care, set out by the incoming Conservative and Liberal Democrat Coalition Government elected in 2010, were pregnant with implications for IPE and collaborative practice as the chapter foreshadows.

Learning objectives

This chapter will cover:

- how change generates stress which prompts workers to be defensive and to withhold collaboration when it is most needed as their roles and relationships are redefined and reassigned
- how IPE can help them to understand the adverse effects of such behaviour as they review policies and their implications for practice within and between professions
- the fact that structural solutions fall short unless and until the workers are involved constructively and collectively
- how differing perceptions of IPE and common learning have been resolved with difficulty
- the proposals for the reform of health and social care under consideration at the time of writing which reinforce the case for closer collaboration in practice and pose additional challenges for IPE.

Coping with change

Implementing policies effectively depends on collaboration between the parties involved. Change may be exhilarating for some, but disorienting, destabilising or debilitating for others as boundaries are redrawn, responsibilities reassigned, power redistributed, jobs threatened and rivalries sometimes reignited. Stress (inherent for many health and social care workers) may be exacerbated, driving them on to the defensive (Obholzer, 1994) and prompting them to withhold collaboration when it may be most needed. That makes the case for IPE not only more compelling but also more challenging; more compelling to stand back, take stock and weigh the merits of policies, options for their implementation and implications for each of the professions in a spirit of give and take; and more challenging to overcome inertia and resistance. IPE can help participants to understand how stress may be influencing their behaviour in ways which may be counterproductive and does less than justice to their better selves. It can encourage them to put working more closely together to the test, discovering how it can spread the load, ease pressure and release energy to improve care.

The structural fallacy whereby policy makers put their faith in organisational solutions without paying sufficient heed to the human factor has long since been exposed (Carrier and Kendall, 1995), but reactions to recurrent change in health and social care in the UK under successive governments have succumbed to that temptation.

Learning from the past

It is no accident that IPE took root in the UK during a period of change in the organisation and delivery of health and social care. Forty years ago policies were being implemented to develop community-based services as alternatives to institutionally based services. Singleton GPs were extending the range of community-based care as they formed group practices and convened primary care teams. Concurrently, interprofessional teams were being established to provide 'care in the community' for vulnerable, institutionalised and highly dependent patients being discharged from long-stay mental health and mental handicap[1] hospitals earmarked for closure.

Team development was integral to service development in primary and community care to establish closer collaboration in response to more complex needs presented by clients and patients. However, research exposed fraught relationships between GPs, district nurses, health visitors and social workers in the formative stages of team development in primary care. While GPs were enthusiastic about the work of the district nurses, they were critical of health visitors whose role some failed to understand. As for social workers, GPs regarded them as relatively junior employees of the local authority, whose main functions were to find home helps, sort out financial problems and rescue battered babies. Neither GPs nor health visitors thought that social workers were trustworthy. They were hard to contact and slow to take action, did not offer a 24-hour service or remain long in the same post, never made time to discuss individual cases and never provided feedback. Comments about GPs were scarcely less critical. According to the health visitors and social workers, they too were difficult to contact, did not understand the work of other agencies and withheld information of importance (Bruce, 1980; Dingwall, 1978; Jefferys, 1965; cited by Barr, 2010a).

Relationships which had seemingly worked well enough at arm's length became problematic at close quarters in an unfamiliar working environment. That may explain why many of the early IPE initiatives in primary care, and indeed other fields as they spread more widely, were preoccupied with resolving misunderstandings, prejudices, rivalries and tensions between the participant professions. The hazard lay in dwelling on the negatives to the exclusion of the positives in working relations. That might drive participants on to the defensive and generate resistance to interprofessional learning by inducing misplaced guilt. IPE which, however inadvertently, held practitioners responsible for problems which were more structural or systemic than personal or professional was destined to fail where remedial action lay beyond the power of participants to deliver.

---

[1] As learning difficulties was then known.

A closer look

Promoting a regional initiative

A working party was convened in the north-west of England to facilitate discussions between GPs, district nurses, health visitors and social workers in 'dealing with patients'. It soon became apparent that there were both areas of common interest and of misunderstanding. It was agreed that a two-day workshop would be convened to examine problems impeding mutual appreciation of roles and effects on interprofessional relationships. Small group discussion was chosen as the learning medium. Eight representatives were invited from each of the four professions, taking into account their experience of interprofessional relationships and motivation to improve them. Working party members assigned to each group experienced some difficulty in avoiding a tutorial role; lessons remained to be learned about interprofessional facilitation. During day one, each profession in each group presented a paper on its present and future role followed by discussion fed back to a plenary session. Recurrent themes, discussed further on day two, were the inclusion of social workers in health centre teams; status in interprofessional relationships; communications and record keeping; and understanding one another's roles. Observational evaluation and participant feedback were positive.

(Lloyd, Borland, Thwaites and Waddicor, 1973)

Many of the early initiatives reflected these preoccupations. Most were local, ephemeral, work-based and unrecorded, but reviewed during successive national conferences (see Barr, 2007a, Chapter 4). With hindsight, the example above may seem unremarkable. Its significance lies in its exploration of ways of interprofessional learning now taken as read.

College-based IPE initiatives were mostly post-qualifying and part-time. Like the work-based initiatives which they complemented, they were dedicated to change by promoting new models of care, equipping workers with new skills for new roles. Many were multiprofessional rather than interprofessional, i.e. providing generic teaching deemed to be applicable across a number of professions rather than reciprocal

learning between them, but some built in interprofessional perspectives in response to students' needs and expectations (Storrie, 1992).[2]

Prequalifying IPE had yet to take off, constrained by the tighter regulation of qualifying rather than post-qualifying programmes and the conventional wisdom that students needed time to find their respective professional identities and to have experience under their belts before being exposed to learning with others. Passing reference was made in the literature to eight such initiatives during the 1970s, but with a tantalising lack of locations and detail (Mortimer, 1979). Some may have been intra-rather than inter-professional, drawing branches of nursing or social work together (Barr, 2007a). Prequalifying interprofessional initiatives, per se, were few and tended to be assigned to the margins of the professional programmes during extra-curricular activities or shared experiences on placement, avoiding the need to negotiate and validate modifications in crowded curricula.

One which attracted attention was in a new town where the staff of recently established primary and community care teams devised innovative opportunities for interprofessional learning between their students on placement.

Classroom-based initiatives at Moray House College of Education in Edinburgh (McMichael and Gilloran, 1984) and the University of Bristol (Carpenter and Hewstone, 1996) reinforced this emphasis on mutual discovery set within a theoretical understanding of intergroup relationships and subject to systematic evaluation.

While interpersonal and intergroup relationships remained pivotal, IPE was becoming more outward and more forward-looking as an agent to promote service, personal, professional and team development. Nationwide strategies for health education and health promotion driven by the Health Education Authority galvanised team development in primary care (Spratley, 1990a, b). Personal and professional development was reinforced when the Chief Medical Officer for England, under the heading of Practice Development Planning, recommended individualised learning programmes (DH, 1998; Wilcock et al., 2003).

---

[2]Defining IPE, as elsewhere in this book, as occasions when two or more professions learn with, from and about each to improve the quality of care as a subset of multiprofessional education with a wider range of objectives and learning methods.

A closer look

Learning together on placement in Thamesmead

Many and varied arrangements were made between 1976 and 1979 for medical, health visiting and social work students concurrently on placement in the new town of Thamesmead south-east of London to share learning experiences. Lunchtime gatherings were the most common but there were also half-day workshops and a weekend retreat. Students from different professions interviewed and then introduced each other to the group. Games were devised and played. Sentence-completion exercises elicited comments about each profession which were then fed into group discussion. Role play, case discussions, joint home visits, joint supervision sessions, peer teaching, topic groups and action groups were all tried. Evaluation was based on participant observation, students' diaries, trainers' notes and interviews, but generalisation avoided given the diversity of the activities.

(Jacques and Higgins, 1986)

A closer look

Sharing learning between medicine and social work

Final year medical and social work students at the University of Bristol tested conditions necessary to modify reciprocal group relations grounded in the contact hypothesis (Allport, 1979). Students worked cooperatively on shared tasks as equals in pairs and small groups respecting each other's identities. Patients were interviewed jointly, combined treatment plans prepared and reports made to the groups. Facilitators highlighted similarities and differences in attitudes and skills. Subsequent activities included further field visits and videoed case studies introduced jointly by a doctor and a social worker. By the end of the programme, overall attitudes towards the other group had become significantly more positive.

(Carpenter and Hewstone, 1996)

A closer look

Building the team

The Monkfield Primary Care Centre was established in 2000 to serve the new community of Cambourne in Cambridgeshire. The core team comprised two GPs, two nurse practitioners, a child/family nurse, a pharmacist, a well-family services coordinator, an information officer, a service development manager, a research and learning officer, a patient participation coordinator, an information technology coordinator and four further administrative staff.

Team members agreed that they should:
- maintain links with their 'base' professions
- work collaboratively within a flat management structure
- foster curiosity
- use their particular skills with patients
- establish respectful relationships with patients
- optimise internal and external training opportunities.

Everyone was encouraged to share their problems in a no-blame culture. Some team members questioned their capacity to carry the exploratory and developmental roles that they had assumed. Those accustomed to working under greater pressure felt anxious and devalued until workloads built up. One-to-one discussions clarified roles and helped members to contain their anxiety and vulnerability. Where applicable and practicable, external mentors were brought in from member's own professions. Individual appraisal, based on 360-degree reflective professional development, was included for everyone, with appraisers appointed from partner organisations for those, like the pharmacist, who were externally accountable.

(Bateman, Bailey and McLellan, 2003)

Reducing error

Tragedies attributed to lapses in collaboration and communication between professions were, however, all too frequent and painful reminders of the need for interprofessional learning to address the problematic as well as the positive in child protection, psychiatric aftercare and patient safety. IPE was instigated in child protection soon after it took root in primary and community care, prompted by recommendations in the first of many inquiries into the abuse or death of children (DHSS, 1974) for 'joint' or 'interagency' training to include GPs, health visitors, police officers, schoolteachers, social workers and others to improve communication and collaboration between them (reviewed by Birchall and Hallett, 1995). The issues raised were uncannily similar to those in mental health, notably in the case of Christopher Clunis (DH, 1994), when professionals variously responsible for supervision and support lost contact with discharged psychiatric patients and with each other; patients who then neglected to take their medication, relapsed into schizophrenic episodes and put themselves and others at risk. Concern about the incidence of medical error is more recent, highlighted in the UK by the Kennedy report (DH, 2001) into the untoward number of infants dying during or following cardiac surgery at the Bristol Royal Infirmary. The report reinforced the need for IPE, already exposed in the United States by the Institute for Medicine (2000) and in other countries, to improve relationships within and between the professions involved in the face of growing public alarm about the frequency of preventable errors which had hitherto attracted surprisingly little attention.

Comparison between the IPE response in these three fields merits more attention than it has so far received, notwithstanding differences in the configuration of professions involved and in the practice settings.[3] The application of collaborative inquiry (Reason, 1994) child protection discussed in 'A closer look: finding common ground' above would be transferable to the other fields.

A closer look

Finding common ground

The inquiry in Northamptonshire started from the premise that ownership was the key ingredient in catalysing change. Individuals and groups needed to be empowered by active participation to explore options on the basis of their knowledge of a situation. Eleven first-line managers representing education, health, the NSPCC, police, probation and social services met on seven occasions. Baroque guitar music greeted participants at the first as every effort was made to put them at their ease. Priority was given to getting to know each other, by means of interviews in pairs and reciprocal introductions to the group. An 'inquiry map' was devised for subsequent sessions to set limits and point directions. Attention focused during those sessions on the distinctive characteristics of management and supervision in child protection, the need for role clarity between agencies and issues affecting cross-agency communication and cooperation. Outcomes distinguished between the desirable and the achievable. The inquiry culminated in a formal presentation to the Area Child Protection Committee.

(Cosier and Glennie, 1994)

Key learning points

- Lessons learned about the role of IPE during its formative years in the management of change still resonate.
- IPE became less introspective and more outward and forward-looking as it gained momentum, but the need to resolve problematic relationships remained if and when they impeded progress.
- Inquiries into recurrent cases of child abuse and medical error reinforced the need for IPE and the collaborative practice which it promotes.

[3]Child protection and psychiatric aftercare are community-based medical errors more often acknowledged in hospital-based than in community-based care (where the need to address them may be no less great).

Modernising education and service delivery

Much the same preoccupations drove IPE in different fields from the late 1960s through to the 1990s and beyond, drawn together by CAIPE (the UK Centre for the Advancement of Interprofessional Education) into a more or less coherent movement. After the turn of the century one-off developments continued to be overtaken as the Labour Government embarked on a raft of radical reforms to modernise the public sector, including health and social care, and IPE was caught once again in a maelstrom of change. Government was committed to closer collaboration to help implement its plans, but also to the modernisation of the workforce to deploy personnel more flexibly in response to the changing demands of policy and practice. Each of these twin objectives had its own curricular implications held in an uneasy and mostly unacknowledged tension. The Department of Health promoted 'common learning sites' nationwide (DH, 2000, 2004a, b). Reference to 'interprofessional education' was conspicuous by its absence from Departmental documents. New wine, it seemed, was not to be put in old bottles.

The contrast between common learning, as commended by the Department of Health, and IPE, as it had evolved over three decades, was marked. Proposals for common learning were top-down to implement government policy: IPE had evolved bottom-up in response to the exigencies of practice. Common learning would be preregistration, university-based, nationwide and ongoing: IPE had, until then, been predominantly post-experience, work-based, local and ephemeral. Common learning would emphasise common curricula to help develop a more flexible workforce transcending professional demarcations: IPE, albeit including some common curricula, had dealt in differences, valuing and optimising the distinctive contribution which each profession brought to collaborative practice.

Interprofessional activists nevertheless welcomed Government's lead which held the promise to move IPE from the margins to the mainstream of professional education, to embed it more firmly in strategies to improve services and to secure its future. The challenge they faced was to instil accumulated practice wisdom from IPE into policies for common learning. CAIPE clarified, codified and exemplified IPE (summarised by Barr, 2010b) complemented by papers published by the Higher Education Academy (e.g. Barr, 2002, 2007a, b; Barr, Helme and D'Avray, 2011). Numerous interprofessional texts described IPE (e.g. Bluteau and Jackson, 2009; Carpenter and Dickinson, 2008) complemented by theoretical perspectives (Colyer, Helme and Jones, 2005), case studies (Barr, Freeth, Hammick, Koppel and Reeves, 2000; Barr and Goosey, 2002) and guides for programme planners (Freeth, Hammick, Reeves, Koppel and Barr, 2005), facilitators (Howkins and Bray, 2008) and students (Barrett, Sellman and Thomas, 2005; Hammick, Freeth, Copperman and Goodsman, 2009; Pollard, Thomas and Miers, 2010). Findings from systematic reviews (e.g. Barr, Koppel, Reeves, Hammick and Freeth, 2005; Freeth, Hammick, Koppel, Reeves and Barr, 2002; Hammick, Freeth, Reeves, Koppel and Barr, 2007) established the evidence base, while outcome statements (Sheffield Hallam University, 2010) focused on the readiness of newly qualified workers for collaborative practice. The *Journal of Interprofessional Care*–http://www.informaworld.com/jic–stimulated scholarship and became a conduit for exchange in IPE, practice and research nationally and internationally. These and other publications, complemented by countless conference presentations, were seminal in generating a critical mass of support in the professions and amongst university teachers, less so amongst service managers and policy-makers.

Reconciling agendas

The Creating an Interprofessional Workforce Project (CIPW) offered a renewed opportunity to reach them (CAIPE, 2007). Promoted and funded by the Department of Health and working closely with CAIPE, CIPW engaged service managers,

Table 3.1 Comparing IPE and common learning

	Interprofessional education	Common learning
Lead roles	Education and practice	Management and policy
Primary objectives	Collaborative practice	Flexible workforce
Curriculum planning	Outcome-led	Input-led
Curricular content	Common and comparative	Common
Learning methods	Interactive	Unspecified

trainers, policy-makers, service users and carers in dialogue with teachers towards mutual understanding and support for interprofessional education (its preferred term), demonstrating how together they could help to establish and sustain an interprofessional workforce. The opportunity to compare and contrast IPE and common learning perspectives towards defining a coherent policy and practice framework which embraced both was missed, however. Nor were funds found to follow up the two-year project.

Permit me to explore further the similarities and differences between IPE and common learning in a renewed attempt to effect reconciliation (see Table 3.1).

Lead roles

Practitioners had led the early work-based IPE initiatives while teachers had led those which were university-based. The Department of Health clearly envisaged that policy-makers and service management would take the lead in defining objectives and content for common learning. In the event, responsibility for programmes was institutionalised in joint planning and management mechanisms which included representatives of universities, service agencies and other stakeholders. Over time teachers have, however, tended to resume the lead roles, in collaboration with employing agencies to

provide practice placements and (until their demise) Strategic Health Authorities developmental funding.

Primary objectives

Collaborative practice and flexible workforce deployment may seem like two sides of the same coin. Effective collaboration encourages flexible working between practitioners from different professions by common consent within teams, grounded in mutual respect and mindful of the constraints of prescribed roles, statutory requirements and patient safety. Local and regional needs and expectations for flexible working were taken into account when planning prequalifying IPE programmes along with externally generated proposals for skill mix, multi-tasking, lateral and vertical career progression and new occupational groups (DH, 2004b), but alive to potential tension if and when those proposals threatened the identity, integrity, roles and boundaries for one or more profession. Programme planners held the tension between facilitating implementation of workforce strategies and proceeding at the pace and to the extent that stakeholders agreed.

Curriculum planning

Planning prequalifying programmes was complicated by the need to reconcile prescription of inputs for common learning in documentation from the Department of Health and from Skills for Health (e.g. Skills for Health, 2010) with outcomes for IPE enshrined in competency-based statements. Outcome-led planning accorded with that for the qualifying programmes in which the IPE was embedded, easing the harmonisation of professional and interprofessional curricula (Barr, 1998) assisted by the adoption of the capability framework devised by Sheffield Hallam University (Sheffield Hallam University, 2010). By taking benchmarking statements published by the Quality Assurance Agency for Higher Education in England for medical, health and social care professions (QAA, 2000, 2001, 2002) into account, especially the composite statement (QAA, 2006), the framework helped synthesise professional and interprofessional means and ends. Above all, the framework provided a context within which to test the desirability, feasibility and compatibility of expectations of IPE generated locally, regionally and nationally.

Curricular content

Common curricula gradually extended in prequalifying IPE as overlaps between the constituent professional programmes became more evident and pressure mounted to effect economies of scale. Savings made helped to offset resources needed for relatively costly small group learning between participating professions, exploring differences in values, perceptions and practices; as well as complementary learning to inform collaborative practice about the distinctive contribution which each profession brought (Barr, 1996). Boundaries between common, comparative and complementary curricula were flexible, permeable and negotiable in time and place. The case for 'common learning' only became problematic when overstated and imposed without acknowledging comparative and complementary learning, and the distinctive contributions which each profession brought to learning and practice.

Learning methods

IPE employed a repertoire of interactive learning methods (Barr, 1996) which enabled the participant professional groups to learn with, from and about each other (CAIPE, 1997). Common learning was silent on methods. Acceptance of the need for comparative and complementary curricula would, by implication, have acknowledged the need for interactive learning.

The New Generation Project was the most far-reaching attempt at the prequalifying stage to reconcile these two agendas, although it proved hard to sustain.

Key learning points

- Common learning emphasises common curricula for workforce development.
- IPE emphasises comparative curricula for collaborative practice.

A closer look

The new generation project

Launched in 2003, the New Generation Project was a partnership between Southampton and Portsmouth universities with health and social care providers in Wessex and the Isle of Wight. Funded by central government, it grew out of small-scale interprofessional initiatives. The Project Steering Group, including key personnel from service delivery to provide strategic direction, influenced local and national policy, convened task groups, secured resources and promoted quality improvement. The first stage of the developmental process was to identify from each separate professional curriculum where students were learning the same things or working towards the same outcomes, referenced to external benchmarking standards (QAA, 2006). The next was to identify areas within them where students might explore collaborative practice. The resulting curricula distinguished between profession-specific learning; learning in common, i.e. the same content but taught separately; and interprofessional learning together in three units. The first was on collaborative learning, the second on interprofessional team working and the third on interprofessional development in practice. Interprofessional learning coordinators linked with service agencies to establish partnership in the provision of practice placements and close collaboration established with the regional Workforce Development Confederation. Three mandatory and assessed 'interprofessional learning units' were embedded in all prequalifying health and social care programmes.

(Humphris and Macleod Clarke, 2007)

Responding to a new government

IPE is caught up once again in turbulence and change following another raft of proposals for the reform of the NHS, this time by the incoming Conservative and Liberal Democrat Coalition Government (Secretary of State for Health, 2010). Modernisation is re-emerging, but in a different guise with promises to reinstate autonomous professional practice free from bureaucratic constraints. Privatisation, personalisation and localisation are on the agenda – privatisation of some public provision; personalisation of care with self-managed budgets; and localisation of services. Group practice – uniprofessional and interprofessional – seems set to gain ground, presenting not only new opportunities but also new challenges for collaboration. So does the prospect of greater reliance on ancillaries and volunteers, reassigning roles and reorienting relationships under the pressure of budgetary constraints. Better services are to be delivered at reduced cost. Competition and collaboration are once again to coexist as uneasy bedfellows. Not for the first time, relationships within and between professions, and within and between community- and hospital-based care, are being rebalanced. GPs' responsibilities for commissioning services are being reinstated and extended with implications for their powers and status relative to other branches of medicine and to other professions. This much is clear: there is to be a renewed emphasis on joint working with a closer affinity to community and local workers than has been customary (Barr *et al.*, 2011).

Promoting and sustaining IPE will depend critically on how devolved and untried arrangements for planning and funding education and training work out as the Department of Health progressively reduces its role and accords employers greater autonomy and accountability for planning and developing the workforce, alongside greater professional ownership of the quality of education and training (Secretary of State for Health, 2010, p. 40).

Professional education will need to go beyond incorporating IPE to allow interprofessional values, objectives and strategies to permeate qualifying and post-qualifying programmes. Obstacles may need to be surmounted first. Notwithstanding support in the white paper for 'a multi-disciplinary approach' (par 4.33), economic arguments may be reignited for common learning, if not by that name. The case for interactive interprofessional learning may need to be made afresh, balancing arguments grounded in evidence to justify resources for small student groups against economies resulting from didactic teaching in larger classes, and setting the overall cost of IPE against projected savings from more cost-effective models for services which it makes possible. More priority will need to be given to the promotion and development of employment-based IPE than during recent years to ensure immediacy of impact as changes in the organisation and delivery of services gathers momentum driven by workforce reforms.

Key learning points

■ Impending reforms in health and social care at the time of writing (December 2011) reinforce the need for collaborative practice to privatise, personalise and localise services.
■ Protecting resources for interactive learning in small groups is critical.

Conclusion

Entering the third age

IPE has entered its third age. During the first age, *initiatives* had been essentially pragmatic, instigated by and for practitioners in response to immediate needs. Most had been one-off, isolated and ephemeral, dependent on dedicated, visionary and charismatic champions who had taken pride in being practical, treating learning together to improve working together as a self-evident truth in need of neither explanation nor verification. Many had proceeded by trial and error, seemingly unaware of other initiatives from which to learn, without prior knowledge of conditions necessary for success and vulnerable when their champions moved on or 'funny money' ran dry. Most had passed unrecorded, unpublished, underevaluated and undervalued, but enshrined qualities on which subsequent developments built.

During the second age, IPE *programmes* had moved from the margins to the mainstream as they had become more strategic, more systemic and more sustained, with longer periods of interprofessional study, larger intakes and multiple objectives. Leadership had become collective within and between institutions and less dependent on charismatic solo performers. Pragmatic initiatives had remained, but strategic programmes had claimed the limelight. Expectations had run high, to be reconciled with difficulty within crowded profession-specific curricula and demanding much of students still finding their professional identities, exacerbated by the failure to invest also in post-qualifying IPE as part of a continuum of interprofessional learning.

Is IPE as it enters its third age robust enough to withstand upheaval in education and practice to which, paradoxically, it may contribute? Will its exponents enjoy sufficient clout to ensure that it becomes integral to all professional education as an agent of change? Will they muster arguments, experience and evidence cogently and convincingly to demonstrate that IPE is indeed indispensable in implementing more cost-effective policies for education and practice? The jury is out.

References

Allport, G. (1979) *The Nature of Prejudice,* 25th edn, Cambridge MA: Perseus Books.

Barr, H. (1996) Ends and means in interprofessional education: towards a typology, *Education for Health* 9 (3), 341–352.

Barr, H. (1998) Competent to collaborate: towards a competency-based model for interprofessional education, *Journal of Interprofessional Care* 12 (2), 181–8.

Barr, H. (2002) *Interprofessional Education: Today, Yesterday and Tomorrow,* London: Higher Education Academy; Health Sciences and Practice. Occasional Paper No. 1, www.healthheacademy.ac.uk.

Barr, H. (2007a) *Interprofessional Education in the United Kingdom: 1966 to 1997,* London: Higher Education Academy; Health Sciences and Practice. Occasional Paper No. 9, www.healthheacademy.ac.uk.

Barr, H. (ed.) (2007b) *Piloting Interprofessional Education.* London: Higher Education Academy; Health Sciences and Practice. Occasional Paper No. 8, www.healthheacademy.ac.uk.

Barr, H. (2010a) Medicine and the making of interprofessional education, *British Journal of General Practice* 60 (573), 296–9.

Barr, H. (2010b) Interprofessional education as an emerging concept, in P. Bluteau and A. Jackson (eds) *Interprofessional Education: Making It Happen,* Basingtoke: Palgrave Macmillan.

Barr, H. and Goosey, D. (2002) *Interprofessional Education: Selected Case Studies,* London: CAIPE.

Barr, H., Freeth, D., Hammick, M., Koppel, I. and Reeves. S. (2000) *Evaluations of Interprofessional Education: A United Kingdom Review for Health and Social Care,* London: CAIPE; the British Educational Research Association.

Barr, H, Helme, M. and D'Avray, L. (2011) *Developing Interprofessional Education in Health and Social Care Courses in the United Kingdom,* London: Higher Education Academy, Health Sciences and Practice.

Barr, H., Koppel, I., Reeves, S., Hammick, M. and Freeth, D. (2005) *Effective Interprofessional Education: Argument, Assumption and Evidence,* Oxford: Blackwell with CAIPE.

Barrett, G., Sellman, D. and Thomas, J. (2005) *Interprofessional Working in Health and Social Care: Professional Perspectives,* Basingstoke: Palgrave Macmillan.

Bateman, H., Bailey, P. and McLellan, H. (2003) Of rocks and hard places: learning to navigate as an interprofessional team, *Journal of Interprofessional Care* 17 (2), 141–50.

Birchall, E. and Hallett, C. (1995) *Working Together in Child Protection,* London: HMSO.

Bluteau, P. and Jackson, A. (2009) *Interprofessional Education: Making It Happen,* Basingstoke: Palgrave Macmillan.

Bruce, N. (1980) *Teamwork for Preventive Care,* Chichester: Research Studies Press.

CAIPE (1997) Interprofessional education – a definition. *CAIPE Bulletin No. 13.* London: Centre for the Advancement of Interprofessional Education.

CAIPE (2007) *Creating an Interprofessional Workforce: An Education and Training Framework for Health and Social Care,* London: Department of Health in association with CAIPE.

Carpenter, J. and Dickinson, H. (2008) *Interprofessional Education and Training,* Bristol: The Policy Press.

Carpenter, J. and Hewstone, M. (1996) Shared learning for doctors and social workers: evaluation of a programme, *British Journal of Social Work* 26, 239–57.

Carrier, J. and Kendall, I. (1995) Professionalism and interprofessionalism in health and community care: some theoretical issues, in P. Owens, J. Carrier and J. Horder (eds) *Interprofessional Issues in Primary and Health Care,* Basingstoke: Macmillan.

Colyer, H., Helme, M. and Jones, I. (2005) *The Theory–Practice Relationship in Interprofessional Education,* London: Higher Education Academy; Health Sciences and Practice. Occasional Paper No. 7, www.healthheacademy.ac.uk.

Cosier, J. and Glennie, S. (1994) *Supervising the Child Protection Process,* in P. Reason (ed.) *Participation in Human Inquiry,* London: Sage.

DH (1994) *The Report of Enquiry into the Care and Treatment of Christopher Clunis,* London: HMSO.

DH (1998) *A Review of Continuing Professional Development in General Practice: A Report of the Chief Medical Officer,* London: Department of Health.

DH (2000) *A Health Service of All the Talents: Developing the NHS Workforce,* London: Department of Health.

DH (2001) *Learning from Bristol: The Report of the Public Inquiry into Children's Heart Surgery at the Bristol Royal Infirmary 1984–1995,* London: HMSO.

DH (2004a) *The NHS Improvement Plan: Putting People at the Heart of Public Services,* London: The Stationery Office, Cm. 6268.

DH (2004b) *The NHS Knowledge and Skills Framework (NHS KSF) and the Development Review Process,* London: Department of Health.

DHSS (1974) *Report of the Committee of Inquiry into the Care and Supervision Provided in Relation to Maria Colwell,* London: HMSO.

Dingwall, R. (1978) *Problems of Teamwork in Primary Care,* Oxford Wolfson College Centre for Socio-legal Studies.

Freeth, D., Hammick, M., Koppel, I., Reeves, S. and Barr, H. (2002) *A Critical Review of Evaluations of Interprofessional Education,* London: Higher Education Academy; Health Sciences and Practice. Occasional Paper No. 2, www.healthheacademy.ac.uk.

Freeth, D., Hammick, M., Reeves, S., Koppel, I. and Barr, H. (2005) *Effective Interprofessional Education: Development, Delivery and Evaluation,* Oxford: Blackwell with CAIPE.

Hammick, M., Freeth, D., Copperman, J. and Goodsman, D. (2009) *Being Interprofessional,* Cambridge: Polity Press.

Hammick, M., Freeth, D., Reeves, S., Koppel, I. and Barr, H. (2007) *A Best Evidence Systematic Review of Interprofessional Education.* BEME Guide No. 9. Medical Teacher 29 (8) 735–51.

Howkins, E. and Bray, J. (2008) *Preparing for Interprofessional Teaching: Theory and Practice,* Oxford: Radcliffe Publishing.

Humphris, D. and Macleod Clarke, J. (2007) In: H. Barr (ed.) (2007b) *Piloting Interprofessional Education,* London: Higher Education Academy; Health Sciences and Practice. Occasional Paper No. 8 www.healthheacademy.ac.uk.

Institute of Medicine (2000) *To Err Is Human: Building a Safer Health System,* L. Kohn, J. Corrigan, and M. Donaldson (eds), Washington (eds), DC: National Academy Press.

Jacques, D. and Higgins, P. M. (1986) *Training for Teamwork: The Report of the Thamesmead Interdisciplinary Project,* Oxford: Oxford Polytechnic Educational Methods Unit.

Jefferys, M. (1965) *The Anatomy of Social Welfare Services,* London: Michael Joseph.

Lloyd, G., Borland, M., Thwaites, M. and Waddicor, P. (1973) An interdisciplinary workshop, *Journal of the Royal College of General Practitioners* 23, 463.

McMichael, P. and Gilloran, A. (1984) *Exchanging Views: Courses in Collaboration,* Edinburgh: Moray House College of Education.

Molyneux, J. (2001) Interprofessional teamworking: what makes a team work well? *Journal of Interprofessional Care* 15 (1), 29–36.

Mortimer, E. (1979) Interdisciplinary learning at the qualifying and post-qualifying stages, in H. England (ed.) *Education for Co-operation in Health and Social Work: Papers from the Symposium in Interprofessional Learning,* London: University of Nottingham, July 1979, Royal College of General Practitioners.

Obholzer, A. (1994) Managing social anxieties in public sector organisations, in A. Obholzer and V. Zagier Roberts (eds) *Individual and Organizational Stress in Human Services,* London: Routledge.

Pollard, K., Thomas, J. and Miers, M. (2010) *Understanding Interprofessional Working in Health and Social Care,* Basingstoke: Palgrave Macmillan.

QAA (2000) *Social Policy and Administration and Social Work: Subject Benchmarking Statements,* Bristol: Quality Assurance Agency for Higher Education.

QAA (2001) *Benchmarking Academic and Practitioner Standards in Health Care Subjects,* Bristol: Quality Assurance Agency for Higher Education.

QAA (2002) *Benchmarking Standards in Medicine,* Bristol: Quality Assurance Agency for Higher Education.

QAA (2006) *Statement of Common Purpose for Subject Benchmarks Statements for Health and Social Care Professions,* Bristol: Quality Assurance Agency for Higher Education.

Reason, P. (1994) *Participation in Human Inquiry*, London: Sage.

Secretary of State for Health (2010) *Equity and Exclusion: Liberating the NHS*, London: Department of Health.

Sheffield Hallam University (2010) *The Interprofessional Capability Framework: Mini Guide*, London: Health Education Academy, Health Science and Practice.

Skills for Health (2010) *Key Elements in the Careers Framework*, Bristol: Skills for Health.

Spratley, J. (1990a) *Disease Prevention and Health Promotion in Primary Health*, London: Health Education Council.

Spratley, J. (1990b) *Joint Planning for the Development and Management of Disease Prevention and Health Promotion in Primary Health*, London: Health Education Council.

Storrie, J. (1992) Mastering interprofessionalism, *Journal of Interprofessional Care* 6 (3), 253–259.

Wilcock, P., Campion-Smith, C. and Elston, S. (2003) *Practice Development Planning: A Guide for Primary Care*, Abingdon: Radcliffe Medical.

Chapter 4
Keeping interprofessional practice honest: fads and critical reflections

Hugh McLaughlin

Chapter summary

This chapter aims to challenge the reader to consider more critically whether interprofessional practice is always the best way to work. In particular the chapter identifies the case for interprofessional practice, the difficulties of defining interprofessional practice and its differing forms. These forms include both organisational and practitioner examples and the evidence of their effectiveness. From this we question whether interprofessional practice may actually be a hindrance in certain circumstances and that we need to be more critical and questioning of when it is right to work interprofessionally and when it is not.

Learning objectives

This chapter will cover:

- the level of interprofessional practice relevant (if any) to work effectively and to achieve the agreed outcomes in this case
- it is just as wrong to work mono-professionally when an interprofessional perspective is required as it is to work interprofessionally when a mono-professional perspective is required
- is our interprofessional practice making a difference, and if so for whom, and how do we know?

Introduction

I have increasingly become concerned about the way interprofessional practice is talked about. Interprofessional, interagency, partnership, collaborative or even multi-agency working is uncritically promoted by agencies and government alike. All five terms significantly overlap and often become conflated. For the purpose of this chapter we will use the term interprofessional while being aware there are other terms used by other workers, organisations and government which mean much the same thing. Terms like 'partnerships' and 'empowerment' and in this case 'interprofessional practice' are intoned in such a way in our public policy discourse(s) that they are like 'mother love and apple pie'. No sane person would wish to be heard raising queries or doubts about whether it was right to promote partnerships, or to empower service users or to work interprofessionally. This chapter seeks to question the implied assumption that 'interprofessional practice' is inevitably 'a good thing'. Just as Sheldon and Chivers (2000, p. 2) stated in relation to social work and social care in general:

> It is perfectly possible for good hearted, well-meaning, reasonably clever, appropriately qualified, hard working staff, employing the most contemporary approaches available to them to make no difference at all to or even on occasion to worsen the condition of those whom they seek to assist.

Sheldon and Chivers's salutary comment is a reminder that just because we are qualified professionals who are trying to make things better for our service users there is no guarantee that this will happen, and in fact in certain circumstances our good intentions can even make matters worse.

This chapter will identify some of the key drivers for interprofessional practice. I will argue that it has its place within practice but that there is more to practice than just interprofessional practice and that we need to rediscover that mono-professional practice still has its place within the delivery of services. Let's be clear from the very outset: I am not against interprofessional practice, in fact in certain situations I would insist it was essential, but that is a very

Exercise 4.1

Thinking about your practice experience, can you think of an example (a) where your practice would have been improved by involving a colleague from another profession; (b) where it would have been better not to have had a colleague from another profession involved. Write down the reasons for both of your answers as they may prove helpful to understand and critique this chapter.

different type of statement from saying that it is always the most effective, the only way or the best way to practice.

The case for interprofessional practice

Human services do not exist in a vacuum. This effective practice can often only be achieved when different professions work together, whether this is the anaesthetist with the surgeon during an operation, the health visitor with family worker in a case where a parent is having difficulties parenting their young child or a GP with a social worker in commissioning a care package with an elderly person. The Roe Commission in Scotland summed up this position in relation to social work:

> Social work services don't have all the answers. They need to work closely with other universal providers in all sectors to find new ways to design and deliver services across the public sector. (Roe, 2006, p. 8)

This position is not peculiar to social work and 'social work services' could quite easily be replaced by any of the other human services. Galvani (2008, p. 105) highlights this situation in relation to people with substance misuse problems:

> Many have a number of problems that precede, coincide with and/or result from the problematic substance use. These problems commonly include experiences of child abuse, domestic violence, financial difficulties, housing problems, trouble with the police, family breakdown, loss of employment, and physical and mental health problems. No one professional can be an expert in all these things. No one agency can provide

all the services that a person may need. Multi-agency working is therefore essential.

Galvani provides a compelling case while Wilson and colleagues (2008) identify both political and professional imperatives for the development of interprofessional practice. Citing Pollard and colleagues (2005) they note it is important to understand both sets of drivers and how they interact. While interprofessional practice in some form or other has been around for a long time, it became an imperative under the Conservative government of Thatcher with her emphasis upon breaking down professional bureaucracies, reducing the power of the professions, fragmenting services and promoting a mixed economy of care. Under such circumstances it could be argued that if interprofessional work did not exist it would have had to be invented. This direction of travel was further reinforced under Blair's New Labour government which helped push the debate and practice into the foreground with a focus upon partnership working and modernisation as the means to address the 'wicked' social problems which were beyond the scope or ability of individual agencies to address (Department of Health 1998a). It is too early to say how the Conservative Liberal Democrat coalition will approach this issue but it would be very surprising if they were to change the direction of travel.

Governments have come to view professional boundaries as barriers to meeting patient or service-user needs that as such are in need of being knocked down and replaced by workers working in partnerships or joint teams. As Dame Denise Platt stated when Chief Inspector of Social Services:

The present government is committed to reforming public services. Its vision is of public services where the services are designed around the needs of the people who use them, rooted in the values of the community.
(Platt, 2002 para 1.4–1.5)

Incorporated within this is the idea of a 'seamless service' or 'joined-up thinking' which many within the human professions would support and which is also evident within the academic literature (Leathard 2003b, Morris, 2008. Joined-up thinking would reduce the overlap between services, promote the

pooling together of resources including expertise and thus result in more effective and economical services. Behind these views there is also the suggestion that interprofessional work should provide added value where 'the whole is greater than the sum of the parts'. Associated with this is an acknowledgement that some services are interdependent and that actions in one part of the system will necessarily have consequences or 'knock-on' effects in other part of the system (Littlechild, 2008). Interprofessional practice is made up of a range of different professions who, if pooling their expertise in a joined-up manner, will address human problems in a way that no single agency or worker would be able to do. There is also a belief that such work would develop a natural reciprocity whereby the interprofessional relationship was seen to be of mutual benefit to each of the partners helping them to achieve their goals while reducing risk and resources (Glasby and Dickinson, 2008).

The failure of professions to work together is a common theme in modern child abuse deaths, ranging from the death of Maria Colwell in 1974 to that of Baby Peter in 2007. The issue of interprofessional working reached a new zenith with the death of Victoria Climbié (2000) whose public inquiry identified the failures of interprofessional working as a significant contributor to her death (Laming, 2003). This case, and the following inquiry, provided a stimulus for improved information sharing, the development of a common assessment framework and greater collaborative working and laid the groundwork for the 2004 Children Act and review of social work by the Social Work Taskforce in England.

Public policy in adult social services has been moving in similar directions with the Department of Health stating in 1998:

All too often when people have complex needs spanning both health and social care good quality services are sacrificed for sterile arguments about boundaries. When this happens people, often the most vulnerable in our society . . . and those who care for them find themselves in the no man's land between health and social services. This is not what people want or need. It places the needs of the organisation above the needs of the people they are there to serve. It is poor organisation, poor practice, poor use of taxpayer's money – it is unacceptable.

(Department of Health, 1998b, p. 3)

Wilson and colleagues (2008) note that although there has been no single tragedy as significant in adult services as those in children's services, there has been an equivalent emphasis on improving interprofessional and interagency working. This has led to the point where they claim:

> The direction of public policy for the delivery of health and social care is therefore clear: interprofessional working is regarded as a key requirement of its delivery, a statement that holds good in relation to work with children, families and adults. (Wilson *et al.* 2008, p. 389)

While we have described a direction of travel towards greater interprofessional practice, this has been against the backdrop of an increased number of mandates and legal mechanisms for promoting cooperation between health and social services while at the same time we are experiencing a greater fragmentation between children and adult services. In England, in particular, children's services are responsible to the Department for Education and adult services to the Department of Health. This trend has increased with the establishment of adult trusts (Glasby and Peck, 2003) and, to a lesser extent, children's trusts, furthering the fracture lines between adult and children's services. As this split becomes more embedded we need to begin to talk openly of developing interprofessional practice between adult and children's workers. This is made more complex when we consider the example of parents with mental health problems who may require adult services from a specialised health and social care mental health team. However, they may also require children's services colleagues to assess and address any issues of the parent's condition which may have an impact upon either the parent's ability to care for their children or the extra support children may require, for example as a young carer. It is ironic that the push towards increased interprofessional practice in adults and children's work has created an extra fault line between adult and children's services which is likely to develop into a chasm in the future, where we will be talking about intergenerational services and the need to develop interprofessional services to reconnect children's and adult services.

Defining interprofessional practice

Interprofessional practice holds much in common with concepts such as partnership, collaboration and multi-agency working, all of which have been notoriously difficult to define. Leathard (2003a, p. 5) suggests interprofessional working refers to 'a team of individuals, with different training backgrounds, who share common objectives but make a different but complimentary contribution'.

On initial examination this definition looks attractive. Its definition neatly sidesteps the issue of which occupational groups can lay claim to be professionals. Hugman (1991) notes that traditionally we have identified professions from a delineation of 'traits' or characteristics that would be held to represent what a profession was. If you could show your occupational group could meet the identified 'traits' you were a profession, if not you were not a profession. These traits were often based upon the time-honoured professions of doctors, lawyers and clerics. It should also be recognised that in today's society many occupational groups claim to be professions, for example 'professional footballers' or the Army, who encourage recruits to 'join the professionals'. Certainly we no longer merely accept that to be a professional is to be a member of a restrictive and restricted set of occupations as exemplified by doctors, lawyers and clerics.

It is a moot point whether social work, nursing, occupational therapy, physiotherapy or teaching can claim to be a profession under the trait approach. While it could be argued that in terms of public confidence it would be better if they were to be viewed as professions, this is probably less important than that the different practitioners should act in a professional manner.

In the human services identifying those with differing training backgrounds is less straightforward than we would first imagine. Most of the occupational groups we have identified earlier – nurses, doctors, teachers, physiotherapists and social workers – would complete modules on human growth and behaviour, ethics, adults and children's safeguarding, research methods and so on. Nursing throws up some interesting examples for our consideration. Do we consider the differences in training between adult and children's nursing branches as sufficiently different to talk of them as being two members of an interprofessional team when they work together? What about social workers who undertake a common qualification course and then may be employed as children's, adults or mental health social workers; do we consider it as interprofessional when these people work together?

One other aspect of the definition worthy of mention here is whether interprofessional work is seen as voluntary in nature or a forced collaboration. Inherent in many of the discussions is the voluntary nature of interprofessional work, suggesting that professionals engage in such work in a spirit of mutual respect and trust, recognising the interdependence of one on the other. Included within this view is the recognition that each can exit from interprofessional practice when this is not meeting the desired outcomes (Glasby and Dickinson, 2008).

We can see that while Leathard's definition has a welcome simplicity, when we probe a bit further the simplicity quickly fades and interprofessional practice becomes a more muddied and contested concept. In fact our analysis would suggest that at its most basic we are talking about a team of individuals with different job titles who 'share common objectives but make a different but complimentary contribution' in a voluntary manner.

On a more critical level, even this rather basic definition along with Leathard's (2003a) definition raises an important issue for us to consider in asking how does this definition help us to identify who is the subject of interprofessional practice? Watson and West (2006, pp. 144–5) highlight this difficulty in relation to multi-agency practice when they write:

> One of the dangers inherent in a multi-agency approach is that a degree of *collusion* begins to emerge between the workers to the detriment of the service user's perspective. This can emerge from an eagerness on the part of the workers to be seen to be sharing a common set of objectives and for the relationships to be working well. (italics in original)

So far we have viewed interprofessional practice in relation to those who are employed to provide a service to someone else without considering the position of those who are to be the recipients of the provided service. Too often the recipient of interprofessional practice is lost behind the need for agencies to work together; success is identified by 'good' interagency practice at the expense of focusing on outcomes and meeting the needs of the service recipient.

Forms of interprofessional work

Thus far this chapter has used the term interprofessional as if it was homogenous rather a term for capturing a continuum. Glasby (2007) has identified a range of relationships between organisations that cover the following activities in a hierarchical format: sharing information, consulting each other, coordinating activities, joint management and partner organisation to a formal merger at the top end of the partnership scale. This partnership scale can also be mapped horizontally in relation to the number of partners to include; these may cover health and social care, health and the wider local authority or health, local authority and wider community as in the example of children's trusts.

From this model it is clear that interprofessional work can take a number of different standpoints while still being termed interprofessional. It should not be assumed that the top of the scale is the most desirable point. In relation to mergers we accept that the police are key personnel in the investigation of child sexual abuse but I do not see many commentators arguing that the police and children's services should be merged. The police, social workers and health colleagues may well work quite effectively at the fourth level in Glasby's hierarchy of coordinating activities to ensure that any child is safeguarded while maximising the opportunities for a successful prosecution should child sexual abuse be confirmed. The usefulness of this model is that it allows us to identify the degree of interprofessional practice currently in place and to ask if this is the degree of interprofessional practice that is best suited to this task to achieve the outcomes of the partnering agencies. This requires organisations to identify which level is most important for them while different levels of interprofessional activity may be best suited to differing activities. It is also possible that different organisations will view this differently and identify different desirable levels of interprofessional practice.

Some thoughts on interprofessional work

We now consider interprofessional practice in health and social care. A similar analysis could be done with other human service organisations like education, or the police with social services or health. Health and social services staff refer to the same person as a patient, customer, client, expert by experience, survivor or service user, with all six terms implying differing power differentials and differing conceptions of the individual and their needs. It could be claimed that health and social care represent two incommensurate traditions based on differing explanatory models, with health based on a medical model and social work on a social model. Glasby (2007) argues that the underpinning difficulties and problems with our understanding of health and social care stem from the assumption that it was possible to distinguish between those who are sick, and by implication have health needs, and those who are identified as being in need of care or safeguarding, who have social care needs. These differences are not always apparent. An individual may come to the attention of social care services when they are unable to hold down employment due to chronic ill health, alcoholism, drug misuse or mental illness. Incidents of domestic abuse, child or elder abuse coming to the attention of social care staff are also likely to require the expertise of medical staff to assist with diagnosis, assessment and treatment. These examples highlight that each service is often the handmaiden of the other.

One other example deserves further consideration and highlights the previous issues, from a structural as opposed to an individual position. This is not to deny that it was individuals who suffered from the 'bed-blocking'. Bedblocking was the term coined to capture the situation whereby hospital discharges, primarily for older patients, were held up because the local authority

was unable to commission or provide suitable care in the community, resulting in the patient remaining in hospital longer than their medical condition required. By doing this the patient 'blocked' the bed and prevented other patients from being admitted to hospital. In response to this the government in England and Wales introduced a system of reimbursement, whereby hospitals were able to recover some of their costs through 'fines' on social service departments. Glasby (2007) questions whether such an incentive unfairly targets and penalises one partner in what is clearly a whole-systems problem as opposed to a case of incompetence on the services side. Policy initiatives imposing structural solutions, far from promoting interprofessional practice, make it more difficult by creating relationships based on an unequal footing whereby one partner is able to financially penalise the other.

Adult services care trusts: interprofessional practice in action

Following the introduction of *The NHS Plan* (Department of Health, 2000), Care Trusts have represented a potential structural interprofessional opportunity for health and social care organisations which has divided opinion. Care Trusts were identified as a key mechanism for delivering improved integrated health and social care services, thus securing better outcomes for users and carers. In particular the Department of Health (2002) identified the following positives in relation to Care Trusts:

- an integrated approach which is shaped around patient and service-user needs supporting and rewarding staff for working together
- clearer and simpler management structures with better working arrangements for staff, and more and varied career opportunities
- a single management structure with multi-disciplinary teams managed from one point with co-location of staff, as well as single or streamlined cross-disciplinary assessments
- a single strategic approach, with a single set of aims and targets
- the potential for financial flexibility and efficiency

- better communication between staff about packages of care. Care Trusts will be in an excellent position to develop a single information system. (DH, 2002, pts 5–7).

The benefits identified above are not agreed upon by everyone. Glasby and Peck (2005, p. 3) identified the following issues from the literature that Trusts need to address:

- the apparent absence of an evidence base to justify the new model
- the perceived threat to social work/care values and to local democratic accountability of local authority services and staff moving into the NHS
- the potential narrow focus of relationships between organisations (i.e. health and social care) rather than on broader partnerships (such as the voluntary sector, Local Strategic Partnerships and wider local authority services)
- the arguably limited capacity of Primary Care Trusts (PCTs) to pursue the partnership agenda given their competing priorities.

Peck and colleagues (2002) and Glasby (2007) suggest that in relation to structural change formal mergers do not necessarily guarantee a better service – by itself structural change rarely achieves its stated objectives. Structural change may give an illusion of change, but is the means to improved services, not the end in itself. Typically the merging of two organisations does not save money, at least not in the short term. Any economic benefits are usually modest and may be offset by negative unintended consequences like reduced staff morale and poorer productivity. Mergers also consume huge amounts of worker and management energy and time and are potentially very disruptive for service users. Glasby and Peck (2005) suggest it may take eighteen months to two years before any significant service development or improvements are recognised.

In order to support public sector mergers Peck and colleagues (2003, p. 49) identified a number of key messages in their evaluation of the integration of the health and social services in Somerset, including:

- be realistic about what can be achieved given the local history and context

- be mindful of the balance between change and continuity
- be creative in the design of personal and organisational development programmes that support managers and teams
- be inclusive
- be careful important objectives are not overlooked in the focus on integration itself
- be prepared for certain things to get worse before they get better.

They also pointed out that it was essential for such mergers to be based on the agreement and voluntary consent of agencies that had an already established trusting relationship. They reported that one care trust which had been established to solve long-standing interagency problems found that rather than being resolved these historical problems were inherited by the new organisation. This raises the important question that all mergers need to consider whether a merger is the most appropriate structural solution to achieve the stated objectives. This brings us back to the challenge of all interprofessional work: interprofessional working with whom and for what purpose? If we accept that a full merger between two services is not necessarily always the best way forward to improve service outcomes for service users we are then faced with the challenge of deciding when structural changes should be considered and when they should not.

Working interprofessionally: practitioner experience

It is also important to consider what it means to be a practitioner and to work interprofessionally. Following the death of Victoria Climbié in 2000, one of the key areas identified for change was the need to improve interprofessional working and communication between the different professions. As the then Health Secretary commented to the BBC (2003, cited in Carpenter and Dickinson, 2008, p. xiii):

> there were failures at every level and by every organisation which came into contact with Victoria Climbié. Victoria needed services that worked together. Instead

the (inquiry) report says there was confusion and conflict. The only sure way to break down the barriers between services is to remove the barriers altogether.

Effective interprofessional practice can thus literally be a matter of life or death. Luckily, most cases are not this serious. There is however a tacit belief that working interprofessionally will prevent such occurrences, and this has helped fuel the development of interprofessional education (IPE), which is discussed more fully in Chapter 3 of this book.

In a discussion of 'interprofessionality' in health and social care Hudson (2002) described a predominately 'pessimistic' or sceptical model of interprofessional practice but also identified research evidence in the north of England representing a more optimistic view. Hudson reminds us that the top-down imposition of government policies and structural arrangements by organisations often fails to acknowledge the influence and impact that front-line staff have on the success or failure of such arrangements. Critically, such change approaches view front-line staff as mere receivers and implementers of policy and structures. This view neglects that front-line workers will interpret any proposed changes and may use their discretion to ameliorate or change the direction of proposed implementation. In extreme cases this may lead to front-line workers trying to block or undermine the changes altogether. This is more likely to be the case where front-line staff have not been involved in the discussions about the desirability of the change and as such are less likely to feel any ownership of the proposals. Individual discretion, professional background and accountability structures can all effect interprofessional working as Quinney (2006, p. 32) notes:

While a strong professional identity, for example as a social worker or as a nurse; might be seen as important, it has also been found that this can create barriers to collaborative working when the different professionals do not share the same beliefs about the contribution that each can bring to the team. This might be expressed as conflicts over beliefs about services being universal or means tested/targeted, about the lack of clarity of team roles particularly where knowledge and skills overlap, misunderstandings about the relative merits of

the medical and social models, polarisations of approaches based on deficit or strengths, and concerns about reduced professional discretion and increased accountability.

From Quinney's comments about the difficulties concerning collaborative or interprofessional work you could be forgiven for wondering whether it is even worth trying because the barriers appear almost insurmountable. From the issues identified it could be argued that it is amazing that any interprofessional work is ever successfully undertaken. It does however begin to explain why so many serious case reviews have exhorted professionals to work together and why this has been much easier to say than to achieve.

In contrast Hudson's (2002) optimistic view is based on three reasons. Firstly, he argues from a normative stance that interprofessionality is inherently a good thing and that the need for organisations to work more closely together is a normal feature of increasing demands and restricted resources. If this is true we can expect even greater calls for more interprofessional practice, given the global financial crisis and the reduced budgets in public services. Workers can be exhorted to work together, or criticised for not doing so without increasing resources and potentially hiding a resources deficit. Secondly, as identified earlier, the policy drivers in health and social care that suggest that this is the only way of tackling the 'wicked problems'. Thirdly, Hudson argues that pessimistic and sceptical academics will need to turn their focus towards making a more constructive contribution to identifying under what circumstances and conditions interprofessionality can achieve positive outcomes for professionals and service users alike.

Quinney (2006, p. 22) summarises the work of Barrett and Keeping (2005) in identifying factors which enable or create a barrier for successful interprofessional working:

- The need to be aware of the role of other professionals as well as having a clear understanding of your own role.
- The need for all to have a motivation and commitment to interprofessional practice.
- The need to be confident, both personally and professionally, about the contribution of your profession.

- The need for open and honest communication, which implies that there is both active listening and constructive feedback to clarify issues and develop a common understanding.
- The time and opportunity to develop trust and mutual respect.
- The need to develop a model of shared power with clear responsibilities and accountabilities.
- Ground rules for the management of conflict while remembering that conflict is not always negative and can be the springboard for energy and creativity.
- The need for senior management support is a prerequisite for effective interprofessional practice.
- Uncertainty is inherent in such practice and needs to be both acknowledged and managed.
- Tensions can and will arise from envy and rivalry between individuals and organisations when competing for resources and power.
- Be aware that working with people with complex problems in a complex structure can create anxiety that can become displaced onto other team members.

There are a number of issues that arise with the above identification of enablers and barriers to successful interprofessional working. There is no view as to how many of this list have to be in place before you can say you worked in an interprofessional way. Alternatively, how many of the factors need to be absent before it becomes impossible to be able to work interprofessionally?

It is hard to disagree with any of the first five points identified above, but when they introduce the concept of 'shared power' this becomes a more complex issue; interprofessional practice does not infer that all partners in the process have equal power. However, this does not answer the question as to when the inequalities in shared power are such that it is no longer feasible to talk meaningfully of interprofessional practice. Practically, shared power may in fact be very difficult to achieve because different professional groups have different mandates, e.g. it is not for the social worker or health visitor to decide upon the quality of criminal evidence in a child abuse case. Each professional will have a view and contribute to a decision but each profession has its own discrete areas of responsibility and accountability that needs to be

negotiated and renegotiated as circumstances and information change. Individual professions are not in a position to delegate their decision-making powers but they have to accept that other people's responsibilities and accountabilities may take precedence over theirs from time to time. While it is easy to see how others' practice can contribute to our own work, it is not always as easy to see how we can contribute to another profession's mandate.

There is an understandable focus on senior management support for interprofessional practice and how without it interprofessional practice is very difficult to achieve. Just as important, I would suggest, are the first-line managers who are responsible for the day-to-day practice and without whose commitment and motivation to promote and develop interprofessional practice it is likely to fail or at least be less effective. All too often the role of first-line managers and their influence on practice is overlooked; senior managers may manage the organisation but it is the first-line managers who manage practice.

Quinney then moves on to highlighting the practitioner's ability to manage uncertainty. This is important because most writings on interprofessional practice appear to suggest that implementation occurs within a stable environment. This is often far from the truth and most workers have experienced differing degrees of continuous change throughout their practice. These changes may have been the result of government initiatives, local policy changes, responses to a crisis or a tragedy or restructuring. Change for professionals has become a constant feature of modern organisational life. This is not likely to reduce in the near future as public service human organisations seek to manage significant reductions in their budgets. Quinney's last two points from Barrett and Keeping's (2005) factors acknowledge that tensions and anxieties are inherent in this form of practice, particularly where there are limited resources or issues of differential power between the organisations.

As previously mentioned in relation to agency and structural solutions to interprofessional practice, Glasby (2007) classified approaches in terms of depth from sharing information, consulting each other, coordinating activities, joint management and partner organisation to a formal merger at the top end of the partnership scale. The first question to ask is, what is the level of interprofessional practice that is required to effectively achieve the agreed outcomes in this case? This question is not peculiar to interprofessional work, but should be a basic question when two or more workers seek to work together whether they are from a different professional background or not. It is quite possible for different professionals to have different views on the answer to this question.

Exercise 4.2 requires the professionals to clarify their roles with the young person, the resources they have available to them and to identify where their mutuality of skills and organisational goals can be split into individual and joint tasks to provide a more effective outcome. What is important here is the ability of the two, or more, workers, to be able to respect each other's contribution, to communicate together in a common language and to clearly articulate the roles and relationships of the individual workers to minimise the chances of misunderstanding or duplication. There also needs to be a mechanism or trigger for reviewing joint working; human interventions rarely proceed exactly as planned and there needs to be a way of responding to a potentially changing situation. These tasks and plans also need to be communicated with and to the service recipient to achieve ownership of the agreed plan and to avoid the service recipient playing one worker off against the other. Even if this is all done, there is no guarantee that the workers will all agree and that there will not be conflict over the proposed outcome, with differing professional representatives espousing mutually contradictory positions.

In response to the question of the level of interprofessional practice required, we should be aware that the question includes an assumption that interprofessional practice is the right thing to do and promotes a temptation to do everything jointly, even if this would not be a good use of limited resources. Similarly, we also need to fight against the opposite temptation of assuming the other worker is doing everything while the service user ends up falling between the different good intentions of the different workers.

The second question relates to our discussion above and asks, is our interprofessional practice making a difference? Throughout this chapter there have been constant reminders about the lack of research evidence to demonstrate a positive outcome for interprofessional practice and it is thus incumbent upon practitioners to assess the impact of their practice to identify what works and what does not. We need to consider if these are generalisable or merely lessons concomitant upon the context and question being addressed or the profession or professions that one is working with. What works with colleagues in health may not work with police officers, social workers or educationalists that come from very different cultures and have differing remits. It is also important to remember that social workers, doctors, teachers and police officers are generally well-meaning people who do not set out to behave in ways that will allow children or adults to be abused. Effective interprofessional practice is not easy and it is therefore important we begin to tease out and understand when we should act in an interprofessional way, when we should not, how we should do it and what outcomes should be expected.

Exercise 4.2

A 15-year-old boy in foster care with a history of offending is causing disciplinary problems in a school and preventing the other pupils in the class to concentrate on their lessons. Consider what a:

- schoolteacher might want from a social worker, youth offending service worker or foster carer
- social worker might want from a schoolteacher, youth offending service worker or foster parent
- youth offending worker might want from a social worker, schoolteacher or foster parent
- foster parent might want from a schoolteacher, youth offending service worker and social worker
- young person might want from the different professionals.

Whose view should take precedence and why? What about the view of the 15-year-old boy?

Conclusion

This chapter has been written to suggest to the reader that they think twice about the nature of interprofessional practice. Interprofessional practice is all around us and sometimes **it can be difficult to see where**

acting mono-professionally and interprofessionality starts and ends. It is often the ubiquitous nature of interprofessional practice that makes it so difficult to identify and measure. The difference between mono-professional practice and interprofessionality is often one of picture size. A social worker might work in depth in a mono-professional way with a child building up a life-story book, but the social worker may also, in the bigger picture, be working with a school-teacher, a foster carer and health professionals. The list will get longer the bigger the picture that we want to view and consider.

This chapter has argued that interprofessional practice is dealt a disservice by its lack of critical attention. We have not only identified compelling arguments why interprofessional practice should be promoted but also raised a number of issues that we need to address if we wish to ensure interprofessional practice remains honest, neither over-claiming, nor under-claiming, what it can achieve. First, there is a need to clarify the language that we are using; interprofessional practice has become enmeshed with similar concepts. There is also **a need to view interprofessional practice as a continuum** identifying a range of positions, both in terms of depth and breadth. Alongside this we have identified the tendency within the interprofessional discourse to neglect and objectify practice recipients. Often effective interprofessional practice is identified by positive working relationships between the differing professionals, neglecting the experience of those they are working with or for.

Interprofessional practice has been championed by government and professional alike at the strategic, organisational and practitioner levels. Organisationally we have looked at the experience of mergers and shown how these should not be considered a panacea. Mergers, like adults or children's trusts, are suitable in very selective conditions, they need to be entered into knowingly and with an awareness that any benefits may take up to 18 months to be realised. Similarly we examined the position of the interprofessional practitioner raising questions as to the depth of interprofessional practice required and when a mono-professional approach may be more appropriate. It was also suggested that it is just as wrong to work mono-professionally when an interprofessional perspective

is required as it is to work interprofessionally when a mono-professional perspective is required. Both are part of the same challenge for practitioners in seeking to identify how best to meet the needs of service users.

Throughout we have identified a paucity of research evidence. Good-quality research is urgently required to understand the extent to which interprofessional practice can lead to better outcomes, in particular what levels and types of interprofessional practice work best for whom, under what circumstances and to achieve which goals. It is only by building the research evidence base that we can we begin to keep interprofessional practice honest.

The aim of this chapter was to question whether it is always best to work interprofessionally. Interprofessional practice can be a very powerful way of addressing difficult situations and it is often seen as an answer to challenges irrespective of the question. However, **to improve, interprofessional practice needs to come under greater scrutiny to identify when it is, and is not, the right way to work or organise services.** We need to **rediscover mono-professional work alongside interprofessional work** to ensure we maximise the opportunities for intervening effectively in people's lives.

Further reading

Glasby, J. and Dickinson, H. (2008) *Partnership Working in Health and Social Care*, Bristol: The Policy Press in association with Community Care. A well-written short introduction to the key issues involved in partnership or interprofessional practice, it is one of a series of books looking at different issues in relation to partnership working.

Quinney, A. (2006) *Collaborative Social Work Practice*, Exeter: Learning Matters, provides an accessible introduction to the key issues.

References

Barrett, G. and Keeping, C. (2005) 'The processes required for effective interprofessional working', in Barrett, G., Sellman, D. and Thomas, J. (eds), *Interprofessional Working in Health and Social Care*, Basingstoke: Palgrave.

Carpenter, J. and Dickinson, H. (2008) *Interprofessional Education and Training*, Bristol: The Policy Press.

Department of Health (1998a) *Modernising Social Services: Promoting Independence, Improving Protection and Raising Standards* (CM4169), London: The Stationery Office.

Department of Health (1998b) *Partnerships in Action*, London: The Stationery Office.

Department of Health (2000) *The NHS Plan: A Plan for Investment a Plan for Reform*, London: Department of Health.

Department of Health (2002) *Care Trusts: Background briefing*. Available from http://www.dh.gov.uk/prod_consum_dh/groups/dh_digitalassets/@dh/@en/documents/digital-asset/dh_4074326.pdf, accessed 03 December 2010.

Galvani, S. (2008) 'Working together: responding to people with alcohol and drug problems', in K. Morris (ed.), *Social Work and Multi-Agency Working: Making a Difference*, Bristol: The Policy Press.

Glasby, J. (2007) *Understanding Health and Social Care*, Bristol: The Policy Press.

Glasby, J. and Dickinson, H. (2008) *Partnership Working in Health and Social Care*, Bristol: The Policy Press in association with Community Care.

Glasby, J. and Peck, E. (2005) *Partnership Working between Health and Social Care: The Impact of Trusts*, Birmingham: University of Birmingham. Available from http://www.hsmc.bham.ac.uk/consult/pdfs/care_trust_dispaper.pdf, accessed 02 December 2010.

Glasby, J. and Peck, E. (eds) (2003) *Care Trusts: Partnership in Action*, Abingdon: Radcliffe Medical Press.

Hudson, B. (2002) 'Interprofessionality in health and social care: The Achilles' heel of partnership', *Journal of Interprofessional Care* 16 (1) 7–17.

Hugman, R. (1991) *Power in Caring Professions* Basingstoke: Macmillan.

Laming, Lord (2003) *The Victoria Climbie Inquiry* Cm 5730, London: The Stationery Office.

Leathard, A. (2003a) 'Introduction', in Leathard, A. (ed.), *Interprofessional Collaboration: From Policy to Practice in Health and Social Care*, Hove: Brunner Routledge.

Leathard, A. (ed.) (2003b) *Interprofessional Collaboration: From Policy to Practice in Health and Social Care*, Hove: Brunner Routledge.

Littlechild, R. (2008) 'Social work practice with older people: working in partnership', in K. Morris (ed.), *Social Work and Multi-Agency Working: Making a Difference*, Bristol: The Policy Press.

Morris, K. (2008) 'Setting the Scene', in Morris, K. (ed.), *Social Work and Multi-agency Working: Making a Difference*, Bristol: The Policy Press.

Peck, E., Gulliver, P. and Towell, D. (2002) *Modernising Partnerships: An Evaluation of Somerset's Innovations in the Commissioning and Organisation of Mental Health Services- Final Report*, London: Institute of Applied Health and Social Policy, Kings College.

Peck, E., Gulliver, P. and Towell, D. (2003) 'The Somerset Story: the implications for care trusts of the evaluation of the integration of health and social services in Somerset', in J. Glasby and E. Peck (eds), *Care Trusts: Partnership Working in Action*, Abingdon: Radcliffe Medical Press.

Platt, D. (2002) *Modern Social Services: A Commitment to Reform*, London: The Stationery Office.

Pollard, K., Selman, D. and Senior, B. (2005) 'The need for interprofessional working', in G. Barrett, D. Selman and J. Thomas, (eds), *Interprofessional Working in Health and Social Care*, Basingstoke: Palgrave Macmillan.

Quinney, A. (2006) *Collaborative Social Work Practice*, Exeter: Learning Matters.

Roe, W. (2006) *Report of the 21st Century Social Work Review: Changing Lives*, Edinburgh: Scottish Executive.

Sheldon, B. and Chivers, R. (2000) *Evidence-Based Social Care: A Study of Prospects and Problems*, Lyme Regis: Russell House Publishing.

Watson, D. and West, J. (2006) *Social Work Process and Practice: Approaches, Knowledge and Skills*, Basingstoke: Palgrave Macmillan.

Wilson, K., Ruch, G., Lymbery, M. and Cooper, A. (2008) *Social Work: An Introduction to Contemporary Practice*, Harlow: Pearson Education Limited.

Zwarenstein, M., Reeves, S. and Perrier, L. (2005) 'Effectiveness of pre-licensure interprofessional; education and post-licensure collaborative interventions', *Journal of Interprofessional Care*, 3 148–165.

Chapter 5
Working in partnership to develop local arrangements for interagency and interprofessional services: a case study

John Hughes and Sue Urwin

Chapter summary

This chapter will examine formalised interprofessional working arrangements through a case study from one geographical area, Hertfordshire, in which partnership working has been shaped by government policies and local partnership arrangements over a number of years. It will look at the drivers for such interprofessional working, the effects on local working practices with one particular group that often creates great interest and debate in the media, that of people who commit crimes and who also have mental health needs; a group which raises immediate images in professionals and the public mind about risks posed by, and for, those who are categorised in such a way.

In doing so, it uses the learning from the Hertfordshire experience to look at the ways in which agencies involved in any form of interagency partnership working can best work together in such environments where there are different cultures and practices which require them to work together closely, and sharing information to a great degree, and in their assessments, practice, reviews and monitoring.

The development of the Hertfordshire partnership arrangements and the issues raised by it are set out as a case study which looks at the issues as they arose over the time it was developing, and how considerations from the influential National Audit Office (NAO) work on partnership working was applied in this case example, for others to potentially learn from. The chapter outlines the challenges and possibilities of such structured interagency working, providing a reflective account of the problems faced and how they might in practice be overcome. These points are set out so that they can be generalised for any form of such systematic interagency planning and development.

At the end of the chapter, four anonymised case studies of individuals are set out to demonstrate practically how the interagency system worked with service users.

▶

Learning objectives

This chapter will cover:

- the aims of policy on interprofessional working from central government, which is explained in terms of its aims, what is intended from it and how these aims can actually work out in practice.

- the potential benefits of formal interagency developments and agreements to provide effective arrangements.

- the main drivers from policy which have driven and defined multi-agency working in one area – mentally disordered offenders – across the main providers for adult services. The nature of the relationships involved between the different providers of services are discussed in relation to how at various stages the concerns of each of the agencies involved were addressed and resolved, within a case study which explains how theory and policy can be worked through in practice.

- a model we set out to aid the development of interagency agreements and arrangements for interprofessional working, based on key elements from government bodies and guidance from other sources, how these were used in this area of interprofessional and interagency working, and how the lessons from this can be applied to any area of formal interagency arrangements.

The nature of public sector partnerships

Partnership working is often presented as a good thing. It invokes images of organisations coming together for selfless reasons to promote the public good. It includes ideas of equally valuable and valued contributions, long-standing commitment and a willingness to go the distance despite problems along the way. It is not an area of work that fits in easily with the idea of a quick turnaround, results-oriented public sector management. Partnership is viewed by government as a means of increasing responsivity to service users by establishing new forms of accountability. This can include local delivery plans, management boards with local representation and a wide range of public engagement mechanisms which can be combined with local engagement, whereby it serves as a focus for local voluntary effort.

The Labour government's (in place until May 2010) view expressed here is that if only public sector organisations would serve the higher public good by working together across boundaries, service users and the public as a whole would be much better served. Individual agency boundaries may be seen as getting in the way of public accountability by providing a shield for the pursuit of narrow provider self-interest. No announcements or stated intentions of the coalition government formed in 2010 have contradicted this. Partnership is therefore necessary to provide a higher level of accountability, because individual providers cannot be trusted to deliver on behalf of service users and the public. Partnership also represents an optimistic and managerialist way of dealing with social issues that have traditionally been seen as intractable.

A key element of the government's belief is the idea that partnership can promote the public interest by providing joined-up solutions to complex social problems.

Developing local partnerships: the example of criminal justice

Criminal Justice Partnership working has been a good example of what government policies have been trying to achieve in interagency working, which has been a key theme of government service delivery since The Crime and Disorder Act 1998 required crime and disorder partnerships to be set up in local areas. Crime and Disorder Reduction Partnerships (CDRPs) bring together various interested partners including the police, local authorities, health authorities, the voluntary sector and community representatives in order to develop a cycle of three-year strategies to tackle crime and disorder (Gibson, 2007, page 62). CDRPs are a major vehicle through which additional government funding has been bid for and have had success in reducing crime and anti social behaviour through this joined-up approach; CDRPs have not been successful in addressing the needs of offenders with mental health needs, as evidenced by the findings of the Bradley report (Department of Health, 2009). This may be because of the size and complexity of the issues involved, but whatever the reason offenders with mental health needs and learning disabilities have often fallen through the cracks of joined-up working.

As a model of partnership developed 10 years ago, Modernising Government needs to be revised in the light of knowledge and experience. For example:

■ the belief that partnership is a disinterested and technical process, and that working together to serve the public in this way comes naturally to organisations. In reality there is often a trade-off to be had between objectives

■ in complex areas of work much longer timescales may be required to 'grow partnership,' especially if they are to have a tangible impact on local areas

■ the public themselves may not necessarily have an active interest in public service delivery and those that do have such an interest may have some concern for the public good but may also be pursuing a personal agenda

■ there is a belief that partnerships are likely to save organisational resources and add value and that there is therefore a limited requirement to measure the public resources that working in partnership can take up. In reality more of a cost and potential benefit assessment may be required at an early stage

■ that there is a degree of equality between partners and therefore no necessity for one partner to put more into the arrangement than any others, or that an unequal contribution from one organisation will not skew the objectives of the partnership.

A closer look

Key areas for public sector partnerships

Underpinning details on the government's thinking about the public sector and public sector partnerships were set down in the Modernising Government White Paper (HM Government, 1999) which was published in March 1999. Modernising Government spoke of a long-term programme of improvement and modernisation with a purpose with three broad aims:

■ ensuring that policy-making is more joined up and strategic

■ making sure that public service users, not providers, are the focus, by matching services more closely to people's lives

■ delivering public services that are high quality and efficient.

These aims were centred on five key commitments:

■ policy-making will be forward-looking in developing policies to deliver outcomes that matter

■ responsive public services to meet the needs of citizens with a commitment to deliver a big push on obstacles to joined-up working, through local partnerships, one-stop shops and other means and to involve and meet the needs of all different groups in society

■ quality public services: a promise to deliver efficient, high-quality public services and not tolerate mediocrity

■ information-age government: to use new technology to meet the needs of citizens and business that trail behind technological developments

■ public service: we will value public service, not denigrate it.

The first three listed commitments are closely linked with the former government's belief in joined-up partnership. Later in the policy there is reference to integrated services, policies and programmes, both local and national, that tackle the issues facing society such as crime, drugs, housing and the environment in a holistic way, regardless of the organisational structure of public sector organisations.

The National Audit Office (NAO) report *Joining up to improve public services* (National Audit Office, 2001) was based on fieldwork carried out amongst five large-scale partnership projects looked into the practical results to date of Modernising Government. Overall the report was positive and identified five potential benefits of partnership working:

1. Taking a wider view so that agencies make a contribution to cross-cutting programmes for client groups such as the elderly or children
2. Tackling intractable social issues such as drug abuse, rough sleeping or juvenile crime by promoting the design of programmes which are better interconnected and mutually supportive, thus increasing their chance of success
3. Improving delivery, e.g. the one-stop shop
4. Promoting innovation by bringing together people from different backgrounds and expertise
5. Improving cost-effectiveness of public services by removing overlaps and realising economies of scale.

The report stressed that similar systems of target setting and accountability to those that are applied internally to the management of effective organisations are equally essential for partnerships. The objectives of the partnership should support the objectives of the organisation; it should have clear objectives that meet SMART criteria – specific, measurable, achievable, relevant and time-bound.

In designing joint working arrangements the NAO report recommended that consideration is given to the following:

- Who needs to be involved?
- What incentives are needed to support joint working?
- What support is needed to improve the capacity of organisations to work together?
- How can funding be provided in ways that promote joint working?
- How long should the joint working partnership last?
- What accountability and regulatory framework will best support joint working?

The NAO report was positive about the benefits of partnership working. Its findings provide a useful framework for a model of partnership working that addresses government objectives and fits the performance delivery framework, and this will be developed later in this chapter.

A closer look

Requirements to be met for effective joint working

The NAO found that there were five requirements to be met for effective joint working:

1. Setting clearly defined, mutually valued, shared goals. If objectives are unclear or not shared, partners may work towards different, incompatible goals and fail to achieve desired outcomes.
2. Progress must be measured: evaluating progress towards achieving the desired goal and taking remedial action when necessary. Joined-up initiatives are no different from other activities in that their progress must be monitored and remedial action taken when performance is less than satisfactory.
3. Sufficient and appropriate resources must be made available for the partnership. Without sufficient resources including appropriate skill, a joint working initiative will not be capable of being sustained in the longer term and value for money and propriety may be put at risk.
4. Leadership. Directing the team and the initiative towards the goal. Joined-up initiatives can be difficult to keep on track because of the additional complexity arising from the number of players involved. Good leadership is important as part of the 'glue' that holds the initiative together.
5. Working well together to achieve a shared responsibility. If organisations do not establish good working relationships based on mutual support and trust, acknowledging their difference and sharing information openly, then joint working will fail and improvements in public services will not be achieved.

Interagency working issues: the example of offenders with mental health needs

Following the NAO model the first element in partnership is to establish that there is an issue to be addressed which has relevance for all partners. An issue will often not be defined and may be only partly understood, such as with offenders with mental health needs.

Becoming involved in a formal interagency agreement about offenders with mental health problems can be affected by agencies having preconceived views and concerns, for example:

■ as a potential risk of serious harm to the public who can only be safely managed in a secure or semi-secure setting

■ as a health service problem rather than a multi-agency problem

■ as a potential waste of resources (an example of this is the untreatability myth which still surrounds personality disorders)

■ as a powerless group of people who have traditionally been neglected and their needs unmet.

The traditional term 'mentally disordered offender' encompasses some of this type of thinking. It is not clear what the term 'mental disorder' actually means; it sounds like someone who is out of control, dangerous and has a permanent condition rather than the

reality that about one in four of the population has mental health needs at some time or another and given proper treatment many of them make a full recovery. The term can also distance organisations from offering a service to individuals who are identified as being in this category by placing them in the '*too difficult*' box.

Mentally Disordered Offenders (MDO) Partnership in Hertfordshire: applying the model

The next sections present a case study of a project in which interagency and interprofessional working arrangements were set up to respond to government policy on this, the recognised needs and difficulties of such offenders themselves and of the risk they may present to others. The case study is presented to provide key learning points for other such developments, and reflecting considerations of the NAO and other government guidance on generic issues in interagency working from the experience of setting up one of the first such set of working arrangements in the UK. It will do this by looking at the issues as they arose in the actual timeline of the development in the following six sections:

1. Is it the right time for partnership?
2. Understanding the issue stage
3. Deciding on the organisations and agencies who can contribute
4. The problem definition stage
5. The action plan
6. Action plan review.

Is it the right time for partnership?

The NAO model makes no reference to the predisposition in potential partnership organisations towards developing a new partnership. Neither do the nature and extent of existing pre-partnerships appear often in the literature as a success factor, but in the Hertfordshire experience it is of importance. If there have been successes they can be built on, while failures or previous bad experiences can be overcome. Both good and bad partnership experiences can

---

Exercise 5.1

1. Consider how the different agencies might view an offender with mental health needs: as a risk? As someone who is need of help and support? How might these be reconciled in interagency approaches?

2. Do the same task with other service-user groups served by your agency or that you have an interest in. What are the agendas/prejudices/preconceived ideas in agencies/professional groups which may might affect any interagency working plans? How might these be overcome, with who, in those agencies?

become mythologised within organisational cultures. All of this can be included as part of the issues stage and as part of an initial cost and potential benefits assessment.

With regard to criminal justice mental health partnerships, Hertfordshire already had a track record of achievement. Mental health panels had been launched in the county in the 1980s and following on from the government's Reed report on these matters (Department of Health/Home Office 1992) a mental health strategy, *Plan for Mentally Disordered Offenders in Hertfordshire,* was launched across the county based on partnership between the police, probation service and the health service. Some of the leaders of these panels had gone on to more senior and influential positions in their organisations and were supportive of developments in this field.

Dr Reed summarised his main findings as:

1. Mentally disordered offenders should be considered as individuals.
2. Their needs should be assessed and should be met by joint working from different professions.
3. People should be diverted to Health and Social Services as soon as possible.
4. The need for an increase in the range of services.
5. The need for ensured continuity of care.
6. The need for agency research and evaluation.

These principles provided the basis of the Hertfordshire Psychiatric Assessment Panel System.

At the time of the development of the current partnership initiative there were three active assessment panels and one was defunct. All three were chaired by probation staff. However, there was no overarching or unifying protocol/statement of objectives and there was a lack of consistency with regard to the storage and transfer of relevant information, e.g. the means of suggesting to the Crown Prosecution Service how to proceed, which was a key purpose of the panels. The key partners were the NHS, police and probation service. In the 1990s, Hertfordshire panels had a national reputation for the quality of work that they produced and they were seen by the key partners as adding value. This, together with the existing panels, provided a good basis for future developments.

Understanding the issue stage

Under the NAO model the preliminary questions for potential partner organisations to address include:

- What is the issue?
- What is the evidence for it?
- Who is it relevant to?
- Why is it important?

These are the questions that have to be addressed in any interagency initiatives or developments against the core duties and purposes of each organisation involved. This may necessitate taking what the NAO describes as a wide view. Taking a wide view, in accordance with this, for example, probation aims can be interpreted as identifying those offenders who have mental health needs that are linked to their offending as a subgroup of offenders, ensuring that these needs are met by the most appropriate agency and any risks of harm they may present to themselves or others are appropriately managed. The rationale for this approach, apart from the humanitarian one which is important, is that it is likely to be the most effective way of managing such offenders. If their mental health needs are being met they will be able to properly contribute to sentence planning and accredited programme work, and of the small number that are imminently dangerous will be less likely to harm themselves or others because of the specialist intervention. A minimum level of 'sign-up' from all agencies had to be negotiated for any such plans to be taken forward.

With regard to the NHS (and this can be an issue in any form of interagency planning and developments, as the NHS is almost always a key player in such developments), the narrow view would wish to maintain a strong boundary between mental health and criminal justice. In this instance, the grounds for this are the potential drain on resources through being asked to take on work which other organisations are currently doing (or not), concerns about the impact on staff, especially with regard to potentially violent offenders, and a belief that mental health interventions are often ineffective, especially with personality disordered offenders.

The broad view would acknowledge considerable overlap in service users, that core agencies are often dealing with the same people in similar contexts and may be working in contradictory ways. It would consider whether it is possible to intervene earlier in some cases and to work with others in a more integrated way so that rehabilitation plans which may include accommodation, work/training and counselling resources are more likely to succeed. This could potentially save NHS resources over a period of time.

In Hertfordshire the initial issue had come from the police and probation service through the Hertfordshire Multi-Agency Public Protection Arrangements (MAPPA). MAPPA have the police, probation and the prison service as statutory authorities and the health service, housing, NHS and Children Schools and Families as 'duty to cooperate' bodies.

A close alliance between police and the probation service had already been established through the existing MDO Panel system. The emphasis on criminal justice panel involvement (along with health) and the adoption of risk to the public as a crucial determinant of the advice given to the Crown Prosecution Service has been a defining element of the Hertfordshire Panel system.

The issue that gave impetus to setting up the partnership concerned what was perceived as a lack of community mental health engagement with a severely personality disordered offender who represented an imminent risk of serious harm and who could not be safely managed in the community. The case was eventually resolved but there were deficiencies in joined-up practice delivery and lessons to be learnt. At an initial stage advice was sought from the Head of the Dangerous and Severe Personality Disorder Unit (DSPDU) Unit of the National Offender Management Service (NOMS). The advice received began to move the issue away from a narrow view towards a wide view, working to set up a multi-agency strategic group with a remit for mentally disordered offenders.

At this stage in the autumn of 2006 the probation service and the police had not given much consideration to the issues other than a joint concern about a particular individual and several others who represented a potential serious risk of harm. The importance of the narrow view was to achieve greater NHS ownership of a fairly low number of high-risk cases as part of MAPPA arrangements. Although the narrow view was quickly developed into a broad view, it is important to note that a key element in mental health partnerships is about working in a joined-up way to manage risk. This is recognised in NHS practice guidance (NHS/Dept of Health, 2005).

The NAO stresses leadership in getting effective partnerships off the ground. Leadership was found to be important but had to be spread amongst the partners to be effective and had to be focused on developing and promoting a partnership identity that was separate from individual organisational interests.

Deciding on the organisations and agencies who can contribute to an understanding of the issue and ensure appropriate buy-in

Without the assistance of the Head of the DSPDU this would have been a more difficult task involving individual networking and developing a wide range of helpful relationships. The Head of the DSPDU approached the NHS to get their commitment to attending an initial meeting and generated interest at senior levels. He was clear that the initiative needed an NHS commissioner on the group and ideally that the NHS should chair it.

At the first meeting chaired by probation with senior managers from the NHS (commissioner level), police, community mental health, adult care, the Crown Prosecution Service and the Regional Offenders Managers Office, the Head of the DSPDU gave a keynote address and a brief paper prepared by the probation service which set out the main rationale for partnership working was delivered.

The initial meeting agreed a need to establish a strategic group with quarterly meetings. It was agreed at a later meeting that it would be chaired by the NHS at commissioner level and that a probation service senior manager would provide the deputy chair and administrative back up.

Buy-in for the partnership was secured from most of the key agencies at senior manager level and a framework agreed for future meetings. An area of relative weakness was a shortage of data to make the case for partnership, an important feature in the NAO

- In developing formal arrangements for interagency and interprofessional working, previous partnership working experiences can become mythologised within organisations, so predispositions, prejudices and old issues between potential partnership organisations need to be taken into account. Previous successes can be built on, and failures or previous bad experiences need to be acknowledged and overcome.
- To start work on proposed formal arrangements, questions for potential partners include:
  - What is the issue?
  - What is the evidence for it?
  - Who is it relevant to?
  - Why is it important?
  - All then need to have a basic agreement on these four elements before work can start.
- Leadership may come from one agency initially, but this must develop quickly to ensure other agencies feel equal partners, perhaps by being offered the lead in the plans if that will aid the successful development of the proposed arrangements.

model, as data usually costs money and organisations collect data for their own purposes.

The problem definition stage

Problem definition is probably the most complex and important stage in multi-agency partnerships. The NAO refers to setting clearly defined, mutually valued, shared goals. This is not a simple process for the following reasons:

- There is a significant 'run in' required which can be described as a 'getting to know you' phase. This requires an effort from the point of view of partners to see things through the perspective of other partners, to understand their core business, their targets and their strategic priorities.
- The availability and sharing of data. Organisations collect data for their own purposes to support their performance objectives and an important part of problem definition involves finding out what data is available and collating it in different ways.
- The problem may cut across traditional 'ways of doing things' and may require rethinking across

existing policies and processes which can have implications within the organisation. Partnerships may either sit outside these structures or be integrated into them at some level. Unless they are integrated into organisational structures they are not likely to be effective.

- The problem may be defined in such a way that there are heavier resourcing implications for one organisation compared to another. This may be a matter of sequencing, for example, investing more in police cells diversion may have knock-on benefits for health because it will enable cheaper joined-up interventions to be applied at an early stage instead of more expensive interventions later on. However, this may require up-front investment and the benefits may not be realised for several years.
- Problems are subject to definition and redefinition and often evolve as different things are tried and more information is collected.
- It is not likely that there will be one simple defined problem – something messier is more probable, a number of problems ranging from the highly complex and expensive to the simpler and cheaper. This generates a range of possible problems for the partnership to decide on and prioritise.

The problem definition is the basis of the partnership and this had to be agreed by the partnership agencies. It should include a clear understanding of of what success will look like.

Work on problem definition went on over several months, and the outcome was formal terms of reference which were signed up to by the key partners.

These were as follows:

1. To provide strategic leadership and policy direction on a range of mental health/learning disability issues which impact upon the criminal justice agencies. This will be through a business plan reviewed every three years which all partnership agencies will sign up to.

2. To define and develop a cost-effective, coordinated package of services to meet the care needs of individuals.

3. To measure the demand for service by implementing agreed methods of data collection which will

be brought together into regular reports for the Hertfordshire Mentally Disordered Offenders Strategic Board and, where necessary, agreeing service priorities.

4. To share needs assessment information across health, social care and criminal justice agencies.

5. To identify gaps in current systems and procedures in relation to managing risk of harm and securing diversion from the criminal justice system where appropriate and propose methods of resolution to agencies including bidding for additional resources.

6. To stimulate more creative approaches to problems and develop new and revised policies for adoption within or between agencies.

7. To develop and support the work programmes of the local mentally disordered offenders Panels.

8. To provide a forum for discussion of issues irresolvable at local level and sponsor further work to assist policy direction and development.

9. To enhance confidence and greater understanding of roles and responsibilities between partner agencies.

10. To ensure that services for mentally disordered offenders meet and, wherever possible, exceed national requirements.

11. To ensure the criminal justice system has access to the most appropriate information and assessments of individuals needs.

12. To develop better understanding of local mentally disordered offender groups and how they work.

It was soon recognised within a multi-agency partnership context that the term 'mentally disordered offenders' was not a helpful term and the National Association for the Case and Resettlement of Offerders (NACRO) terminology of 'offenders with mental health needs' was used instead. 'Mentally disordered offenders' was viewed as an imprecise term that carried pejorative overtones. This change in thinking is one indicator of how attitudes started to change at senior levels within the partnership organisations.

A needs-based service does not mean that there are no offenders who represent a significant risk of harm to the public and who require secure mental health treatment; this was always and still is a key part of the work of the panels. Risk of harm to self and others is an overarching context for all work with offenders, whether or not there are mental health needs present. The difference is that perceived risk does not define the whole service for offenders with mental health needs.

The problem definition stage that the NAO put forward assumes a degree of knowledge and data that was not readily available in Hertfordshire and is unlikely to be available in many areas with regard to offenders with mental health needs. Their needs are complex and there is likely to be a range of problems that have to be addressed. The experience of the Hertfordshire partnership has been that terms of reference are important and are a good way of gaining multi-agency buy-in.

The action plan

The action plan should operationalise the problem definition into a series of SMART objectives with individuals identified to lead on them. The basic format usually includes the objectives, a timescale, a lead person and a review date.

The initial energies of the strategic group were taken up with working out terms of reference. When this was in place a strategic planning day was held in the summer of 2008. Four key themes which it was decided should form the basis of the initial action plan were identified on the day. These were assessment processes, reinvigorating local panels, developing a protocol for information sharing and setting out a broad strategic pathway for providing services for offenders with mental health needs.

Each of the four themes was led by a different member of the strategic group; the theme lead recruited a multi-agency working group whose first task was to submit a work plan to the strategic group for signing off.

The assessment processes working group was concerned with how and where appropriate assessments could be commissioned. It was chaired by an experienced probation service mental health practitioner and included a probation offender manager, the consultant forensic psychiatrist for Hertfordshire, a chartered forensic psychologist from the prison service, a mental health social worker, a community psychiatric nurse, an NHS planning and commissioning manager and a detective sergeant from Hertfordshire police.

Reinvigorating local panels was concerned with finding out what was happening with local panels on the ground and making proposals as to how they should be managed in the future across Hertfordshire. The working group was chaired by a detective chief inspector from Hertfordshire police and included two forensic liaison nurses who had worked closely with the panels, a community psychiatric nurse, a mental health social worker and a senior probation officer.

The protocol for information sharing was intended to pull together a range of different protocols, local and national, and produce a written document that the partner agencies would be able to sign up to which would enable information to be shared regarding different service users. The working group was chaired by a senior adviser in adult care services and included a senior crown prosecutor, a senior probation officer and a mental health social worker.

The strategic pathways theme was concerned with working out mental health pathways at each stage of the process from the perspective of the service user from pre-court to post-release. It was intended to provide an overall template for future service development. The working group was chaired by a probation assistant chief officer and included a prison service forensic psychologist, a NOMS commissioning manager, a representative of the Hertfordshire housing departments, a senior probation officer, a mental health nurse, a detective sergeant and an NHS commissioning manager.

The intention was that the working groups would produce recommendations to the strategic group which would then be amended as appropriate and monitored. It was also intended that they would foster sharing of knowledge and start to grow multi-agency involvement at the operational level.

Setting up an operational arm of the strategic group is a key success factor and the working group format, whereby a body of different people come together from different parts of the partnership organisations to produce a focused, time-limited piece of work, was found to be a good way of achieving this.

Action plan review

The working groups took longer to set up and get working than anticipated. The problem was one of getting busy people together. This did have one advantage in that it focused minds on achieving the task with as few meetings as possible. It placed a lot of responsibility on the group chairs who had to ensure that group members who were not able to attend were consulted with and had a voice.

The assessment processes working group redefined some of the issues in a different way. A good example of this was that what had been defined as a problem of getting reports for court on time was redefined into a problem of how reports had been requested. This resulted in the development of a standard referral form and a single point of contact for requests who would screen them and then attend a weekly meeting with the forensic team. The system has been rolled out and has been found to work well in reducing the numbers of reports by clarifying when and where reports are needed and in setting up a system which promotes joint working at an early stage. This has been of significant use in the management of risk of harm by providing diversion without the use of the MAPPA process.

The local panels were in place in two out of three centres in Hertfordshire and in the two centres that were operational they had developed in different ways. One of the panels had recently been commended by an external audit and had been referred to nationally as an example of good practice, it was adopted across Hertfordshire. The probation service had used additional temporary funding to pay for a forensic mental health worker, one of whose roles was to chair all the panels as a way of producing consistency and sharing learning. The NHS also increased the numbers of community mental health nurses to support this initiative.

The 'protocol for information sharing' theme proved more complex than originally anticipated. It was concerned with differing professional values and what it was appropriate to share without the service user's consent. It also cut across a similar piece of work this was being carried out by the MAPPA strategic board so it made sense to combine both pieces of work. The report *Safe and secure. Managing and sharing information across the health and criminal justice systems* (Offender Healthcare Strategies, 2005) provided an excellent base for developing a protocol which was achieved and has been adopted, and is the subject of Chapter 6 in this book.

The main task of the pathways working group was to map existing services against the good practice template included in the offender mental health care pathway document (NHS/Dept of Health, 2005). It was intended to provide the basis for future work plans but has now largely been superseded by the Bradley report. The benefit of the pathway approach is that it takes a whole-systems view of the field and encourages creative thinking across organisational boundaries. As a result of this work additional NHS funding was made available for women prisoners in order to pilot a care programme approach which would be carried forward in the community post-release.

Outcomes

One of the most worthwhile outcomes to come out of the mentally disordered offender partnership has been a closer understanding of the field of work; each partner agency has added something to the mix. This is a key positive for all interagency initiatives. This has sometimes involved the sharing of written documentation which partners would not otherwise have been aware of, sharing objectives and priorities and having discussions about values. The sharing and development of values which was viewed by the NAO as a key success factor has proved important and the wide view of partnership has changed the definition of offenders with mental health needs, at least at the strategic level. The partnership has placed Hertfordshire in a strong position when it comes to implementing the recommendations of the Bradley report, as the appropriate structures are already in place.

Key learning points

- In order to move any proposed formal arrangements forward, each agency has to agree to try to view matters from the point of view of other partners, to understand their core business, targets and strategic priorities and to share relevant data.
- Working groups on specific topics/issues can be valuable as long as key personnel at appropriately senior levels from the different agencies commit to them, and the main group ensures that the work of all is coordinated effectively.

Exercises 5.2

- What are the key features from the case study that would you consider to be important in planning for an interagency project such as this in your own area of practice?
- What are the key features you would consider to be important in ongoing maintenance of inter-agency projects such as this in your own area of practice?
- What in professionals' and agencies' beliefs and approaches might militate against setting up and maintaining such close working relationships as those set out in this chapter? What needs to be done, by whom and how, to overcome these?

Case study 1

A male offender in his early 30s was referred to the Hertfordshire MDO Panel on the grounds of an offence of harassment of his neighbour over the course of several months by banging on their party wall and shouting and screaming abuse at the neighbour. He had no previous convictions but had been cautioned previously for a similar offence against the same injured party. He had not been under the auspices of the mental health services, but as a direct result of the Panel referral, the MDO liaison worker member of the Panel referred him for an outpatient assessment by his local Community Mental Health Team who diagnosed a likely underlying psychotic illness, probably schizophrenia. The assessment was that he had lost insight and was delusional at the time of the offence. A robust care plan was put in place including regular monitoring and anti-psychotic medication. The Panel recommendation therefore was that both criteria for diversion had been met, i.e. a direct causal link between the mental illness and the offence and a care plan likely to obviate a recurrence, and diversion to the mental health care plan took place.

Case study 2

This offender has a diagnosis of severe depression/anxiety and has reported ongoing virtually permanent suicidal ideation. He has attempted overdose and set light to his flat. He has discussed ambivalence as to how far he genuinely wants to end his life by his own hands, and one of his convictions, possession of an imitation firearm, involved trying to provoke a situation where police firearms officers would call and he would be killed. He has been subject to a number of pre-sentence reports and statutory supervision, which have in turn precipitated the involvement of the local psychiatric services through a panel referral, leading to Section followed by intensive outpatient treatment which has stabilised his condition, although a tendency towards impulsive offending remains.

The revised panel systems which built on earlier work on mental health issues with offenders has proved valuable and the following case studies illustrate something of the breadth of their work.

Further consequences

A spin-off result of the Criminal Justice Board sponsorship of a forensic probation officer has been a better understanding of risk of harm from the perspective of each agency and closer working relationships. This has started to spread beyond forensic services and is leading to a greater understanding of the contribution each partner can make to risk assessment and management and a quicker response to mental health concerns. It has enabled some cases to be dealt with without recourse to the panel. This has been built on further with the appointment of a specialist mental health worker in one of the Hertfordshire courts to promote diversion where appropriate and to serve as a source of advice.

Case study 3

This man, aged 50, has an extensive history of offending dating back 25 years. The offending pattern was mixed, including theft, damage, public order, violence both male on male and against female sexual partners, and indecent assault on a prison officer. A common thread throughout the offending was poor impulse control, emotional instability, grandiosity, a sense of entitlement and lack or remorse or ability to take a perspective on his behaviour. There was a previous hospital order on his record, but during latter years he had been subject to pre-sentence reports and statutory supervision by the probation service on a single-agency basis, his behaviour and demeanour causing concern, particularly in a domestic violence context. The relatively low level of seriousness of his offences as charged, combined with a convincing and plausible demeanour in court, did not exemplify the risk which the probation service felt he posed. Eventually a high P-Scan score, which is a version of the Hare Psychopathy checklist developed by Hare for social workers and probation officers to use (see www.hare.org/scales), followed by intensive liaison and information sharing with the local forensic psychiatric team and community mental health team led to a fresh assessment and a diagnosis of personality disorder with dissocial and emotionally unstable traits and with a tendency to become violent when under stress. He was sentenced for his most recent offences, common assault on a stranger and public order (after arguing with a police officer), and by imposition of a Section 37 under the Mental Health Act in a medium secure setting when he became eligible for discharge. MAPPA and public protection police were involved to formulate a risk-management plan to protect the public including any partner.

Case study 4

A male offender, 33 years of age, has a succession of convictions dating back to his late teens, including theft and damage. The primary offending pattern is a series of unsolicited approaches to members of the public begging for money, sentenced under public order legislation, and dealt with by ASBOs successively breached. One of these instances led to a conviction for assault on the victim. The offences took place in the context of his need for money to feed a Class A drug habit, this in turn linking back to a deprived and abusive childhood. His father died during his childhood and he reports being verbally and physically abused by his mother's subsequent partners. Following deterioration in his mother's health he was placed in care and then lived on the streets during his latter teenage years. Prior to probation service involvement under the terms of a community order he was receiving intervention from the community drug and alcohol team, but not from mainstream mental health services. Insofar as there was a mental health diagnosis it was in relation to personality issues which were not regarded as a mental health diagnosis amenable to treatment. When the probation service became involved under the terms of a community order he was living with a relative but his behaviour was placing an intolerable strain upon the relationship. The Probation Officer made a MAPPA referral, which in turn precipitated the involvement of the local forensic psychiatric services. Intensive efforts were made over an extended period to liaise with the community mental health service through to panel with a view to revisiting the diagnosis and this subsequently led to a diagnosis of schizophrenia and hospital admission on Section. Supported accommodation was found for him on discharge, and although further offending and emotional instability have followed (virtually inevitable in a young man with this degree of damage) there is now an infrastructure in place including ongoing mental health support.

An excellent example of added value by providing additional services mediated through the NHS is the involvement of the Revolving Doors organisation and the Hertfordshire Criminal Justice Board in setting up a multi-agency project to provide services for low-level offenders with mental health needs called the Navigator project. The project attracted additional funding and a pilot based on screening admissions to police cells in Watford polilce station has been recently completed. The screening tool, based on eight questions completed by the police, was started in April 2009 and completed in April 2010. This showed that there were 300 relevant cases. The project has been developing a comprehensive local directory of services and is moving into the second phase where volunteer 'navigators' will be appointed across Hertfordshire to support people identified through screening and put them in touch with local services. A real strength of the project has been the way that local community groups have been engaged from the start, with the aim of focusing their efforts on the needs of low-level offenders with learning disability and/or mental health needs. Over 120 organisations are involved with the project in the Watford area alone.

Protocols have been developed to enable more effective targeting of cases for psychiatric report preparation from probation staff. Guidance notes have been distributed to probation staff.

In terms of results there are elements that have been less successful and are still on the developing agenda for the future. Stable accommodation, ideally which should range from fully supported to semi-supported to independent, is a major issue. The housing department has agreed to give some priority to offenders with mental health needs which addresses an element of the problem, but there is more to do. All partners are aware that a programme of work with an offender who has mental health needs is likely to involve two steps forward and one step back. Unless intermediate options between accommodation and prison and medium security and prison are developed with different levels of community support there will be an over-reliance on the most expensive options. In addition, in working with offenders with mental health needs it is important to minimise the possibility of failure as far as is possible, because failure makes it harder for the offender to succeed next time.

Developing targeted employment and training opportunities for offenders with mental health needs is an area that requires further development. The strategic board increased to include a representative of the Criminal Justice Board and the housing department but were not successful in recruiting a representative from the Job Centre. The strategic board has not been as data-driven as the NAO model recommends – this may be inevitable at an early stage of development. Data collection is improving but is nowhere near the sophistication achieved by local Crime and Disorder Partnerships, for example. It is likely that this is due in part to the difficulties of definition and measurement.

Conclusion

There is a tension between identifying 'problems in living' associated with personality disorder such as anger, depression and antisocial behaviour with a formal diagnosis. **A two-strand approach may be required, working to address 'problems in living' at an early stage, reserving formal diagnosis for the minority who exhibit persistence** and for whom earlier work has not worked. This would be problematic in so far as the diagnosis is the trigger for providing or refusing services. An example of this is borderline learning disability: such individuals can often not cope on their own but slip under the radar for services.

An approach based on 'problems with living' could be justified if there was evidence that it worked in preventing more serious and expensive problems later on. It would require a **coordination and development of existing services in local areas, especially voluntary sector services and training across the partnership agencies** to provide consistency of approach.

Further reading

Barrett, G., Sellman, D. and Thomas, J. (eds) (2005) *Interprofessional Working in Health and Social Care: Professional Perspectives,* Basingstoke: Palgrave MacMillan.

Wilson, K., Ruch, G., Lymbery, M. and Cooper, A (eds), (2011) *Social Work: An Introduction to Contemporary Practice*, 2nd edn, Harlow: Pearson Education. The Interprofessional working chapter is very useful in looking at these issues in various practice areas.

Useful websites

www.nao.org.uk

The National Audit Office website has a number of reports on partnership working, including *Joining up to Improve Public Services, Reducing Crime, Promoting Well-Being for Older People.*

www.dh.gov.uk/en/index.htm

The Department of Health website has a number of reports on partnership working, including building on a successful **partnership working** model for a Health and Wellbeing Board, and on how to do this in the area of Learning Disabilities, amongst other areas.

References

Department of Health/Home Office (1992) *A Review of Health and Social Services for Mentally Disordered Offenders and Others Requiring Similar Services*, Cmd 2088, London: HMSO/Department of Health/Home Office.

Department of Health (2009) *The Bradley Report. Lord Bradley's Review of People with Mental Health Problems or Learning Disabilities in the Criminal Justice System*, London: Department of Health.

Gibson, B., (2007) *The New Home Office: an Introduction*, Hook, Hampshire: Waterside Press.

HM Government (1999) Modernising Government: White Paper, Cm 4301, London: HM Government, publications.parliament.uk/pa/. . ./cmwib/wb990403/wgp.htm.

National Audit Office (2001) *Joining Up to Improve Public Services. Report by the Comptroller and Auditor General.* London: The Stationery Office nao.org.uk/idoc.ashx?docId=c3890996-944e-4cf5-b682-0e3b6f.

NHS/Dept of Health (2005) *Offender Mental Health Care Pathway,* London: Department of Health.

Offender Healthcare Strategies (2005) *Safe and Secure: Managing and Sharing Information Across Health and Criminal Justice Systems*, London: HM Prison Service/Department of Health.

Chapter 6
Information-sharing agreements between agencies and professionals: making use of law, policy and professional codes

Sue Urwin and Stephanie Sadler

Chapter summary

A number of chapters in this book raise the issues about the way information is shared – or not – in different areas of work as set out in Part 2, across professional groups and agencies as set out in Part 3, and with service users and carers. This chapter explores in detail some of the professional, ethical and practice issues involved in information sharing between agencies, including police, probation officers and social and health workers, in the specific context of the Hertfordshire Mentally Disordered Offenders (MDO) Panel Scheme. During the course of the writing of the Information Sharing Agreement (ISA) and consultation with the signatories, issues arose which have a universal relevance and application across different service-user groups and agencies, including issues about informed consent from service users or carers for professionals to judge when considering sharing such information.

The chapter then uses the example of different professional groups' situation and requirements, including medical personnel, social workers and nurses and midwives, in relation to sharing information with others based on their professional, ethical and legal requirements.

The chapter uses a variety of anonymised case examples to illustrate the use of such considerations in practice.

Learning objectives

This chapter will cover:

- decisions about sharing information on individual service users between agencies and professionals are based on their different professional, ethical and legal requirements, and have to take into account individual patients/service-user circumstances – there is no protocol which can provide definitive guidance on every possible set of factors in one individual's circumstances

▶

- as a general rule, informed consent should be sought from the patient/service user wherever practicable and safe to all to do so; this information sharing should meet the twin requirements of necessity and proportionality.

- the chapter examines these requirements, using the examples of medical personnel, nurses and midwives and social workers as illustrative case studies representative of the challenges and concerns of different agencies and groups for the areas that need to be addressed in any information-sharing protocol, and in any forms of information sharing between professionals and agencies.

- professionals need to actively check out at the beginning of contacts how other professionals, interprofessional panels or agencies will treat information they share with these latter groups in order to avoid problems caused by unfounded assumptions about the use of such information.

- issues about informed consent from service users or carers, within considerations of capacity for such service users to consent and what to do if they are judged not to have such capacity, are important for all professionals and agency policies to judge when considering sharing such information.

Background to the case example

The Hertfordshire Mentally Disordered Offenders Panel Scheme originated in the 1980s, but an operational policy was first formalised following the then government's Reed Report (Department of Health/ Home Office, 1992). The Panel scheme is central to several recommendations in the April 2009 Government-commissioned Bradley Report (Department of Health, 2009) – a review of people with mental health problems or learning disabilities in the criminal justice system – including those relating to intervention with offenders with mental health problems at the earliest possible point of their journey through that system, diversion from the system for those who do not belong in it by virtue of mental health issues, and provision of good-quality information to courts sentencing mentally disordered offenders who have to be prosecuted, requested from, and agreed by, the Panels. The Panels are an important element in the Hertfordshire Multi Agency Public Protection Arrangements, (MAPPA) as set out in Chapter 5 of this book.

The scheme has been developed for use by all those who work within the criminal justice system or are affected by it – police, probation officers, social workers and health workers, Crown Prosecution Service, magistrates, court officers, solicitors and the prison service.

The aim of the scheme is to identify appropriate care for offenders with mental health problems, which can include mental illness, personality disorder or learning disability. This may be achieved by putting a care plan in place alongside any community or custodial sentence or by diverting the individual from the criminal justice system entirely.

The core Panel members are police, probation and specialist police cell-based Criminal Justice Mental Health Practitioners. Other professionals specifically involved with any individual referral are invited on an ad hoc case-by-case basis to give an opinion. The Panel has no formal authority; it acts in an advisory capacity to suggest an appropriate course of action to the police, Crown Prosecution Service and, where prosecution takes place, the courts. Any agency can refer a case to the Panel but in practice the majority of referrals are made by the police at or shortly after arrest. At the Panel meeting, all available appropriate information is shared relating to the offender and the offence. The police representative would give details of the latter along with previous convictions/antecedents. Crucial to the Panel decision-making process is the view of mental health professionals as to whether criteria for diversion are, or are not, met (see below).

The Panel discussion revolves around the two criteria for diversion both of which have to be met if diversion is to be advised:

1. A direct causal link between the mental disorder and the offence.
2. The availability of a new or amended mental health care plan sufficient to minimise/significantly reduce the risk of further offending.

The Panel is therefore primarily risk-based, diversion only being recommended if it is felt to be in the public interest to do so. In reality a relatively small number of referrals meet both criteria for diversion, but an equally important role for the Panel is to seek to ensure that, when offenders are prosecuted, magistrates and judges receive appropriate advice with regard to possible mental health intervention, either alongside any sentence imposed by the court or as an integral part of it such as a Mental Health Treatment Requirement attached to a probation supervised community order or, in some cases, a Mental Health Act disposal.

The Panel coordinator, at present the probation service representative, writes to the Crown Prosecution Service and/or relevant police officer giving the Panel's advice. If diversion is recommended, either that no further action should be taken or that the offender should be cautioned (if the offence is admitted), the letter contains details of the proposed care plan supporting the contention that the defendant can be appropriately and safely managed in the community short of prosecution. If the advice is that it is in the public interest to prosecute, an indication is given where appropriate as to the information/reports the court should commission, in the event of a plea or finding of guilt, before proceeding to sentence.

Information-sharing issues

The Panel operated for a number of years without a formal information-sharing protocol or procedure for obtaining consent from the referred person. This may have been because the Panels have traditionally been probation service- and police-led, and the criteria and 'setting of the bar' for sharing information are determined by issues relating to prevention/investigation of crime which are met per se in terms of the route by which a referral reaches the Panel, i.e. an allegation that an offence has occurred. There is a public interest element in most of the referrals; offences where there is little or no risk to the public and no forensic history usually do not reach the Panels but are disposed of by the police in some other way. However, while there is usually some element of risk to the public in Panel cases, the level of this varies and will not always be classified as imminent or serious.

A key issue for any form of interprofessional and interagency working became clear as part of the developing set of working relationships in the Panels; that assumptions are frequently made that all understand each others' ethical and professional codes, when this is not the case. It became increasingly clear that mental health professionals and other professionals work to separate and specific professional codes of ethics in relation to confidentiality which overlaps to some extent with those binding criminal justice agencies, but which contains imperatives particular to them. Accordingly, the ISA, the first iteration of which resulted from a multidisciplinary working party and which has subsequently been rewritten and refined during the consultation process, lays stress on guidance to and safeguarding the position of mental health professionals disclosing patients' information to the Panel, and also safeguarding, as far as is possible, the privacy and integrity of the

Key learning points

Never make assumptions about how other professionals or interprofessional panels or agencies will treat the information you share with them.

■ Find out what may happen to such information with the chairs of panels, professionals and agencies you are sharing with, as unfounded assumptions can be made that all understand each other's ethical and professional codes, and/or how they expect to be able to make use of this information.

patients/service users concerned. The signatories to the Hertfordshire MDO Panel ISA are Hertfordshire Constabulary, Hertfordshire Probation Trust, Hertfordshire Partnership NHS Foundation Trust (mental health) and Hertfordshire County Council (Adult Care Services). All have actively engaged with the consultation process and suggested amendments from their own organisation's point of view.

Individual Panel members' current professional guidance can be summarised as follows:

1. *Psychiatrists:* the General Medical Council (GMC) position is that confidentiality can be breached only in exceptional circumstances, i.e. to prevent serious harm or if there is a clear indication that failure to disclose would be more detrimental to the patient than not disclosing. There must have been an attempt to obtain consent even if it is subsequently dispensed with.

2. *Police:* have a general duty of care to the public. Emailing the original intranet referral and sharing information at the Panel (including witness statements and antecedents from the file) are sanctioned by the Crime and Disorder Act and Criminal Justice Act. Panel discussions can be defined as coming under the heading of prevention/investigation of crime given that the discussion centres on how best MDOs offending behaviour can be dealt with through a mental health care plan and/or a sentence of the court. Information must be shared for a specific policing purpose being:

   - the administration of justice
   - maintaining public safety
   - the apprehension of offenders
   - the prevention of crime and disorder
   - the detection of crime
   - the protection of vulnerable members of the community
   - protecting life and property.

3. *Probation service:* information can be shared according to similar criteria as the police, sanctioned by the Data Protection Act, Criminal Justice Act and Crime and Disorder Act – as needed for the prevention/detection of crime and/or in the public interest. Consent is not required under

these circumstances and, as with the police, these criteria could be argued to apply to all Panel cases.

4. *Community mental health teams/emergency duty teams/hospital nurses/residential care workers:* the guidance seems to be somewhat more general. Sharing of information can occur without consent where disclosure is required by law or order of a court (not relevant to MDOs) or when disclosure is considered to be necessary in the public interest, including child protection. It would be prudent however to set the bar at the same level as doctors, and seek where practicable to obtain consent in every case.

5. *Criminal Justice Mental Health Practitioners:* could be seen as having a dual responsibility to the local Mental Health NHS Trust and the Criminal Justice System. As with police and probation, their involvement with the MDOs referred to Panels will be as the result of an offence. However they may still feel bound by health criteria for disclosure. Their dual role is particularly sensitive as, at least in Hertfordshire, they have immediate access to electronic patient records, i.e. the medical notes.

MDO panel protocol

It has proved virtually impossible to develop a protocol to cover every conceivable situation. The overarching principle is that all colleagues should initially consult, on a case-by-case basis, their own professional protocols/guidance and take their own steps to ensure that information is shared with the Panel in accordance with them. However, the two overriding principles by which we are guided are that:

1. Informed consent should be sought from the referred person wherever practicable.

2. Information sharing should meet the twin requirements of necessity and proportionality. The necessity criterion requires that there is a pressing public protection need. The proportionality criterion requires that the information shared must be *only* that information which is necessary to achieve the purpose for which it is being shared. These twin requirements should be met even if consent has been obtained from the referred person.

Public interest versus patients' rights to confidentiality

This debate becomes relevant in cases where it has not been possible, for whatever reason, to obtain informed consent from the referred person for disclosure of medical information to the Panel. Attempts will have been made to obtain this, using the MDO Panel information sheet and consent form, ideally discussed directly with the referred person/patient by their own medical practitioner if there is one appointed, otherwise by post or face-to-face by the Criminal Justice Mental Health Practitioner. Seriousness/public interest is necessarily on a spectrum and the MDO Panel point on that spectrum varies from case to case. We have had lengthy discussion during the development of the ISA relating to the definition of 'public interest'. In terms of impact on actual or potential victims of actions carried out by the referred person, we tend to define public interest in terms of serious physical or psychological harm, particularly in relation to children or other vulnerable people. Public interest issues can also arise in relation to the patient referred to the Panel, if for example it is precipitated by or associated with mental disorder not proving amenable to treatment placing them in jeopardy of conviction of increasingly serious offences and increasingly severe court sanctions. There is also of course the additional issue of capacity, any doubt about which needs to be adjudicated upon by the relevant medical practitioners. A lack of capacity invokes a 'best interest' concern and there is a separate legal framework for addressing this, as set out in the Mental Capacity Act 2005 (see ico.gov.uk/.../document_library/data_protection. aspx).

Exercise 6.1

What are the considerations with regard to informed consent and the passing on of information to other professionals and agencies that you need to take into account for your agency/service-users group?

Key learning point

In the absence of informed consent from the referred person, sharing information without consent can leave professionals open to legal challenge even where the public interest test is felt to have been met, although this is a very rare occurrence in the Panel context.

There is ongoing discussion about what constitutes the potential for serious harm to others. In the case of, for example, abuse of a child, or serious life-threatening violence to a partner in a domestic situation, the public interest element is clear. There may however be room for debate in relation to violence of a lesser ilk – for example someone charged with assault occasioning actual bodily harm as against grievous bodily harm with intent. As indicated above, the seriousness and victim implications of each case needs to be judged alongside the mental state and capacity of the alleged perpetrator.

The difficulties of incorporating the ethical, professional and practical requirements of an ISA that both promotes public safety and defends patients' rights are self-evident. A point came during our deliberations in the development of the Agreement where we wondered if it was actually an achievable objective. Our final conclusion, however, was that while every possible effort should be made to share

Key learning points

Key principles in information sharing

The existing protocols relating to health, police and probation Panel colleagues have, broadly speaking, the following principles in common.

- Proportionality, i.e. the minimum information must be given to achieve the desired outcome.
- Consent should be obtained if at all possible and an attempt should be made to obtain this.
- Whether or not consent has been obtained disclosure should only be made in the public interest.
- Absence or withholding of consent can be overridden in cases where there is serious/imminent risk to the person (adults) or child protection concerns.
- In the case of Health Service colleagues it should be able to be demonstrated that all practicable attempts have been made to obtain informed consent.

information ethically and in accordance with professional protocols, in order to respect the rights of the referred MDO, the existence of a viable Panel scheme is in itself in the public interest. The scheme would not remain viable were there to be regular or protracted delays in obtaining consent and all Panel signatories recognise that a test of common sense may need on occasion to be applied. Examples of legislation under which information can be disclosed are given at the end of this chapter. It should be noted that this list is not necessarily exhaustive.

Case vignettes

Cases where consent could be and was obtained:

1. A male offender in his 30s was referred to the Hertfordshire MDO Panel on the grounds of an offence of harassment of his neighbour over the course of several months by banging on their party wall and shouting and screaming abuse at the neighbour. He had no previous convictions but had been cautioned previously for a similar offence against the same injured party. He had not been under the auspices of the mental health services, but as a direct result of the Panel referral, the MDO liaison worker member of the Panel referred him for an outpatient assessment by his local community mental health team (CMHT) who diagnosed a likely underlying psychotic illness, probably schizophrenia. The assessment was that he had lost insight and was delusional at the time of the offence. Consent was obtained via the CMHT assessment instigated through the Panel. A robust care plan was put in place including regular monitoring and anti-psychotic medication. The Panel recommendation therefore was that both criteria for diversion had been met, i.e. a direct causal link between the mental illness and the offence, a care plan likely to obviate a recurrence, and diversion to the mental health care plan took place.

2. A woman in her early 40s was referred to the Panel in respect of racially aggravated public order and assault matters. Consent for disclosure of information was obtained by the referred person's care coordinator who was present at the Panel. As far as could be ascertained, the trigger to the offences was alcohol. Although the referred person was currently a

psychiatric inpatient, inpatient admissions had not previously resulted in care plans in the community being able to obviate reoffending, and there was a history of similar matters. This was the not uncommon situation whereby a patient with a psychotic illness is stabilised when in hospital, but relapses through lack of compliance with a care plan on discharge, and in this case the referred person was not eligible for a Community Treatment Order and had been self-medicating with alcohol. We advised that the criteria for diversion were not met, but that pre-sentence and psychiatric reports should be obtained in the event of a prosecution and plea or finding of guilt.

Cases where consent was not obtained through lack of capacity:

1. The offender had a diagnosis of severe depression/anxiety and had reported ongoing virtually permanent suicidal ideation. He had attempted overdose and set fire to his flat. He had discussed ambivalence as to how far he genuinely wanted to end his life by his own hands, and one of his convictions, possession of an imitation firearm, involved trying to provoke a situation where police firearms officers would call and he would be killed. He had been subject to a number of pre-sentence reports and statutory supervision, which had in turn precipitated the involvement of the local psychiatric services through an MDO Panel referral from the police, leading to Mental Health Act Section followed by intensive outpatient treatment which stabilised his condition although a tendency towards impulsive offending remained. He did not have capacity at the point of referral to give consent but his responsible clinician was of the view that public interest issue justified disclosure of information, including possible 'suicide by police' risk to himself, and potential risk to bystanders and police officers were there to be a siege situation.

2. An elderly man, resident in a care home, was subject to an allegation offence of assault on staff. When the MDO Panel meeting convened, involving community and residential professionals, each with some piecemeal knowledge of the MDOs history, it transpired that a series of events, over years, had taken place against staff and other residents, some with life-threatening implications. As a result of the Panel a properly coordinated care plan could be drawn up to protect others as well as to meet the offender's clinical needs. The clinical judgement was

that his mental state represented incapacity to give informed consent to involvement in the Panel but public interest issues were felt to predominate in terms of risk of serious possibly fatal injury to potential victims, including other vulnerable residents in his care home, and also risk to himself of long-term detention in a secure hospital as a penalty of the court should such an incident occur. This case also raises other implications in terms of the prosecution versus diversion decision-making process in the context of risk balanced against clinical need. It was considered in this case that once all the information was known, protective measures could be put in place such as to protect the public and the patient himself. Had this not been the case, however, and more especially had the current allegation represented serious harm to the victim, the patient's lack of capacity to understand court proceedings would not have prevented prosecution. In that instance fitness to plead issues, and possibly ultimately a trial of the facts, would have arisen. The Law Commission has recently issued a consultation paper that seeks to examine the issue of unfitness to plead within the broader context of the law relating to vulnerable defendants, the Mental Health Act 1983 as amended by the Mental Health Act 2007, and the Mental Capacity Act 2005 (see ico.gov.uk/.../document_library/data_protection.aspx).

3. A young male was referred on three successive occasions to the MDO Panel by a secure facility where he was detained under the Mental Health Act. On each occasion he had been referred in respect of an assault against a member of staff or another patient. On each occasion the Panel recommended prosecution, on the grounds that, on the advice of the responsible clinician (RC), he was aware of the consequences of his actions, and the care plan would be bolstered by a prosecution. On the first occasion he was cautioned and a decision had not been taken in respect of the second matter when the third occurred. The RC's view was that in the event of a plea or finding of guilt he would probably meet the criteria for a court order under the Mental Health Act 2007. Prosecution did subsequently proceed, by which time the consensus was that he was unfit to plead. There was an anomaly in that the offences could only be tried at the Magistrates' Court where fitness to plead could not be determined, so in fact the Crown Prosecution Service (CPS) would have to discontinue the offences unless the defence, whom they approached, would agree to proceedings with a

view to Section 37 of the Mental Health Act 2007. A Section 37 order was made.

Cases where consent was overridden by risk issues

1. A male in his mid-50s was referred to the Panel in respect of an offence of domestic violence, an assault on his wife. He was detained under Section 2 of the Mental Health Act but the assault had occurred while he was on home leave. The discussion at Panel revealed a history of assaults on his wife that had so far not been 'crimed' or prosecuted, due to his mental health problems, one of them involving the use of a knife. He had a diagnosis of psychotic illness and when floridly unwell, as he tended to become if he failed to take medication while on home leave, he lost insight into his behaviour and the dangerous implications of it. A planned period of leave to coincide with his wedding anniversary was approaching at the point of the Panel referral, and due to the imminent danger attaching to home leave at a potentially emotionally fraught time, the RC agreed to disclose relevant information immediately. A Panel discussion precipitated a Multi Agency Risk Assessment Conference (MARAC) meeting (the domestic violence equivalent of MAPPA) and a full protection plan was put in place in respect of the referred person's wife. His care plan was amended and his home leave was curtailed with hospital contact with him during the course of it. While the causal link test between his psychiatric condition and his offence could be said to have been met, it was not possible to ensure under the current circumstances that the care plan would obviate risk of further harm and prosecution was recommended. (In high-risk situations such as this the Panel advice letter to the CPS can include a recommendation that in the event of a plea or finding of guilt, or it having been proved at a trial of the facts that the defendant committed the offence, consideration should be given to a court sentence under the Mental Health Act 2007.)

2. A male in his early 20s was referred to the Panel for offences of affray and ABH committed against his aunt. They involved attempted strangulation and the referred person was narrowly prevented from an attempt to stab her. There were also a series of already prosecuted assault offences going through the court against his grandmother. There was felt to be acute risk to these two individuals and the public in general. His care coordinator attended the Panel and

divulged the necessary clinical information without consent due to the imminence of risk. The diagnosis was that his condition arose from a degenerative brain condition that was producing psychotic-type symptoms. Due to a previous address being in northern England, he was last known to a psychiatrist no longer available. The consultant psychiatrist sitting as a permanent Panel member was willing to take ownership of the case, given that the patient was now living in her catchment area in Hertfordshire. The consultant's recommendation to the CPS was that while the causal link criterion for diversion was probably met, it was not possible to formulate a care plan such as to obviate risk to the public short of compulsory detention in hospital which was more likely to be achieved via the court process than through civil sectioning powers. Prosecution was recommended and he was ultimately dealt with by disposal under Section 37.

Information sharing across agencies: the particular case of medical personnel

The sharing of information with others may pose more of a difficulty for a doctor than for any other profession. It could be argued that the duty of a lawyer is to uphold and apply the law within due process and that their clients' interests must be

Exercise 6.2

1. You are working as a social worker/nurse/doctor in a local community mental health team: your service user has been identified for discussion at the next MDO Panel. What criteria would you each apply in deciding whether to share information?

2. You are working as a social worker/nurse/doctor in a local community mental health team: your service user has been identified for discussion at the next MDO Panel due to allegations of child abuse, which the local child protection team are inquiring into under the Children Act 1989 and the *Working together to safeguard children* regulatory guidance (Department for Children, Schools and Families, 2010). What criteria would you each apply in deciding whether to share information?

considered within this framework; a social worker or probation officer will seek to facilitate their service users' well-being but always within a wider spectrum of the greater good and public protection. A doctor's primary responsibility is to their patient, and both professional tradition and legal doctrine in the UK have decreed that the cornerstone of this duty is medical confidentiality. In Hertfordshire this became apparent when, in devising guidelines for information sharing amongst professionals on Mentally Disordered Offender (MDO) Panels in place in Hertfordshire (see Chapter 5 in this book), we found that the highest thresholds for sharing information were set by the General Medical Council (GMC). If we could draft an Information Sharing Agreement (ISA) that met the stringent conditions of the GMC it would automatically satisfy the criteria for all other health and social services bodies such as the Nursing and Midwifery Council and the General Social Care Council. In order for psychiatrists to bring information to the MDO panel a complex maze of decision-making had to be negotiated, even though it might be apparent to everyone involved that the sharing of information was in the interests of all, including the patient.

These ethical dilemmas have become a commonplace consideration in the delivery of modern day mental health services. Every working day the community mental health team receives requests for information and interagency working from disparate sources:

- **Example 1** A housing officer with the local council telephones for information concerning a council tenant who has been disturbing neighbours with loud music at night. Information has reached the housing officer to suggest that this man may be a client of local mental health services. The council officer would like to know if this man is 'open' to our services, what is his diagnosis and may they have a copy of his risk assessment?

- **Example 2** A social worker with the statutory child protection team is requesting diagnostic information and a copy of the risk assessment on a male who is the father of an eight-year-old child. On the basis of information they have received

Exercise 6.3

With the issues of information sharing in mind, consider the issues arising from the above two very typical requests to CMHTs from your own agency/ professional group perspective, and consider what you would take into account in considering what content would be included/how and with whose consent the information sharing would take place.

they are gathering data to determine possible risks to the child.

Over the last 25 years the response from mental health services to requests such as the two examples above has changed, sometimes in response to advice and direction from professional bodies, but often as a direct result of serious untoward incidents that have reached national attention, resulting in formal inquiries with ensuing recommendations for practice. Staff working on the front line therefore find themselves having to deal with requests for information in the context of a busy working day, and seek to make decisions while juggling to recall the guidance of their professional body, their particular employer's guidelines, national directives about information sharing to ensure public safety and permeating all these – the memory of recent headlines in the national press about professionals failing to communicate adequately resulting in the death of some unfortunate and usually vulnerable person.

Two decades ago, doctors, nurses and social workers kept separate records and each professional group determined what information they would share in various circumstances. Recommended good practice now dictates that all these professional groups working together in mental health services share one set of notes, and thus, from a doctor's perspective, these constitute medical notes and normal standards of medical confidentiality apply. Hertfordshire Partnership NHS Foundation Trust, for example, has addressed this issue by informing patients at the beginning of their involvement with mental health services who their information will be shared with in the Trust, i.e. medical personnel, nurses, occupational therapists, social workers etc., and the limits of confidentiality. The situation has been rendered

more complex still by the introduction of electronic patient records and related legislation – the Data Protection Act, the Human Rights Act and the Medical Records Act.

The case of medical personnel and their professional ethics in relation to information sharing

In the past a doctor's response to requests for information was straightforward – the patient's written consent was essential in the absence of a legal requirement to divulge information, e.g. a court order. As the delivery of health and welfare services became more multifaceted and intricate, the momentum for information sharing between various agencies gathered pace, often accelerated by the findings of serious incident inquiries and new legislation to safeguard children and vulnerable adults (The Children Act 1989 etc.). This move towards a more general openness has been welcomed by many and may have facilitated an holistic (and possibly safer) approach to mental health care. However, even as staff were being trained in information sharing and justifying their actions to each other, complaints and sometimes lawsuits started to emerge as a result of patients considering that their confidential medical information had been shared without consent. A general multi-professional response that information sharing was now considered 'a good thing' proved inadequate for the doctors involved and the GMC issued a carefully constructed document outlining its position on good medical practice as it applied to confidentiality (GMC, 2009).

The basis of good medical practice is that the duty of confidentiality that a doctor holds towards a patient is not simply an historical notion now embedded in current practice merely as a consequence of tradition and professional whimsy, but that such a duty exists for the 'clear public good' and 'confidential medical care is recognised in law as being in the public interest' (GMC, 2009). Without such an exclusive relationship with their doctor a patient may fail to seek appropriate help or disclose information that may have a direct bearing on the wider public health, e.g. communicable diseases such as tuberculosis. In the case of X v Y (1988) when a national newspaper was seeking to publish the HIV status of doctors, Mr Justice Rose ruled in his judgment:

> In the long run, preservation of confidentiality is the only way of securing public health . . . future individual patients will not come forward if doctors are going to squeal on them. Consequently, confidentiality is vital to secure public as well as private health, for unless those infected come forward they cannot be counselled. (All England Law Reports, 1988)

The public appeared to be in broad agreement with this if the results of a MORI poll, commissioned by the GMC, are to be believed (MORI Social Research, 1999). A sample of the public were asked to consider which, of a number of offences committed by a doctor, should lead to their definitely being struck off the medical register. 'Not respecting and protecting confidential information' came top of the list and trumped other offences such as 'their personal beliefs prejudicing the care of their patients' and 'not keeping their professional knowledge and skills up to date'.

The GMC recognises that the right to medical confidentiality is not absolute and may be overridden in stipulated circumstances. It is clear as to the general principles that underlie a permitted breach of confidentiality but there is a requirement for clinical and sociological judgement when these principles are applied to individual cases.

The GMC guidance is very clear that information cannot be shared if a competent person has explicitly refused consent, where the risk is only to that individual alone.

Interestingly the GMC guidance on confidentiality makes no specific reference to the protection of children but subsumes them in the general category of 'others'. However, it does publish separate guidance for the care of children and young people up to 18 years. Where a person under the age of 18 is considered to be at risk from abuse or exploitation, but is specifically refusing consent to share information, the decision for the doctor is not whether this individual is a child but rather whether they are 'Gillick competent' and have the capacity to decide for themselves.

If it is clear that the disclosure of information is in the public interest consent should still be sought from the individual concerned unless it is not practicable to do so, e.g. they are not competent to do so, might put the doctor or others at risk of serious harm. If consent is explicitly withheld but disclosure remains in the public interest then the patient should be informed that disclosure is to be made – unless there are practical reasons not to do so – as above.

As two further examples, we will look at the professional codes for social workers and nurses and midwives.

Social workers under their professional registration body, the General Social Care Council (GSCC), are required to comply with the GSCC Codes of Practice (see www.gscc.org.uk/codes/) as follows:

- protect the rights and promote the interests of service users and carers;
- strive to establish and maintain the trust and confidence of service users and carers;
- promote the independence of service users while protecting them as far as possible from danger or harm;
- respect the rights of service users whilst seeking to ensure that their behaviour does not harm themselves or other people . . .

A closer look

General Medical Council Principles governing disclosure of personal information

The GMC advises doctors that they can disclose personal information in the following circumstances:

1. It is required by law, such as a result of a specific statute, e.g. infectious diseases or in response to statutory powers of various regulatory bodies.
2. The patient consents – either implicitly for the sake of their own care or expressly for other purposes.
3. It is justified in the public interest i.e. to protect individuals or society from risks of serious harm, such as serious communicable diseases or serious crime, or to enable medical research, education or other secondary uses of information that will benefit society over time.

More specifically, in the following sections:

1.4 Respecting and maintaining the dignity and privacy of service users;

2.1 Being honest and trustworthy;

2.2 Communicating in an appropriate, open, accurate and straightforward way;

2.3 Respecting confidential information and clearly explaining agency policies about confidentiality to service users and carers;

4.3 Taking necessary steps to minimise the risks of service users from doing actual or potential harm to themselves or other people; and

4.4 Ensuring that relevant colleagues and agencies are informed about the outcomes and implications of risk assessments

these duties are set out in ways which mean that meeting these differing and potentially conflicting demands requires a depth of understanding to be able to consider the best way forward in any particular situation.

The professional registration body for nurses and midwives, the Nursing and Midwifery Council, requires them to work under the *Standards of conduct, performance and ethics for nurses and midwives* (www. nmc-uk.org/aArticle.aspx?ArticleID=3056) as follows:

The people in your care must be able to trust you with their health and wellbeing

To justify that trust, you must:

- make the care of people your first concern, treating them as individuals and respecting their dignity
- work with others to protect and promote the health and wellbeing of those in your care, their families and carers, and the wider community
- provide a high standard of care at all times
- be open and honest, act with integrity and uphold the reputation of your profession.

As a professional, you are personally accountable for actions and omissions in your practice, and must always be able to justify your decisions.

Respect people's confidentiality

5. You must respect people's right to confidentiality.

6. You must ensure people are informed about how and why information is shared by those who will be providing their care.

7. You must disclose information if you believe someone may be at risk of harm, in line with the law of the country in which you are practising.

As can be seen, these specific duties mean that social workers and nurses and midwives have to carefully consider their professional duties in sharing information about service users under their codes, taking into account the areas raised in this chapter.

The new age of information sharing and inter-agency working is a daily reality in modern mental health services and front-line workers are generally cognisant and understanding of the principles that guide their practice. Such familiarity with the involvement of agencies other than their own, e.g. housing, child protection and probation services, especially at a local level where there may be a working personal acquaintance with the staff involved, may run the risk of a less than robust approach to each individual case – a general application of the 'information–sharing subculture' rather than a rigorous testing of the evidence and criteria for this particular patient and their right to confidentiality.

Example 1, p. 83. Playing loud music at night is unlikely to constitute per se a serious risk to anyone. Granted the individual concerned may find themselves at risk of confrontation with their neighbour, or in the longer term possibly at risk of losing a tenancy. However, applying the GMC principles and weighing up whether these risks are sufficient to override the 'public good' of maintaining the confidential relationship between doctor and patient there would not seem to be sufficient risk for the duty worker to disclose without consent immediately.

The patient was seen in the outpatient clinic the next day – he had paranoid delusions that his neighbour had been replaced by an imposter who had

---

Exercise 6.4

Check your own professional codes in relation to information sharing with patients/service users, and other agencies and professionals. Consider the types of issues set out in this chapter that you need to prepare for with your own agency and service-user group in order to meet your own profession's requirements in these areas.

stolen the patient's girlfriend away. He was playing loud music to drown out the spells that the neighbour was supposedly casting and kept a baseball bat behind the door in case the imposter-neighbour came to call.

This was now a high-risk case requiring immediate intervention – the patient left the clinic before the conclusion of the appointment and the decision was rapidly made to contact the Housing Department and to alert the neighbour. It was impractical to seek consent and the risk of serious harm to others was considered sufficiently high to justify breaching medical confidentiality.

After a period of treatment in hospital the patient agreed that the breach of his confidentiality was justified and requested that the Housing Department be included in future care planning.

Example 2, p. 83. The duty worker receiving the call considered it highly likely that information would need to be shared, even if the patient's consent could not be obtained, given that this was a child protection issue. They immediately conferred with the consultant psychiatrist clinically responsible for the patient. However, on obtaining more information from the Child Protection Officer it emerged that this father had not had any contact with his child for seven years and in that time had not sought to make contact with the child or wider family, neither had he demonstrated any untoward behaviour. He was not now seeking to make contact, was wholly compliant with his care plan and engaging regularly with mental health services.

The Child Protection officer had been accumulating information about the family for reasons other than the father and was conscientiously compiling background information as appropriate – in fact he was doing his job. The CMHT, however, while recognising

Exercise 6.5

Consider the team within which you work and whether and how your practice might be enhanced by the existence of an Information Sharing Agreement relevant to your own particular situation. How might you go about setting up such an Agreement? What are the issues you would plan to address, with whom, and how, in setting up such an Agreement?

that the safety of a child is paramount, could find no evidence that this child was in any way at risk from this individual and any postulated theoretical risk did not amount to 'serious'. It therefore declined to breach confidentiality without the consent of the patient – which the patient subsequently refused.

Conclusion

The Hertfordshire MDO Panel scheme illustrates specific information-sharing issues appertaining to the interface between mental health care and the criminal justice system. It highlights in a specific context the potential conflict between medical ethics and clinical need on the one hand, and on the other the management of risk to the public and the promoting of appropriate sentencing or diversion.

The need to produce an Information Sharing Agreement for the Hertfordshire MDO Panel reflects the reality of interagency working in modern mental health care provision. The fact that it turned out to be a complex and tortuous process over many months involving numerous agencies, their employers and regulatory bodies indicates that there are no simple directives or guidelines for interagency working; every step required respect and understanding of the different perspectives and objectives of colleagues. The regular advice from the Hertfordshire Constabulary Information Sharing Agreement Administrator who guided this work on legal and procedural matters and who circulated countless drafts to signatories to fine tune the Agreement was invaluable. While none of the agencies were required to compromise on essential tenets of our practice, there were a number of areas where we resorted to the possibly platitudinous maxim of 'each case must be considered in its own right'. This seemed to us a reasonable position given that matters of social work, health and law may be hugely significant for any given individual and may have profound consequences for them – all areas have the wherewithal to remove an individual's liberty.

We have been guided throughout by the unanimously agreed overarching principle that the worst outcome for the public and the patients/offenders would be to sacrifice the Panel scheme altogether on the grounds that it was impossible to achieve an exactly prescriptive ISA covering all eventualities. The challenge of managing some 'shades of grey' in it prompts the ongoing reflection and consultation that is an essential part of the process.

This chapter has used the example of one very high-profile and risk-laden area of practice that has meant agencies and professionals have often been very worried about how to make decisions about sharing information across the different agencies and professionals involved in that area. The chapter has examined some key areas of law, professional ethics, and how to balance rights to service users, and risks to the public, which are similar in many other areas of interprofessional working, e.g. child protection, and other areas of mental health work, in order to provide ideas and guidance for all areas of interprofessional practice. It has provided discussion and analysis of key points for consideration for professionals on how to judge when to share, and determine what might be too much or too little, based on the law, agency policy and professional codes to meet the different requirements to minimise risk to the service user or others, against the right of the service user to not have information shared about them when this is not justified by law, professional codes or agency policy.

Useful websites

Your own professional Codes on your professional body's website.

ico.gov.uk/.../document_library/data_protection.aspx

The Information Commissioner's Office website contains advice on the laws and practice in these areas.

www.workingtogetheronline.co.uk/index.htm

Working Together to Safeguard Children (2010) Government guidance and regulations on interprofessional and an interagency child protection working, including on information sharing.

connectingforhealth.nhs.uk/systemsandservices/infogov/codes)

Confidentiality: the NHS Code of Practice.

ico.gov.uk/.../document_library/data_protection.aspx

Legislation under which information can be disclosed includes but is not limited to the following. All can be found on the ico.gov.ukwebsite.

Children Act 1989
Mental Capacity Act 2005
The Data Protection Act 1998
Common Law duty of confidence
Freedom of Information Act 2000
Mental Health Act 1983
Health and Social Care Act 2001
NHS and Community Care Act 1990
Sex Offences Act 2003 Part 1, Part 2 Sch. 3
Criminal Justice Act 2003 Part 1, 2 of Sch. 16
Human Rights Act (Articles 2, 3 and 8)
Violent Crime Reduction Act 2006
Crime and Disorder Act 1998 (S115)
Human Rights Act 1998
Mental Health Act 2007

References

All England Law Reports (1988) X v Y [1988] 2 All ER 648, gateway.nlm.nih.gov/MeetingAbstracts/ma?f=102180956.html.

Department of Health (2009) *Lord Bradley's Review of People with Mental Health Problems or Learning Disabilities in the Criminal Justice System,* London: Department of Health, dh.gov.uk/en/Publicationsandstatistics/.../DH_098694.

Department of Health/Home Office (1992) *A Review of Health and Social Services for Mentally Disordered Offenders and Others Requiring Similar Services,* Cmd 2088, London: HMSO/Department of Health/Home Office.

Department for Children Schools and Families (2010) *Working Together to Safeguard Children* Nottingham: DCSF Publications.

GMC (2009) *Guidance for Doctors: Confidentiality October 2009,* www.gmc-uk.org/guidance/ethical_guidance/confidentiality.as.

Law Commission (2010) *Unfitness to Plead Consultation Paper No 197,* justice.gov.uk/lawcommission/areas/unfitness-to-plead.htm.

MORI Social Research (1999) *From Attitudes Towards Doctors and Their Codes of Conduct,* London: MORI Social Research.

Part Two
INTERPROFESSIONAL AND INTERAGENCY WORKING WITH DIFFERENT SERVICE-USER GROUPS

Chapter 7
Mental health

Di Bailey

Chapter summary

This chapter will explore the interprofessional context of integration at practice and professional levels of the health and social care systems when working with people with mental health needs. It will cover the key policy changes that have framed the development of interprofessional working (IPW) in the mental health field, the different professionals who work within it, and the challenges of the coordination and management approaches needed in this current period of IPW. The chapter will draw out the key points from these areas, and give a case study to illustrate some of them.

Interdisciplinary working forms the bedrock of contemporary mental health care in Britain following the introduction of the National Service Framework in 1999. Community-based services in particular have been subject to unprecedented change including the introduction of specialist teams, new roles and new ways of working for existing professionals. The latest Mental Health Act (2007) reflects the political ideology that modern mental health care is predicated upon a greater degree of service integration that draws from a range of disciplines combining skills, theories and expertise. The flurry of recent policies such as the Care Programme Approach (2008), Achieving Excellence (Department of Health (DH), 2010) and Our Health, Our Care, Our Say (DH, 2006) are amongst the strongest drivers for an era characterised by collaborative practice between professionals and service users working in partnership.

The move towards increased care integration in mental health is inevitable because of the cost and complexity of services together with the more informed demands and expectations of the people who use them and their families. By bringing together professionals from the range of disciplinary backgrounds in mental health it is expected that they will engage in an open exchange of ideas and skills to solve service users' problems in cost-effective ways (Colombo et al., 2002). The alternative, according to Horder (2003), is confusion, duplication and inefficiency.

While in principle there are few counter arguments to this approach there are a number of challenges associated with its implementation as a result of:

- the absence of a shared philosophy of practice between mental health workers largely due to the tensions between social, psychological and medical explanations for mental distress

▶

- the growth of the survivor movement in psychiatry that has encouraged the recovery model as an alternative to more traditional explanations for signs and symptoms
- the lack of a common language by which mental health workers can define and describe interdisciplinary working, including how their unique professional contributions can be augmented by shared approaches to practice for the benefit of service users
- the relatively brief historical development of community services compared with the domination of institutional care between the 1800s and the 1980s.

This chapter will consider these challenges and offer some suggestions for developing interdisciplinary working that supports rather than undermines contemporary practice and service development.

Learning objectives

This chapter will cover:

- how laws such as the Mental Health Acts, and recent policies such as the Care Programme Approach (2008), Achieving Excellence (DH 2010) and Our Health, Our Care, Our Say (DH 2006), have shaped the nature of, and requirements upon, collaborative practice between professionals and service users working in partnership
- how the significant growth of the survivor- and recovery-based movements have helped shape mental health services, and how these can be incorporated into interprofessional and interagency practices
- how the effects of historical developments have meant a lack of a common understanding and language about mental heath amongst professionals and how this negatively affects services
- the need for interdisciplinary teams, and the leaders within them, to openly acknowledge different viewpoints and to debate which models of mental distress are informing their practice, and how they might jointly develop a more inclusive philosophy that emphasises a 'being-with' rather than 'doing-to' approach when working with service users
- the real potential for conflict within interdisciplinary teams arising as a result of role rivalry, power dynamics, professional stereotyping and competition between disciplines that needs to be addressed rather than allowed to undermine collaboration.

Defining interdisciplinary working in mental health

Without a common language it becomes difficult to articulate what is meant by interdisciplinary working in mental health and how this incorporates the range of complementary but different practice philosophies. Within the general literature on collaborative working, terms tend to be used interchangeably. For example, Marshall *et al.* (1979) use both inter- and multidisciplinary to refer to teams of individuals with different training backgrounds. Lethard (2003) suggests that multi-professional and multidisciplinary are preferable descriptors for wider teams of professionals and that interprofessional refers to *interactions* between these groups.

The limitations with the use of terms like multi- or interprofessional working is the assumption that this lies exclusively within the domain of professionals, qualified as such because of their recognised training route and in some disciplines being licensed to practice by a professional body. This negates the contribution to contemporary mental health care by the growing numbers of non-professionally affiliated staff such as Support Time and Recovery (STR) workers and graduate Primary Care Mental Health Workers and excludes the experience of those who use services. Increasingly families and carers play a crucial support role in community care and therefore also contribute to what works in respect of care provision. Multi-or interprofessional working also colludes with tensions and power struggles inherent in services that attempt to transcend the hospital and community interface.

For these reasons the term 'interdisciplinary' is suggested as a more accurate reflection of the type of mental health care being aspired to in the twenty-first century. A 'discipline', as defined by *The Oxford Popular English Dictionary and Thesaurus,* is 'a branch of instruction or learning, shaped by the mental, moral and physical training undertaken'. Such learning could be acquired on professional training programmes but also through a person's experiential learning of using mental health services.

Lethard helpfully points out that Latinists translate *'inter'* as between and *'multi'* as many, thus it is this 'between-ness' and interaction that delineates interdisciplinarity in contemporary mental health services as distinct from the more traditional ways of working. Integrated working in mental health thus involves going a step beyond *many working together* to *many interacting to work collaboratively* to respond to the complexity of mental health needs within the spectrum of care provision.

Historical developments in interdisciplinary working

The journey towards interdisciplinary working can be considered an evolutionary process that has involved the range of mental health professionals in different ways at different times. A mental health professional is a person who provides care and treatment for the purpose of improving an individual's mental health and in Britain mental health services have traditionally included a range of professionals.

The nineteenth century marked the beginning of uniprofessional mental health care, professional because it lay in the hands of professionals and uni because of the dominance of the medical or disease model for understanding mental distress. In 1828 the Madhouses Act saw mentally ill people moved from depraved, poverty-stricken communities where the emphasis previously had been on containing criminal insanity, into a closed but more humane and disciplined asylum environment that aimed to cure disorder. By the late 1800s, doctors openly recognised mental disorder as a form of illness and the symptoms of schizophrenia were first described by Kraepelin in the 1890s. The 1930 Mental Treatment Act consolidated the medical model approach through the option of voluntary treatment and psychiatric outpatient clinics.

Between the 1940s and the late 1970s there was ongoing support for hospital care. The National Health Service Act of 1948 defined hospitals as places of treatment for people suffering from illness or defectiveness: the NHS inherited a system of over 100 'mental hospitals' with an average population of 1000 people in each. By the mid-1950s, however, bed numbers had risen to an unsustainable peak and financial constraints, alongside the introduction of drugs like chlorpromazine and imipramine, supported moves to reduce the hospital population. Despite this trend the medicalisation of mental disorder dominated, legally recognised by the Royal Commission on the Law Relating to Mental Illness and Mental Deficiency which resulted in the Percy Report in 1957. The key themes were that mental disorder should be regarded

Exercise 7.1

Think about the team you work in currently or a team you are familiar with. To what extent do team members share duties but retain their own specialist areas of practice? Are there any good examples of where team members interact, bringing their disciplinary expertise together to achieve better outcomes for service users?

'in much the same way physical illness and disability' and that mental hospitals should be run as nearly as possible like hospitals for physical disorders. This message was reinforced by Enoch Powell's famous Water Tower Speech in 1961 and the ensuing Hospital Plan in 1962 that increased the role of psychiatry in District General Hospitals and emphasised re-institutionalisation albeit in different settings, not community care.

The 1959 Mental Health Act provided the legal framework for compulsory admission to any hospital facility, thereby retaining medical decision making. This Act also introduced informal admission for psychiatric disorders and separated out social care for people who did not need inpatient treatment by handing over this responsibility to local councils. This marked the beginning of a shift towards collaborative working at a strategic level, reinforced in the 1970s by visiting multiprofessional teams whose aims were to feedback poor practice to a Department of Health and Social Services working group. The outcome of this process, the Nodder Report (DH, 1980), underlined joint planning at a strategic level between health and the local authorities, together with the involvement of community groups such as Community Health Councils and voluntary organisations. This, together with the emergence of psychological treatments, was perhaps the first suggestion that uniprofessional working in mental health was on the wane.

However, the psychiatric social work departments that had developed as a result of this increasing local authority involvement continued to remain separate and occupational therapy was largely confined to hospital workshops notoriously associated with basket weaving or work-based schemes concerned with menial tasks. Whilst a more psychologically oriented discourse on mental distress emerged from the work of Freud, Jung and Skinner psychologists were still rarely involved in treatment plans. Patients[1] were passive recipients of a regime of containment and medical interventions such as electroconvulsive therapy (ECT) and psychosurgery. This approach rests on the premise that once the illness is medically treated the need for other forms of intervention diminishes because the signs and symptoms will improve. Thus contributions from other professionals still remained subsumed within the disease model, reflecting their differential status relative to psychiatry (Figure 7.1).

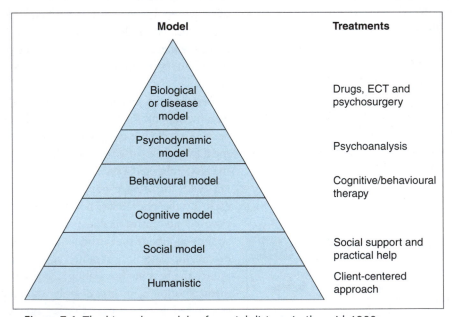

Figure 7.1 The hierarchy models of mental distress in the mid-1900s

---

[1]This term is used here intentionally to reflect the powerless status of individuals receiving mental health treatment from 1900–1980s.

The introduction of a multi-professional approach

From the 1980s onwards the configuration of mental health services reflected the developments of the previous 30 years with a mix of old, unclosed, large psychiatric hospitals, purpose-built units for acute care in new general hospitals and designated psychiatric wards in older general hospitals. Community provision included residential services, such as hostels, group homes and therapeutic communities, community mental health centres and day centres run by the NHS and local authorities. Treatment for individuals at high risk of offending, who also had mental health needs, was provided in regional secure units and special hospitals.

Against this backdrop the 1983 Mental Health Act (MHA) influenced a significant move from uniprofessional to multi-professional working because as Rogers and Pilgrim (1996, p. 88) point out, its main accomplishment seemed to be 'the formal codification of existing professional roles and practice in relation to compulsory detention of patients'. This was achieved in a number of ways.

Firstly, the 1983 MHA introduced the right for patients to apply to a Mental Health Review Tribunal that would review the legality of their detention. Tribunal panels included representatives from lay professions as well as legal advocates and doctors. This gave a clear mandate to a multi-professional panel of individuals to combine their expertise from different backgrounds to ensure the safeguard of patients' rights.

Secondly, the delineation of professional roles, both within and between disciplines, was made more apparent by the legislation. Under section 5 registered mental nurses in addition to doctors were given new 'holding powers' in order to prevent patients detained informally from leaving hospital. These orders allowed for compulsory detention for short periods of time (up to 72 hours) so that further assessment for compulsory admission could be undertaken.

Finally the Act specified in detail how professional roles and responsibilities should be exercised. For example, Approved Social Workers (ASWs) were required to make the application for admission under section while two medical doctors had to recommend that this course of action was in the best interests of the patient. ASWs were required to interview people being assessed under the Act in a suitable manner to ensure that detention was the most appropriate way of providing the care and treatment they needed. By specifying professional responsibilities in this way the 1983 MHA provided a much clearer demarcation of skills and roles of the professional groups than previously and contributions other than the medical perspective were acknowledged.

The 1983 MHA also reinforced multi-agency working, primarily between health and social services, by formalising in section 117 the provision of 'aftercare' for patients being discharged from compulsory treatment in hospital. Providing joint aftercare was identified as a shared responsibility between health and social services who were required to coordinate packages of care on discharge. Similar messages regarding multi-agency working were echoed by the subsequent 1990 National Health Service and Community Care Act (NHSCCA) that changed the traditional territory of psychiatric services, setting out more clearly the responsibilities of local authorities for providing community mental health care.

Despite these changes, professionalisation of mental health care in the 1980s was still clearly demarked from a more inclusive approach that sought contributions from service users to their care and treatment. As Perkins and Repper (1998, p. 3) point out, service users were excluded from service planning meetings and were 'only invited to ward rounds to demonstrate their symptoms and hear the doctor's prescription'. Thus while joint working between professionals could be deemed to have moved on a stage, the involvement of service users remained at an impasse.

Multidisciplinary working in the 1990s

The Care Programme Approach guidance (DH 1990), coinciding with the NHS and CCA (1990), encouraged multidisciplinary working because both emphasised the need to involve people who used services in the ways in which they were designed and delivered. Even though involvement in the 1990s continued to be rather tokenistic there was an emerging acceptance that service users could no longer be regarded as passive recipients because they had a distinct perspective to offer about mental health services, based on their direct experience of using them. While Community Mental Health Teams (CMHTs) emerged the models of implementation varied from integrated Community Mental Health Centres (CMHCs) to fragmented teams with Community Psychiatric Nurses (CPNs) and social workers being separated geographically undertaking their own referral and assessment procedures. This diversity of multidisciplinary provision was reflected in the extent to which service-user involvement was integrated into CMHTs.

Not surprisingly a number of mental health inquiries began to highlight the flaws in this multidisciplinary approach, including the problems with professionals recording and passing information, poor risk management and a lack of integration between hospital and community care. The 1995 Mental Health (Patients in the Community) Act, alongside a renewed emphasis on Care Programme Approach (CPA), attempted to strengthen coordinated aftercare on discharge. While there was some evidence that multidisciplinary working in the CMHTs was evolving from the early stages in the mid-1990s in response to the critics, there was a political view that mental health and social care needed more radical modernisation (DH 1998a, 1999). This led to the National Service Framework (DH 1999) and related Mental Health Policy Implementation Guide (DH 2001) as the blueprint for modern-day standards in mental health, the service models of Crisis Resolution and Home Treatment (CRHT) Assertive Outreach Teams (AOTS) and Early Intervention in Psychosis (EIP) that would embody a new way of working.

Values and power in interdisciplinary working

Professional power is a key contributing factor to the success or failure of interdisciplinary working. Power is maintained by the language and models the different professional groups use to understand and describe mental distress, together with the different value systems that influence the knowledge and skills of the mental health workforce. It influences the relative importance attached to professional versus service-user contributions to care and treatment approaches.

Since the introduction of the mental health National Service Framework in 1999 the government has been dedicated to a parallel process of changing the workforce and occupational culture in mental health (DH, 2007), whilst strengthening the mandate for service-user involvement and 'personalisation' (DH, 2006).

Paradoxically then, as professional/service-user relationships are redefined it becomes even more

A closer look

Key professionals in mental health work

- Psychiatrists are medical doctors specialising in the treatment of mental illness using a biomedical or disease model approach to understand signs and symptoms.
- Clinical psychologists have an undergraduate degree in psychology and post-doctoral training to understand and intervene with people with psychologically based distress and dysfunction.
- Traditionally for many years mental health social workers have received additional post-qualifying training with a focus on social causation and labelling as explanations for mental distress, some of whom will have completed additional training to become 'approved' to undertake statutory duties as defined by the 1983 Mental Health Act (although other professionals can now undertake this role after changes in the Mental Health Act 2007).
- Psychiatric nurses specialise in a branch of nursing that provides skills in psychological therapies and the administration of psychiatric medication.
- Occupational therapists assess and treat psychological conditions using specific, purposeful activity to prevent disability and promote independence and well-being.

Key learning points

Key developments as a consequence of these policy changes:

- service users have political support in their quest for services that promote recovery and are therefore much less accepting of services that fail to listen and take account of their individual needs
- psychiatrists are being encouraged to prioritise their 'consultant' role and delegate hands-on care and treatment decisions to other team members
- new roles for non-professionally affiliated staff such as Support Time and Recovery Workers and Carers' Support Workers are being introduced in the existing mental health workforce
- the ASW role has been extended to other professionals (occupational therapists, nurses) who will become the approved mental health professionals of the future.

important for workers to develop a clear sense of their unique identity and disciplinary contribution in order to be confident about their role when working collaboratively with others. The New Ways of Working initiative is not about all professional groups being able to do the same thing. It is about each group having a basic foundation of shared skills, knowledge and values that coexists with an openly acknowledged disciplinary/professional contribution. It is these discipline-specific contributions that allow for an interdisciplinary response to the increasing diversity of need within the service-user population, who seek help and assistance for a whole range of mental health problems.

Teams such as the one above that are attempting increased integration and collaboration will also need to revisit the tension between managing and containing mental illness on the one hand and collaborative approaches to fostering the promotion of mental

Case study

An example of interdisciplinary working

Initially a CMHT, North P Team has specialised further to work with individuals with psychosis. The team comprised social workers, community psychiatric nurses (CPNs), occupational therapists (OTs), a consultant psychiatrist and consultant psychologists. Team members also include support workers and link workers who work under the guidance and direction of professionally qualified staff. The team has a team manager who is a CPN by background, and several administrative staff. The team adopts an interdisciplinary approach in that all CPNs, social workers and OTs are first and foremost care coordinators and service users are often unaware of their disciplinary contribution. As a result case-load size is similar across disciplines and averages at 35.

The team manager is responsible for the overall day-to-day running of the team and the allocation of clinical work is done weekly through allocation meetings which all team members attend.

Service users who need their medication by injection are normally allocated to CPN care coordinators, but this depends on CPN availability and their case-load size. Each individual care coordinator is responsible for designing a care package in collaboration with the service user. All care coordinators provide a combination of psychological therapies and learn basic skills in cognitive behavioural therapy and dialectical behaviour therapy. Where more specialist therapeutic skills and/or assessment is needed service users are referred to the consultant psychologists and staff members from other disciplines who have advanced skills and expertise in therapeutic interventions.

The consultant psychiatrist adopts the New Ways of Working approach and acts mainly as a consultant to other team members when there are more complex issues with service users' medical treatment and or diagnosis. Some CPNs are promoted as advance practitioners and nurse consultants and take a more specialist professional role in prescribing and managing medication.

The role of the Approved Mental Health Professional (AMHP), although having been opened up to other disciplines as a result of the 2007 MHA, remains exclusively undertaken by social workers. Because of their specialist role in respect of mental health act assessments, AMHPs get a lower case load than other care coordinators, currently around 20. One senior AMHP has been promoted to the role of 'expert practitioner' and provides supervision to some of the social workers. Where professional support is provided in addition to workload management this system seems to work well. However, in a 'sister' team in the same locality where both the team manager and expert practitioner roles are held by CPNs, social workers express significant concern about the lack of disciplinary-specific supervision, particularly in relation to their statutory social work duties.

Feedback from interviews with team members as part of a current study reveals increasing support for interdisciplinary working within the team because this lends itself to practice that is more responsive to the service user with psychosis and enables good relationships and communication.

The involvement of service users and their carers in decisions about care and treatment is mainly through their collaborative relationship with their care coordinator. Within the team it would appear there is further scope for interagency working at a more strategic level with service-user organisations who may also be supporting people collectively on a locality basis.

Exercise 7.2

Put yourself in the position of a service user receiving care and treatment from the above team. What concerns would you have about your care in the light of how these professionals work together? What suggestions might you make to your care coordinator in respect of effective interdisciplinary working?

health on the other. If professionals invest negative energy in their approach, working against each other as a means of retaining professional superiority, this will detract from any benefits of others trying to working collaboratively. This phenomenon has been demonstrated in practice by Colombo and colleagues (2002) who explored why shared clinical decision-making undermined collaboration as an outcome.

Colombo *et al.* asked participants from different professional groups in mental health (including social workers, service users, carers, nurses and psychiatrists) to respond to 12 open-ended questions after reading a case resumé for a person called Tom whose behaviour suggested that he may have schizophrenia. The 12 questions sought to establish which models of mental distress the different groups used to make sense of what was happening to Tom. Not surprisingly Colombo *et al.* found that psychiatrists and

nurses clearly favoured the medical approach, which received most overall support. In contrast social workers showed support for the social model to explain Tom's signs and symptoms. Amongst the service users, there was some degree of consensus across a range of perspectives and carers endorsed the medical and family models.

These findings led Colombo *et al.* to conclude that as a consequence of such implicit models competing for recognition the interdisciplinary decision-making process can become highly contested. The likelihood then is that cooperation between colleagues and with service users and carers is undermined. For this reason interdisciplinary teams need to openly debate which models of mental distress are informing their practice, being guided by a more inclusive philosophy that emphasises a 'being-with' rather than a 'doing-to' approach when working with service users (Hinselwood 1996).

The recovery model, with its emphasis on psychosocial interventions in contemporary mental health services, places equal value on social, psychological and medical interventions from different disciplinary groups, including the person using the service and their family. This approach allows for a more holistic perspective about how best to intervene and solve the difficulties being experienced by the service user.

This is perhaps most clearly articulated by Perkins and Repper (1998, p. 25), who assert that:

Case study

Meet Sharon

Sharon is 42 years old, has retired from work on grounds of mental ill health and lives alone in a flat about a mile away from her family who reside in the same village. Sharon has bizarre thoughts of persecution, demonstrates some self-harming behaviours and is reluctant to engage with mental health services or take medication. Sharon's mother has hinted that Sharon was abused as a child by her uncle but will not go into any detail. Sharon has a very ambivalent relationship with her mother and gets very angry when questioned about her childhood. All she will say is that all the other children in the village were victims of incest but she 'was special'. Sharon has a good relationship with her niece and on a good day presents as very intelligent and engaging. She enjoys ten-pin bowling and likes the company of animals. Sharon's GP has tried to intervene in the past but Sharon has resisted visits from a CPN for depot medication.

As a support worker, how might you work with Sharon to promote a more holistic approach to her mental health which draws on relevant input and advice from a range of professionals but does not 'over-medicalise' signs and symptoms that may be the result of traumatic life events?

Different people adopt different models for understanding what has happened to them . . . organic constructions . . . psychological, social, religious or spiritual formulations. People have a right to define their own experiences for themselves and it is rarely helpful and more likely to be alienating for the clinician to insist that their understanding is correct.

Interprofessional education to support interdisciplinary working

One way to support interdisciplinary working is through the provision of interprofessional education (IPE), which has been reinforced by a raft of policy developments since the mid-1990s. Interprofessional education becomes interdisciplinary when service users, carers and non-professionally affiliated groups in the workforce interact with professionals to learn with, from and about each other to improve collaboration and the quality of care delivered. Interdisciplinary learning is different from shared learning approaches in that it should be planned, designed and delivered with the explicit aim of enhancing collaborative practice.

A commitment to the importance of IPE as a necessary ingredient to support new ways of working in mental health was underpinned by the NHS Workforce Strategy (DH 2000) which called for genuinely multi-professional training to promote:

- teamwork
- partnership and collaboration between professions, agencies and with service users
- skill mix and flexible working
- opportunities to switch training pathways to expedite career progression
- the introduction of new types of workers into the health service workforce.

These priorities have been realised in different ways in mental health. First, in the late 1990s a number of shared or joint learning programmes began to develop with a focus on psychosocial interventions for people with severe and enduring mental health problems (Brooker *et al.* 2001; Milne *et al.* 2000; Carpenter *et al.* 1999, 2000). IPE has been supported nationally by the Mental Health in Higher Education Project and through joint events between the Higher Education Academy subject centres. The funding of two interdisciplinary Centres for Excellence in Teaching and Learning in Mental Health in 2005, (at Birmingham and Middlesex Universities) was a deliberate attempt by the Higher Education Academy to support education developments that dovetailed with increased integration in mental health practice.

Attempts to develop an increasingly shared skill mix among mental health professionals began in 2001 with The Capable Practitioner framework (Sainsbury Centre for Mental Health, 2001). This set out a list of capabilities that were linked to the NSF standards and covered the knowledge, skills and values deemed necessary for contemporary mental health practice across all professions. This framework evolved into the more succinct Ten Essential Shared Capabilities (DH 2004) that is now recognised as the underpinning blueprint for the curriculum of all mental health training initiatives. A series of learning materials to support the implementation of these capabilities has also been designed and made available through the Centre for Academic Workforce Innovation at the University of Lincoln. Teamwork has been explicitly encouraged through the Creating Capable Teams Approach launched at the New Ways of Working (NWW) Conference in April 2007. Packs to support the development programme are available via the National Centre for Mental Health.

The new types of worker roles in mental health services have gathered momentum over the last 10 years with a significant increase in the numbers of non-professionally affiliated staff such as Support Time and Recovery Workers and Gateway Workers in Primary Care Mental Health. An overview of the development of these roles is provided by Dickinson *et al.* (2008). Mental health training programmes that have developed to support these new roles such as the one for Graduate Primary Care Workers at the University of Birmingham have a module or parts of their curriculum dedicated to teamworking. An evaluation jointly undertaken by Newcastle and Durham Universities has sought to establish how the introduction of these roles alongside the new ways of working for other professionals has been implemented nationally and the implications this has for future IPE developments.

Managing interdisciplinary mental health

Managers of interdisciplinary mental health teams and services face a challenge which involves two sets of complementary activities; managing increasingly complex models of service delivery and creating the organisational climate to foster people from different disciplines working more effectively together.

The ultimate aim of change in mental health services has been to reorientate the culture of care delivery,

away from the traditional model of medical treatment towards the promotion of mental health and well-being. Responsibility for staying mentally well is increasingly shared between mental health professionals, carers and service users and implemented through collaborative care planning. Colleagues need to be attuned to the psychological impact of working with people with mental health problems, because as Scheid (1996) points out their role requires commitment at a deeper emotional level, to be caring, as well as practicing in a caring way. This is echoed by Ramon and Williams (2005 p. 15) who advocate replacing a distanced 'hands-off' approach with a more 'hands-on' way of working in mental health that demonstrates emotional closeness to the service user and an interest in their everyday concerns.

Responding to this complex agenda affords the potential for conflict within interdisciplinary teams arising as a result of role rivalry, power dynamics, professional stereotyping and competition between disciplines (Onyett *et al.*, 1995, Onyett, 2003). While addressing these issues can pose a challenge for managers, it is important that they are addressed rather than allowed to develop as a subculture that can undermine collaboration. According to West and Farr (1989) successful organisations manage rather than suppress conflict, and everyone in the team needs to take some responsibility for conflict management. Onyett (2003) notes that well-defined responsibilities within teams together with clear lines of accountability will make conflict resolution easier.

In addition to the interpersonal challenge, managers will also need to manage issues relating to effective time management, workload prioritisation/allocation and ensure that safety standards for practice are met. Managing the way in which clinical team meetings operate and how work is allocated is an opportunity for managers to foster collaborative interdisciplinary learning.

In this climate Onyett (2003) highlights the need for a combination of transactional and transformational leadership. The former is concerned with the organisation and planning of the use of resources, dealing with problems as they arise and monitoring activities aimed at meeting targets. The latter involves 'challenging the status quo and is about creating new visions and scenarios to stimulate the creative and emotional drive in individuals to innovate and deliver excellence' (p. 162). An effective manager of an interdisciplinary team or service will be adept at delivering a leadership approach that ensures the task is achieved and that individuals collaborate to achieve it. Onyett (2003) claims that interdisciplinary teams will also need a manager who can cope with being used both by the team members in the way the manager represents the team to the organisation, but also how they in turn represent the organisation to the team. Managers will also need to be able to operate at an interagency level to work with different organisation's systems and structures and facilitate opportunities for interdisciplinary practice across agency boundaries. Statutory organisations are likely to be characterised by a very top-down, vertically aligned, and multilayered hierarchy which contrasts with the independent sector where 'flattened' management structures and 'bottom-up approaches' that hinge on service-user contributions are more common.

Conclusion

Legislation, recent policies and long-standing histories – and sometimes rivalries – of the different professions involved in work with mental health service users have shaped the nature of, and requirements upon, collaborative practice between professionals and service users working in partnership. **Interdisciplinary working goes with the territory of contemporary mental health care delivery**. Beset with challenges, it is not easy to achieve, requires support from IPE and good interdisciplinary leadership and management in order to deal with the real potential for role rivalry, power dynamics, professional stereotyping and competition between disciplines. There has been a significant growth of the **survivor- and recovery-based movements which have challenged these old constructions**, and helped shape mental health services and concomitant interprofessional and interagency practices.

The qualitative difference between inter- and multidisciplinary working is the effective interaction between groups of professionals, service users and carers to achieve improved outcomes through the process of active collaboration. **The recovery model of mental health provides a framework for a less hierarchical and more inclusive way of working**. This, together with organisational systems and structures that facilitate good communication and effective partnerships in the planning and delivery of coordinated care, will underpin increasing interdisciplinarity in the future.

Further reading

Bailey D. (2012) *Interdisciplinary Working in Mental Health: from Theory to Practice*, Basingstoke, Palgrave Macmillan.
Journal of Interprofessional Care.

Useful websites

http://www.mhhe.heacademy.ac.uk/
Mental health in higher education project
http://www.caipe.org.uk/
Centre for the Advancement of Interprofessional Education

References

Brooker, C., Saul, C., Robinson, J., King, J. and Dudley, M. (2001) *Is Training in Psychosocial Interventions Worthwhile?* Report of a psychosocial intervention trainee follow-up study, Sheffield: ScHARR.

Carpenter, J., Barnes, D. and Dickinson, C. (1999) *Birmingham University Programme in Community Mental Health.* Progress Report 1 from the external evaluation team, Durham: Centre for Applied Social Studies, University of Durham.

Carpenter, J., Barnes, D. and Dickinson, C. (2000) *Birmingham University Programme in Community Mental Health.* Progress Report 2 from the external evaluation team, Durham: Centre for Applied Social Studies, University of Durham.

Colombo, A., Bendelow, B., Fulford, B. and Williams, S. (2002) Evaluating the influence of implicit models of mental disorder on processes of shared decision making within community based multidisciplinary teams, *Social Science and Medicine* 56, 1557–70.

DH (Department of Health) (1980) *Organisation and Management Problems of Mental Illness Hospitals (The Nodder Report)*, London: HMSO.

DH (Department of Health) (1990) Caring for People. The Care Programme Approach for People with a Mental Illness referred to the specialist mental health services. Joint Health/Social Services Circular C(90)23/LASSL(90)11. London: Department of Health.

DH (Department of Health) (1990) *NHS and CCA,* London: HMSO.

DH (Department of Health) (1995) The Mental Health (Patients in the Community) Act, London: HMSO.

DH (Department of Health) (1998a) *Modernising Mental Health Services: Safe, Sound and Supportive,* London: HMSO.

DH (Department of Health) (1998b) *Modernising Social Services,* London: HMSO.

DH (Department of Health) (1999) *National Service Framework for Mental Health: Modern Standards and Service Models,* London: HMSO.

DH (Department of Health) (2000) *A Health Service of All the Talents: Developing the NHS Workforce,* London: DH.

DH (Department of Health) (2001) *The Mental Health Policy Implementation Guide,* London: The Stationery Office.

DH (Department of Health) (2004) *The Ten Essential Shared Capabilities: A Framework for the Whole of the Mental Health Workforce.* National Institute for Mental Health in England, the Sainsbury Centre for Mental Health Joint Workforce Support Unit in conjunction with the National Health Service University (NHSU), London: DH.

DH (Department of Health) (2006) *Our Health, Our Care, Our Say,* London: DH.

DH (Department of Health) (2007) *New Ways of Working for Everyone*, London: Department of Health.

Dickinson, C., Lombardo, C., Pearson, P., Barnes, D. and Bailey, D. (2008) Mapping new roles in mental health services; the development of four new roles from 2004–2006. *Journal of Mental Health Training, Education and Practice* 3 (1) 4–11.

Hawker, S. and Hawkins, J.M. (eds) (1995) *The Oxford Popular English Dictionary and Thesaurus*, Bath: Paragon.

Hinselwood, R. D. (1996) Creatures of Each Other: Some historical considerations of responsibility and care, and some present undercurrents, in A. Foster and V. Zagier Roberts (eds) *Managing Mental Health in the Community, Chaos and Containment,* London: Routledge.

Horder, J. (2003) Foreword, in A. Lethard (ed.) *Interprofessional Collaboration: From Policy to Practice in Health and Social Care,* Hove: Brunner-Routledge, pp. xiii–xiv.

Lethard, A. (2003) Introduction, in A. Lethard (ed) *Interprofessional Collaboration: From Policy to Practice*, Hove: Brunner-Routledge.

Marshall, M., Preston, M., Scott, E. and Wincott, P. (eds) (1979) *Teamwork For and Against: An Appraisal of Multidisciplinary Practice,* London: British Association of Social Workers.

Onyett, S. (2003) *Teamworking in Mental Health,* Basingstoke: Palgrave Macmillan.

Onyett, S., Heppleston, T. and Muijen, M. (1995) *Making Community Mental Health Teams Work,* London: SCMH.

Perkins, R. and Repper, J. (1998) Principles of working with people who experience mental health problems, in C. Brooker, and J. Repper, (eds) *Serious Mental Health Problems in the Community, Policy, Practice and Research,* London: Balliére Tindall Ltd.

Ramon, S. and Williams, J. E. (2005) Towards a conceptual framework: the meanings attached to the psychosocial, the promise and the problems, in S. Ramon and J.E. Williams (eds) *Mental Health at the Crossroads: The Promise of the Psychosocial Approach,* Aldershot: Ashgate.

Rogers, A. and Pilgrim, D. (1996) *Mental Health Policy in Britain,* Basingstoke: Macmillan.

Sainsbury Centre for Mental Health (SCMH) (2001) *The Capable Practitioner: A Framework and List of the Practitioner Capabilities Required to Implement the National Service Framework for Mental Health,* London: SCMH.

Scheid, T. L. (1996) Burned Out Emotional Labourers: An Analysis of Emotional Labour, Work Identity and Burnout. Paper presented at the American Sociological Association Meeting, New York.

West, M. A. and Farr, J. L. (1989) Innovation at work: psychological perspectives. *Social Behaviour* 4, 15–30.

Chapter 8
Learning disabilities

Michelle Culwick and Carolyn Wallace

Chapter summary

This chapter explores the interprofessional context of integration at practice and professional levels of the health and social care systems when working with people with learning disabilities. In order to achieve this we must first define what we mean by interprofessional. Hammick *et al.* (2009, p. 10) say 'being interprofessional is learning and working or working and learning with others: as appropriate, when necessary and sometimes both'. The level of working together generally required in this context is that of coordination, which is a form of integration (Leutz, 1999, 2005). Integration is defined by Demers and Lavoie (2008, p. 6) as occurring 'when a comprehensive range of services is co-ordinated so that each user receives the right service at the right time by the right person without having to find it by him- or herself'. Practice (or clinical) integration is the context of interaction between professional and service user, and sometimes the informal carer, while professional integration is the act of registered and non-registered professionals working together in various forms in order to deliver seamless care (Wallace, 2009).

Hammick *et al.* (2009, p. 8) state that being interprofessional 'is an active rather than passive practice-related behaviour'. It means:

- knowing what to do
- having the right skills to do what needs to be done in a competent and capable manner
- conducting ourselves in the right way which means with the right attitude, appropriate values and beliefs.

The context of interprofessional working within this chapter will provide a clear contextual framework for the reader. Knowledge and skills debates around interprofessional working will be provoked through the inclusion of research-informed activities and interactive exercises. Points of reflection will assist the reader in exploring the benefits and potential barriers to interprofessional working. Dilemmas will be explored and practice debate enthused. To give as real life an insight as possible the application of working models to case study material is included.

Therefore this chapter takes a systems thinking approach to care. It takes the view that the demand for services originates from the service-user perspective of their need. As a result, this service-user focus or 'value demand' impacts on all levels in the care system by demanding various forms of working together in order to meet and satisfy the holistic needs of the individual (Seddon, 2008; Wallace, 2009). However, in this chapter we are concerned only with the practice and professional levels within the whole system (Delnoij *et al.*, 2002). Supporting the view that in order to work together effectively with the service user across health and social care means it is important to learn collectively what is and how to work together (Barr, 2000; Braithwaite *et al.*, 2007).

Learning objectives

This chapter will cover:

- services for people with learning disabilities provided from across a range of agencies and professional groups. These must start from the key concepts that they are planned and delivered from service-user perspectives, and work together to provide holistic services for their needs

- concepts about social inclusion and person-focused approaches. These provide key areas from which interprofessional agency and interagency working can be explored as part of care management and person-centred planning, in order to ensure the rhetoric of individualisation and empowerment are realised in practice

- the development of the 'interprofessional willingness condition' – to do whatever is required to enable effective interprofessional working – thereby placing needs of the service users and carers as equal to if not higher than the needs of individual professionals and agencies as key to these processes

- an early appreciation of the dynamics within interprofessional teams such as community learning disabilities and between agencies in order to deliver these services more effectively.

Case Study

Meet Phillip

Phillip Lewis is a 33-year-old man who has a moderate learning disability. Phillip has always lived at home with his mother Joy. He has a part-time job in a local café that supports adults with learning disabilities to work there and develop skills. Over recent months Phillip has expressed the wish to move out and live independently. Joy is apprehensive about this and does not think it could be a possibility due to his support needs. Phillip and Joy have had many in-depth discussions over this and Joy is concerned he will become lonely and potentially isolated, leaving him vulnerable. Phillip has never financially been independent and Joy is worried he will not be able to budget or support himself. Joy has contacted Social Services for further advice and assistance. A social worker from the local team for adults with learning disabilities undertook an initial assessment.

Barr and Gates (2008) have explored the perceived need for improving the educational needs of people in learning disability services. They argue that shared learning and partnership between education and services are required, with a change in curriculum to reflect the change in policy objectives. Examples from the authors' experiences will illustrate how by learning together we can help eradicate the 'silo' thinking.

To illustrate this, an invitation is given to follow Phillip Lewis' care journey, which begins in the Case study 'Meet Phillip'. Phillip has a moderate learning disability and is a recipient of services. Concepts around social inclusion, a person-focused approach, and a variety of forms and degrees in which we can work together will be explored. The relationship between service user and professional, professional role and service provision will be critiqued.

Key learning points

- The interprofessional context of integration at practice and professional levels generally requires the act of coordination.
- Being interprofessional is an active, not passive, behaviour.
- In order to meet the needs of the service user, education and service provision should work together.

Cultural change and the context of service provision

The World Health Organization's definition of learning disability is

a state of arrested or incomplete development of mind. Moderate or mild learning disability is seen by the Department of Health as having an IQ of 50–70 as opposed to 20–50 for severe and less than 20 for profound.

(Northfield, 2004a)

With the move from institutionalisation to community living, professionals aspire to a fully inclusive service. Professional practice and education across health and social care is constantly debating the concept of interprofessionalism. Bringing the rhetoric

Exercise 8.1

Consider the 'interprofessional willingness condition'. How would you promote an interprofessional willingness condition in order to support Phillip and his family through the assessment process?

into reality is the challenge for policy makers, education- and service-providers alike.

Sellman (2010) argues that a person's behaviour is fixed and consistent with their individual character. In the past it has been argued that at the centre of an individual's culture are values which are affected by generational, gender and class differences (Hofstede, 1991).

Macro developments around social inclusion, anti-discriminatory practice and combating stereotypes are needed to encourage inclusion. Systems theories assist us in understanding the person in their situation. To truly acknowledge and appreciate the importance of the degrees of working together coupled with joined-up thinking, it is essential to understand the impact this can have on service provision and the inclusion of people with learning disabilities in decision making and their ultimate rights as equal citizens.

Care management is the predominant practice of statutory adult social care services. Methods of

A closer look

Core values for systems development

Attwood *et al.* (2003) identified ten core values which were essential to the success of whole-system development. They were:

- optimism
- empathy and humility
- tenacity and courage
- learning
- relationships
- a whole-system perspective
- local knowledge for local solutions
- building social capital
- celebrating small steps
- the long view.

Sellman (2010, p. 159) takes this a step further and discusses a 'willingness condition' which an individual must have in order that the team can most effectively meet an individual's needs. It is described as 'the willingness to do whatever is required to contribute to effective team working. This includes a willingness to put the needs of the team on an equal, if not higher, footing than their personal needs'.

Adapting this concept further, the interprofessional willingness condition is the willingness to do whatever is required to enable effective interprofessional working that will meet the needs of Phillip and his family, so placing their needs equal if not higher than the needs of individuals within the interprofessional team. Phillip's and Joy's experience of team working has been ad hoc when different members of the team have responded individually.

A closer look

It is sometimes the reality that families encounter a different professional each time they make contact with the team. Professionals themselves may see this as inconsistent and service users/carers may feel this impacts on their interaction with the service. A recent document called the 'Triangle of Care' (Worthington and Rooney, 2010, p. 3) included six elements which are required to ensure that collaborative care is achieved along the care journey between service user, carer and staff. The fourth principle states that 'defined post(s) responsible for carers are in place'. This is to ensure that carers have a single person identified to them with whom they can discuss any issues or potential concerns they have with their caring role. Although this document was written with mental health services in mind it is worth looking at and considering practices that could be transferable across to your services.

Exercise 8.2

Consider the impact on families that a constant change in the worker dealing with their case would have.

A closer look

A review of day services for people with learning disabilities, 'Having a good day?' (Cole *et al.*, 2007), ascertained this group to have experienced least benefit from the 'modernisation' of services for people with learning disabilities. It is often the case that people who have extensive needs are offered expensive packages to pay for services within their community (Swift and Mattingly, 2009). The White Paper 'Valuing People' (Department of Health, 2001) emphasised the improvement of service provision for people with learning disability by identifying four key principles to ensure a fully inclusive service. Rights, independence, choice and inclusion underpin service ethos when aspiring to meet the needs of people with learning disability. Valuing People raised expectations of local decision makers to prioritise improvements in support for the key principles. Access to services is often dependent on service-user-assessed eligibility and the availability of resources.

assessing and planning the care needs of adult service users are based on 'Person-Centred Planning' (PCP). This practice aims to ensure the rhetoric of individualisation and empowerment principles are actualised in care management processes. The Community Adult Learning Disability Team (CALDT) constitutes a team of health and social care professionals who provide an array of services and help that support people over the age of 18 with a learning disability. Support is also provided to carers, such as family and friends, who assist people with a learning disability.

Interprofessionalism: the role of assessment and information sharing

As informed by the NHS and Community Care Act 1990, local authorities have a duty to ensure the assessment of need for people with learning disabilities. Community care services have predominantly adopted a procedural model of assessment when eligibility criteria are taken into consideration (Lymbery, 2005; Welsh Assembly Government, 2002). The Department of Health (2009a) has identified the link between the act of working together and the quality of care, i.e. receiving services which meet identified need. The issues of how to manage people's complex needs in respect of which levels and forms of working together (i.e. cooperation, collaboration, coordination, intensive case management, co-location, multidisciplinary, trans- or interdisciplinary assessment or a full integrative team) has not truly been addressed. A person-centred or person-focused approach to assessment requires professionals who work together to exchange assessment information in such a way as to maximise the opportunity for problem solving while enabling 'the service user and carer to be the centre of the act of care and treatment' (Wallace and Davies, 2009, p. 12). Information-sharing is a mechanism for enabling the act of working together. Very often this is achieved through the act of joint assessment and the blurring of professional boundaries across roles and agencies (Lloyd and Wait, 2005).

Standardised assessment frameworks and processes across health and social care are known in England, Wales and Scotland as the Single Assessment Process, the Unified Assessment Process and the Single Shared Assessment (Department of Health, 2002; Scottish Executive, 2001; Welsh Assembly Government, 2002). They prescribe a layered approach to assessment within which staff are required to have a prescribed level of competency in assessment and the impact of risk upon an individual (Wallace and Davies, 2009).

The Single Assessment Process (SAP) in England was viewed as an attempt to provide a seamless approach to assessment and support care management for older people (Department of Health, 2002). However, the SAP implementation approach has been found to be fragmented with local implementation (different assessment tools, different technologies) creating what has been called 'organisational aquariums,' that is exposing challenging organisational behaviour when trying to improve the communication and coordination of assessment information across and within agencies and professionals (Glasby, 2004; Wilson and Baines, 2009; Wilson *et al.*, 2007). The subsequent publication of the Common Assessment Framework has included all adults (Department of Health, 2009b). Certainly the introduction of these standardised assessment frameworks has found inconsistencies in professional practice in respect of process and principles, in addition to professional disengagement and professionalisation (Ridout and Mayers, 2006).

In attempting to achieve consistency across different agencies and professionals, it is necessary to acknowledge and have an understanding of the effects of having a wide variety of potential services involved in the lives of people with learning disabilities. These include:

■ Community Adult Learning Disability Team
■ supported housing
■ day centres
■ family aid support
■ supported employment
■ domiciliary care at home
■ personal assistants.

Exercise 8.3

Community learning disability team – a team experience of sharing information

How would different members of the team implement the policy framework of using a standardised framework? Consider in relation to Phillip.

Commentary

You may have considered the gaps in applying policy guidance into practical experience. This is especially so in respect of information-sharing protocols across agencies. When information is shared effectively the experience for the family such as in Phillips' case is one of uncertainty and duplication. A concern would be that members of the team are not communicating vital information to one another, perpetuating the impression of 'organisational aquariums'.

Key learning points

■ For real inclusion of service users it is essential to work in partnership with them from the outset of their service journey.
■ The sharing of information within teams and across professions is key to effective assessment processes.
■ Interprofessional dilemmas can occur in the assessment information-sharing process if there is not a transparency of role or the existence of the 'interprofessional willingness condition' mentioned earlier in this chapter.

Models of partnership

Partnership is essential to enable working together at both practice and professional levels of the whole system. Policy documents in the UK require a partnership approach, for example in the development of *Supporting People* (Department for Communities and Local Government, 2007). Dickinson (2008) has suggested that this is a catch-all phrase for joint working, multi-agency working and interprofessional working. For some partnership is 'a state of relationship, at organizational, group, professional or interpersonal level, to be achieved, maintained and reviewed'; whereas collaboration is 'an active process of partnership in action' (Weinstein *et al.*, 2003). Flynn (2007) discusses a collaborative spectrum which ranges from 'meetings, no action', joint bid, cooperation, collaboration, joint budgets to 'merger/acquisition', while Fritchie (2002) suggests that collaboration is a level of partnership. These definitions lead us to consider that these terms are about the proactive interaction between people. However, the lack of consistency in the language used around the levels of working together has not aided its legitimacy and value at all levels of the health and social care system. Indeed it may have led to some concept confusion, interpreted by different people at different levels of the health and social care system in different ways (De Long and Seeman, 2000; Wallace, 2009). This lack of standardisation with the meaning of words leads to 'positively valenced concepts', that is, confusion and loss of meaning for

A closer look

Boon *et al.*'s (2004) conceptual framework

Parallel – independent workers in a 'common setting' performing their jobs in accordance with their own professional range of practice.

Consultative – 'expert' advice given to one professional by another.

Collaborative – professionals who normally practice in parallel, share information about a common patient.

Coordinated – a formally gathered team of professionals with a common purpose who have an agreed structure for communication and information sharing. A care coordinator has information-sharing responsibilities.

Multidisciplinary – teams (may be virtual) managed by a non-physician. The team member integrates the decisions and recommendations made by the individual members of the team.

Interdisciplinary – professionals practice consensus decision-making and have regular 'face-to-face meetings'.

Integrative – team with non-hierarchical members who practice person-centred care, with consensus decision-making, mutual respect, shared vision, joint care plan.

students, researchers, educationalists and practitioners alike (Cowen, 2001).

Boon *et al.* (2004) describe seven models of 'team-oriented health care practice' on a continuum from parallel working through to integrative working. Integrative learning disability teams constitute health and social care professionals and support workers who help adults with a learning disability. These are formally gathered professionals who work in a structured way and have formal arrangements for sharing information (see 'A closer look/Boon *et al.*'s conceptual framework' above). People with learning disabilities or their families initiate first contact. This is typically to a social worker or community nurse, usually at the point where support over and above that of family or friends is required. Social workers and community learning disability nurses are predominantly 'care managers' and work with individuals and their families to identify required assistance. The care manager is responsible for locating and ascertaining appropriate services for individuals and their families and aid with the coordination of those services. Integrative services in their truest form should only be provided in proportion to individual need (Leutz, 1999, 2005). Therefore the more complex the service user's health and social care needs, the more likely they will require services which are fully integrated. This will include strategic partnership boards made up of service users, stakeholders and professionals, and they will meet regularly; co-located professionals using interdisciplinary assessment, a single service-user care plan, practicing with joint governance and joint outcome arrangements. Therefore they are integrated at practice level, professional and organisational levels using mechanisms or tools which enable them to achieve full integration, that is a single point of access and shared information systems.

Rhetoric to reality: a service-user journey

Empowerment, which stems from *Valuing People* (Department of Health, 2001), is often associated with person-centred approaches when working with

Key learning points

- To gain some clarity and move on from the current 'concept confusion' we need to practise some consistency in the words we use to define how we work together, such as collaboration, coordination and partnership.
- Boon *et al.* (2004) offers a useful conceptual framework by which we can describe our engagement with one another in practice; however, further work applying it in the work context would be useful to give practitioners some detail on how this works and the skills you need to deliver it in practice.
- Understanding service-user need and their complexity is key to identifying how professionals should engage with each other in the workplace. This may mean that you prastise in different ways for the different people you have on your caseload. Those with one to three comorbidities may require coordination whereas those with more will require you to practise interdisciplinary or integrative working.

people with learning disabilities. Person-centred planning is the process of constant evaluation, listening and learning. Learning disability partnership boards were introduced following the publication of *Valuing People* to oversee and inform service commissioning and delivery.

Person-centred planning is essential to the reviewing process of service provision and delivery focuses on the immediate and futuristic needs of the individual. An individual should be fully included in the process and consulted with on their concerns and opinion. Those in the 'personal network' of an individual will also be included in this process.

What exactly does person-centred planning mean?

In theory, services should be flexible and tailored to the needs of the individual, rather than a homogenous approach of one size fits all. Drawing upon ecological theories 'micro' social work services should be person-centred to address specific needs, for example encouraging choice through direct payments (Northfield, 2004b). The community living experience is fundamental to how people with learning disabilities are valued as people first and core to

them having equal human experience. Interagency collaboration as a minimum is conducive to the actualisation of person-centred planning and its success, thus ensuring that professionals who usually work in parallel are brought together to share information (see 'A closer look/Boon *et al.*'s conceptual framework' on p. 108).

Exercise 8.4

Consider the integrative element of Boon *et al.*'s (2004) model set out previously in this chapter in relation to Phillip's experience.

- What is important here to Phillip and his network?
- How do you ensure Phillip is included in the process?

Comment

For Phillip, the experience of authentic social inclusion is about experiencing equality in expectations of his health, education, employment opportunities, housing, and financial security. He has every right to exert choice along with the right to enjoy positive social relations and roles within his family and community. Phillip is an equal citizen with the right to participate fully in the decision-making processes that concern him. Thus opportunities should be available to Phillip when planning for his family and community living.

It is important to emphasise consideration here to service principles (O'Brien, 1987) which are key for Phillip while designing his care package to ensure that the package is tailored for his individual needs. Applying the following principles will attempt to ensure Phillip's right to live a community life.

Exercise 8.5

Using key service principles (O'Brien, 1987), consider your role in working with people with a learning disability.

Community presence. How would you promote this in your role?

Community participation. How would you encourage Phillip to build relationships within his community?

Encouraging valued social roles. How can we enhance the reputation people have and increase the number of valued ways people can contribute?

Promoting choice. How can we help people have more control and choice in life?

Supporting contribution. How can we assist people to develop more competencies?

It is important that people with learning disabilities are valued as people first. Phillip is entitled to have his preferences and needs heard as part of the assessment process if we are to value him as an individual. Occupational groups such as professionals are dynamic organisational subcultures and strive to achieve a core culture for themselves in which they have control over their unique body of knowledge, education, their work and their evaluation (Trice, 1993). Communication of this knowledge is essential when working toward meeting service-user need. Essentially working together in a coordinated, multidisciplinary, interdisciplinary or integrative fashion (Boon *et al.*, 2004, see 'A closer look/Boon *et al.*'s conceptual framework' on p. 108) requires 'skill, knowledge, values and motives' (Wallace and Davies, 2009). The right environmental ingredients within which any form of working together can be nurtured or professionals are likely to clash with those they interface for fear of deskilling or diluting their uniqueness are required, e.g. joint assessment (Trice, 1993; Wallace, 2009).

Interprofessional agendas and service-user impact

With regard to the aforementioned 'willingness condition' (Sellman, 2010) the Community Learning Disability Team will have the shared knowledge and expertise; however, in reality this is not without dilemmas and barriers to practice. For teamworking with Phillip there is close proximity of working roles as the teams are housed in the same building. However, getting together for meetings concerning Phillip are difficult due to time constraints and conflicting diaries. Staff feel they have less time to spend with people such as Phillip and his family, despite more professionals being involved. It could be argued that they are working in parallel with one another, aware that each professional is there but failing to engage formally at regular times during the week to ensure that they communicate information. As a result communication may happen only with crisis intervention instead of regularly to inform planning and support preventative work. The sharing of expertise is invaluable, but there is sometimes a dilemma over role confusion. The more professionals communicate with one another and share knowledge about their roles – what they do, who they network with on a daily basis, – the more likely it is that this role confusion will gradually disintegrate.

Real inclusion for Phillip would include an exchange of communication at all levels. An understanding of the exchange model (Smale *et al.*, 1993) would assist the social worker in the scenario to work with Phillip when trying to ascertain her needs as a service user or carer. It is likely that standardised tools and assessment documentation will be used by the social worker to ascertain if Phillip is eligible for services. Hence, for the purpose here, Phillip's needs would be assessed in relation to what he could not do (deficit) in order to provide interventions that would support him (Gurney, 2004). Systems influencing professionals such as the social worker may be deemed limiting in relation to the volume and depth of paperwork that requires completion (Coulshed and Orme, 2006). The social worker and learning disability nurse are essential with regard to holism and person-centred approaches. The CALDT will share expertise with regard to meeting the holistic needs of the service user. Hence, the learning disability nurse will have expertise on health and medication issues, while still adopting a social model approach and supporting the service user in their environment. It will be the role of the social worker to primarily assess and evidence the social support needs, such as housing issues for Phillip, as part of the assessment process.

Person-centred planning is a core product of social inclusion principles as informed by the social model of disability. It is vital to service-user need and interprofessional practice that assessment process have grown away from medical model-based approaches. For Phillip and service users in a more general sense person-centred approaches should maintain their focus on the locus of service-user control within assessment and planning (Wallace and Davies, 2009). Cambridge (2008) argues that there is not always a transparent relationship between the care management and person-centred processes.

Care management, person-centred planning (PCP) and direct payments have developed through separate policy strands, with tasks and agency responsibilities blurred. A wide diversity of care management arrangements currently operate, with the relationship between care management, PCP and direct payments imprecisely defined.

(Cambridge, 2008, p. 91)

Adopting exchange model approaches in essence operates to avoid power imbalances between service users and professionals (Duffy and Sanderson, 2005). This is not without conflict of responsibilities, roles and accountability issues, however (Cambridge, 2008). However, let's consider the introduction of direct payments, which was primarily to allow personal choice and purchase power by service users (Department of Health, 2001, 2004a). This, moved away from the influence of the medical model (Oliver, 1990) in defining a person by their impairment, instead valuing them as autonomous citizens. Nonetheless, despite this shift it has been argued that service delivery is now more competency-based (Concannon, 2006), which challenges the shift towards inclusive practice to that of service-user competence versus deficit. Hence for Phillip if eligibility criteria is required for service provision, whether it is support for accommodation or eligibility for direct payments, a questioning model (Smale *et al.*, 1993) could be more in line with the medical model appreciation of disability and has

the potential to disempower Phillip because the expertise and power would lie with the professionals. Beadle-Brown (2002) identified obstacles such as insufficient guidance and limited guidance to support the process as having impeded the successful implementation of direct payments.

This brings us back to the question of exactly how person-centred and autonomous services really are for the service user with a learning disability?

Informing practice: professional role conflict and service provision

Issues surrounding health and social care are more complex today than they have been in the past, and collaborative working is proposed as the new solution offering a multidimensional approach, however concerns remain about the future of integrated working. It is not possible, for example, to anticipate how interprofessional relationships will continue to develop over time.

(Concannon, 2006, p. 202)

The discussion paper 'Inclusion or control? Commissioning and contracting services for people with learning disabilities' (Concannon, 2006) stimulates debate on the cultural shift which has introduced the commissioning and contracting of social care services for people with learning disabilities. The development of the community learning disability team and its multidisciplinary function (Department of Health, 1998) was intended to eradicate multiple points of service entry for people with learning disabilities and provide a one-stop shop approach with direct access to services. Social workers and health professionals were given the opportunity to integrate their expertise and services. Nonetheless, truly joint partnership working requires strong leadership and guidance. Joint funding and the ability to share ownership caused initial objections. However, we now see joint legal contracts, working agreements and the commissioning of services. Concannon raises the issue of how well-supported people with learning disabilities are in exerting their influence in this process, highlighting the lack of substantive evidence to support this. Learning disability partnership boards and direct payments were seen to be essential to the full inclusion of people with learning disabilities.

Exercise 8.6

Person-centredness and Phillip

How significant is the need for Phillip to live independently?

For a comprehensive inclusive assessment experience it is important that as professionals Phillip's understanding of his situation is established fully and then fully explored. What does this mean to him? Does Phillip want to live away from his mother or does he just require more self-autonomy?

His mother thinks his dependency needs are so high that it is safer for him to live at home. How will you weigh this up?

Consider support needs for Phillip in order to encourage his independence and have the opportunity to his right to inform decision making. This may also have implications for the carer's needs. Joy will be entitled to a carers assessment should she wish for this or if the need becomes apparent.

Integrative education equals integrative practice: a micro experience of learning together to work together

Practice is inspired and informed by professional education. Interprofessional education (IPE) is defined as occurring 'when two or more professions learn with, from and about each other to improve collaboration and the quality of care' (CAIPE, 2002). Its purpose is to promote collaboration in practice to meet both service-user needs and those of an evolving workforce which has to be increasingly flexible, responsive and have the ability to plan across health, local authority, voluntary and independent sectors. It engenders mutual trust and support, limits demands on any one profession, reduces stress and improves service-user care. It is a recognised problem-solving strategy which enables the formation of 'working together' values and culture through enhancing knowledge and communication between professionals and agencies within the whole system (Freeth *et al.*, 2002). The components of IPE are identified by Barr (2000, p. 23) as

> The application of principles of adult learning to interactive group-based learning, which relates collaborative learning to collaborative practice within a coherent rationale which is informed by understanding of interpersonal, group, organizational and inter-organizational relations and processes of professionalisation.

This is in contrast to 'shared learning' and 'multiprofessional education' where 'two or more professions learn side by side in parallel' without facilitated interaction with one another. This offers limited formal contact between students and is most often used for the purpose of economies of scale (Carpenter and Dickinson, 2008).

The Welsh Assembly Government has required (through unified assessment) health and social care to work in partnership to ensure that assessment is holistic, person-centred, proportional to needs and outcome-focused, avoids the risk to independence, well coordinated and so avoiding duplication (Welsh Assembly Government, 2002). As this standardised assessment process prescribes a layered approach, staff are required to be competent in assessment and have the ability to think about how risks may impact upon a person's independent living. This demands teamwork which is multidisciplinary and multi-agency in nature, and is consistent with the demands of current Welsh and UK policy and culture, i.e. that professionals and organisations working with people who have complex needs should not work autonomously but with shared awareness and understanding that leads to better communication and enhanced patient/service-user care (Department of Health, 2004b; Martin and Rogers, 2004; Wallace and Davies, 2009; Welsh Assembly Government, 2003).

Using an interprofessional approach to learning in this context gives credence to learning as a social process which is determined by social interaction (Bandura, 1977; Vygotsky, 1962). This ensures that any learning programme developed enhances collaborative working at a minimum through learning about each other's roles and professions within the new process.

Considering the nature and requirements within the guidance, the authors applied Hunsberger *et al.*'s (2000) integrative/partnership teaching model to the context requirements of unified assessment (Welsh Assembly Government, 2002). It required using two lead lecturers from both health and social care backgrounds (a nurse and a social worker) and local managers from the local health board, local health trust and social services. Additional lecturers were included for their given expertise within specifically requested areas of learning. The level of working together required for practice was reflected and reinforced within the model of teaching and learning used within the local setting. The local flavour adopted promoted relationship-building at both organisational and professional levels through its programme development and delivery.

Exercise 8.7

How are you working with others? How are you sharing information with other professionals involved? Consider how you work and reflect on the case of Phillip. Is Phillip central to this process? Is Phillip being consulted? If he is to feel valued in the community and to live an independent life, consider the skills and coping strategies required to achieve this successfully.

In summary, from our experience it is invaluable for professionals to have joint learning experiences.

- *Learning as a social process*
  - social interaction is important to meeting key objectives
  - this approach gives insight into problem solving from health and social care perspectives
  - it enables reflection on current practice
- *Team approach*
  - two lead lecturers from health and social care
  - local managers from health and social care
  - expert lecturers reflected the specialist or indepth assessments identified from practice, e.g. mental health
- *Shared mental models of the new process*
  - role play to re-enact a real-life assessment scenario enabled participants to collectively identify and problem solve the real issues
  - coordinated social interaction – absorbing other perspectives
  - need for respect and valuing interagency/multi-professional contributions
  - a chance to model the new documentation (Krebs, 2000).

This resulted in enhanced understanding of roles and individual perspectives within their professional networks, all of which promoted their ability to work together.

Key learning points

- Learning together enhances the ability to work together.
- Shared knowledge between professional groups can break down barriers and prevent role confusion.
- Planning how we communicate formally with our colleagues on a regular basis is an essential part of working together successfully.

Conclusion

This chapter has explored some of the concepts underpinning services for people with learning disabilities. Interprofessional rhetoric and reality has been acknowledged when identifying the dilemmas of delivering seamless person-centred care across professionals and in true partnership with service users.

A model of working, alongside the understanding of needs of people as individuals, has expectantly given some insight into the importance of interprofessional practice. Furthermore, the application of theoretical underpinnings of service delivery for people with learning disabilities has been explored to enable an understanding of service function.

In order to work together **it is vital that concepts are clarified and opportunities are created to communicate and learn together.** We have provided a succinct insightful example of where shared opportunities can work and ultimately enhance professional practice and the service-user experience.

Further reading

Braithwaite, J., Westbrook, J. I., Foxwell, R. A., Boyce, R., Devinney, T., Budge, M., Murphy, K., Ryall, A., Beutal, J., Vanderheide, R., Renton, E., Travaglia, J., Stone, J., Barnard, A., Greenfield, D., Corbett, A., Nugus, P. and Clay-Williams, R. (2007) An action research protocol to strengthen system-wide interprofessional learning and practice. *BMC Health Service Research* 7 (144), [online] available from **http://www.biomedcentral.com/1472-6963/7/144,** accessed 16 February 2010.

Concannon, L. (2006) Inclusion or control? Commissioning and contracting services for people with learning disabilities. *British Journal of Learning Disabilities* 34 (4), 200–205.

Department of Health (2001) *Valuing People: A New Strategy for Learning Disability for the 21st Century*, London: Department of Health.

Useful websites

http://www.circlesnetwork.org.uk/what_is_person_centred_planning.htm
http://thechp.syr.edu/PCP_History.pdf
Person-centred planning
http://www.learningdisabilities.org.uk
Foundation for People with Learning Disabilites

References

Attwood, M., Pedler, M., Pritchard, S. and Wilkinson, D. (2003) *Leading change. A Guide to Whole Systems Working,* Bristol: The Policy Press.

Bandura, A. (1977) *Social Learning Theory*, New Jersey: Prentice Hall.

Barr, H. (2000) Working together to learn together: learning together to work together, *Journal of Interprofessional Care* 14, 177–179.

Barr, O. and Gates, B. (2008) Education for the future: the changing nature of education for staff in learning disability services, *Learning Disability Review* 13 (1), 18–27.

Beadle-Brown, J. (2002) Direct payments for people with severe learning disabilities: a service case study and implications for policy, *Tizard Learning Disability Review* 7, 8–15.

Boon, H., Verhoef, M., O'Hara, D. and Findlay, B. (2004) From parallel practice to integrative health care a conceptual framework, *BMC Health Service Research*, available from http://www.biomedcentral.com/1472-6963/4/15, accessed 24 October 2009.

Braithwaite, J., Westbrook, J. I., Foxwell, R. A., Boyce, R., Devinney, T., Budge, M., Murphy, K., Ryall, A., Beutal, J., Vanderheide, R., Renton, E., Travaglia, J., Stone, J., Barnard, A., Greenfield, D., Corbett, A., Nugus, P., Clay-Williams, R. (2007) An action research protocol to strengthen system-wide interprofessional learning and practice, *BMC Health Service Research* 7; 144 [online] available from http://www.biomedcentral.com/1472-6963/7/144, accessed on 16 February 2010.

CAIPE (Centre for the Advancement of Interprofessional Education) (2002) *Interprofessional Education: The Definition*, available from http://www.caipe.org.uk/about-us/defining-ipe/?keywords=definition, accessed 1 October 2009.

Cambridge, P. (2008) The Case for New 'Case' Management in Services for People with Learning Disabilities, *British Journal of Social Work* 38, 91–116.

Carpenter J. and Dickinson H. (2008) *Interprofessional Education and Training*. Better Partnership Working Series, Bristol: The Policy Press.

Cole, A., Williams, V., Lloyd, A., Major, V., Mattingly, M., McIntosh, B., Swift, P. and Townsley, R. (2007) *SCIE Knowledge Review 14: Having a Good Day? A Study of Community-based Day Activities for People with Learning Disabilities*, London: SCIE.

Concannon, L. (2006) Inclusion or control? Commissioning and contracting services for people with learning disabilities, *British Journal of Learning Disabilities* 34 (4), 200–205.

Coulshed, V. and Orme, J. (2006) *Social Work Practice*, 4th edn., Basingstoke: Palgrave.

Cowen, E. (2001) Ethics in community mental health care: the use and misuse of some positively valenced community concepts, *Community Mental Health Journal* 3, 3–13.

Delnoij, D., Klazinga, N. and Glasgow, I. K. (2002) Integrated care in an international perspective, *International Journal of Integrated Care* 2, 1 April, available from http://www.ijic.org/, accessed 18 July 2009.

De Long, D. and Seeman, P. (2000) Confronting conceptual confusion and conflict in knowledge management, *Organizational Dynamics* 29 (1), 33–44.

Demers, L. and Lavoie, J. (2008) Integrating services for frail elderly people: the role of local, regional and departmental actors, in R. Hebert, A. Tourigny and M. Raiche (eds) *Integration of Services for Disabled People: Research Leading to Action*, Quebec: Edisem.

Department for Communities and Local Government (2007) *Independence and Opportunity Our Strategy for Supporting People*, available from http://www.spkweb.org.uk/NR/rdonlyres/4E92E1E2-B5EF-42B4-AD0C-FE5B68C4330B/12855/bm07024supportingpeoplestrategy.pdf, accessed 1 February 2010.

Department of Health (1998) *Signposts for Success in Commissioning and Providing Health Services for People with Learning Disabilities*, London: Department of Health.

Department of Health (2001) *Valuing People: A New Strategy for Learning Disability for the 21st Century*, London: Department of Health.

Department of Health (2002) *Guidance on the Single Assessment Process for Older People*, HSC 2002/001, available from http://www.dh.gov.uk/en/PublicationsAndStatistics/LettersAndCirculars/HealthServiceCirculars/DH_4003995, accessed 21 November 2009.

Department of Health (2004a) *Direct Choices: What Councils Need to Make Direct Payments Happen for People with Learning Disabilities*, London: Department of Health.

Department of Health (2004b) *Securing Good Health for the Whole Population: Final Report*, by Derek Wanless and H. M. Treasury. Crown Copyright.

Department of Health (2009a) *Integrated Care*, available from http://www.dh.gov.uk/en/Healthcare/Integrated-Care/DH_290, accessed 21 July 2009.

Department of Health (2009b) *Common Assessment Framework for Adults: Consultation on Proposals to Improve Information Sharing Around Multi-disciplinary Assessment and Care Planning*, available from http://www.dh.gov.uk/prod_consum_dh/groups/dh_digitalassets/documents/digitalasset/dh_093715.pdf, accessed 25 August 2009.

Dickinson, H. (2008) *Evaluating Outcomes in Health and Social Care*, Bristol: The Policy Press.

Duffy, S. and Sanderson, H. (2005) Relationships between care management and person-centred planning, in P. Cambridge and S. Carnaby (eds) *Person-centred*

Planning and Care Management for People with Learning Disabilities, London: Jessica Kingsley Publishers.

Flynn, N. (2007) *Public Sector Management*, 5th edn, London: Sage Publications.

Freeth, D., Hammick, M., Koppel, I., Reeves, S. and Barr, H. (2002) A critical review of evaluations of Interprofessional education. Occasional Paper No. 2, London: The Interprofessional Education Joint Evaluation Team, Learning and Teaching Support Network Health Sciences and Practice.

Fritchie, R. (2002) *The New Health Strategy – Organisation Development and the Leadership Challenge*, available from www.tohm.ie/download/rtf/evpaper_fritchie.rtf, accessed 26 September 2009.

Gates, B. (2003) *Towards Inclusion: Learning Disabilities*, Edinburgh: Churchill Livingstone.

Glasby, J. (2004) Social services and the single assessment process: early warning signs? *Journal of Interprofessional Care* 18 (2), 129–39.

Gurney, A. (2004) Models of Assessment. Open Learning Partnership, University of Central England and RNIB.

Hammick, M., Freeth, D., Copperman, J. and Goodsman, D. (2009) *Being Interprofessional*, Cambridge: Polity Press.

Hofstede, G. (1991) *Cultures and Organisations: Software of the Mind*, Maidenhead: McGraw-Hill.

Hunsberger, M., Bauman, A., Lappan, J., Carter, N., Bowman, A. and Goddard, P. (2000) The synergism of expertise in clinical teaching: an integrative model for nursing education, *Journal of Nursing Education* 39 (6), 278–82.

Krebs, D. (2000) On levels of analysis and theoretical integration: models of social behavior, *Behavioral and Brain Sciences* 23 (2), 260–61.

Leutz, W. N. (1999) Five laws for integrating medical and social services: lessons from the United States and the United Kingdom, *The Millbank Quarterly* 77 (1), 77–110.

Leutz, W. (2005) Reflections on integrating medical and social care: five laws revisited, *Journal of Integrated Care* 13 (5), 3–12.

Lloyd, J. and Wait, S. (2005) *Integrated Care: A Guide for Policy Makers*, available from http://ns1.siteground169.com/~healthan/healthandfuture/images/stories/Documents/integrated%20care%20-%20a%20guide%20for%20policy%20makers.pdf, accessed 2 May 2008.

Lymbery, M. (2005) *Social Work with Older People: Context, Policy and Practice*, London: Sage.

Martin and Rogers (2004) *Leading Interprofessional Teams in Health and Social Care*, Abingdon: Routledge.

Northfield, J. (2004a). *Factsheet – What Is a Learning Disability?* Kidderminster: British Institute of Learning Disabilities, http://www.bild.org.uk/.

Northfield, J. (2004b). *Factsheet – Direct Payments*, Kidderminster: British Institute of Learning Disabilities, http://www.bild.org.uk/.

O'Brien, J. (1987) A guide to personal futures planning, in G. Bellamy and B. Willcox (eds) *A Comprehensive Guide to the Activities Catalogue: An Alternative Curriculum for Youth and Adults with Severe Disabilities*, Baltimore, MD: Paul H. Brooks.

Oliver, M. (1990) *The Politics of Disablement*, Basingstoke: Macmillan.

Ridout, A. and Mayers, C. (2006) Evaluation of the implementation of the single assessment process and its impact on occupational therapy practice, *British Journal of Occupational Therapy* 69 (6), 271–80.

Scottish Executive (2001) *Guidance on Single Shared Assessment of Community Care Needs*, CCD 8/2001, Edinburgh: Health Department, available from http://www.sehd.scot.nhs.uk/publications/DC20011129C-CD8single.pdf, accessed on 20 November 2009.

Seddon, J. (2008) *Systems Thinking in the Public Sector. The Failure of the Reform Regime . . . and a Manifesto for a Better Way*, Axminster: Triarchy Press.

Sellman, D. (2010) Values and ethics in interprofessional working, in K. C. Pollard, J. Thomas and M. Miers (eds) *Understanding Interprofessional Working in Health and Social Care. Theory and Practice*, Basingstoke: Palgrave Macmillan.

Smale, G., Tuson, G., Biehal, N. and Marsh, P. (1993) *Empowering Users to Make Choices: Assessment Care Management and the Skilled Worker*, London: HMSO.

Swift, P. and Mattingly, M. (2009) *A Life in the Community: An Action Research Project Promoting Citizenship for People with High Support Needs*, London: Foundation for People with Learning Disabilities, available from http://www.learningdisabilities.org.uk/publications/?esctl544701_entryid5=32795&q=0%c2%accommunity%c2%ac.

Trice, H. M. (1993) *Occupational Subcultures in the Workplace*, New York: Cornell University.

Vygotsky (1962) *Thought and Language*, Cambridge, MA: MIT Press.

Wallace, C. (2009) An exploration of health and social service integration in a deprived South Wales area. Ph.D. Thesis. University of Coventry in collaboration with University of Worcester.

Wallace, C. and Davies, M. (2009) *Sharing Assessment in Health and Social Care: A Practical Handbook for Interprofessional Working*, London: Sage Publications.

Weinstein, J., Whittington, C. and Leiba, T. (2003) *Collaboration in Social Work Practice*, London: Jessica Kingsley Publishers.

Welsh Assembly Government (2002) *Creating a Unified and Fair System for Assessing and Managing Care; Guidance for Local Authorities and Health Services*, available from http://wales.gov.uk/docrepos/40382/4038212/403821/403821/4038211/4038213/unified_assessing_care.pdf?lang=en, accessed 17 April 2008.

Welsh Assembly Government (2003) The Review of Health and Social Care in Wales. The report of the project team advised by Derek Wanless. Cardiff. Welsh Assembly Government. [online] http://wales.gov.uk/dhss/publications/health/reports/wanlessreview/wanlessreviewe.pdf;jsessionid=tspmPvCR6fCfv2QQ2NSd3WqPR12lZS7ZLQBZKhPnhd2jqX9jPys4!-351825548?lang=en, accessed 26 January 2012.

Wilson, R. and Baines, S. (2009) Are there limits to the integration of care for older people? in B. D. Loader, M. Hardey, and L. Keeble (eds) *Digital Welfare for the Third Age. Health and Social Care Informatics for Older People*, Abingdon: Routledge.

Wilson, R., Baines, S., Cornford, J. and Martin, M. (2007) 'Trying to do a jigsaw without the picture on the box': understanding the challenges of care integration in the context of single assessment for older people in England, *International Journal of Integrated Care* 7, 25 June, available from http://www.ijic.org/, accessed 20 August 2009.

Worthington, A. and Rooney, R. (2010) *The Triangle of Care. Carers Included: A Guide to the Best Practice in Acute Mental Health Care*, available from http://www.ltscmentalhealth.org.uk/home//triangle-of-care-carers-included.pdf, accessed 5 December 2010.

Chapter 9
Safeguarding children and child protection

Mary McColgan, Anne Campbell and James Marshall

Chapter summary

This chapter addresses a number of professional issues related to interdisciplinary working in child protection. At the outset, the reader is introduced to a case study which outlines some of the dilemmas and the tensions experienced by a range of professionals involved in the complex arena of child protection. Specific focus is given to exploring the factors which facilitate effective practice in interdisciplinary working and defining models of good practice.

Drawing on national perspectives, the chapter discusses contemporary structures and practices in one jurisdiction, Northern Ireland, and considers how procedures and processes to safeguard children are framed and at times constricted by interagency structures.

Key findings from research and child protection inquiries, relevant to interprofessional working and to the whole of the UK, are addressed and then applied to the Northern Ireland and UK situation case study.

Learning objectives

This chapter will cover:

- the different child protection professional identities and roles in child protection work
- the fundamental similarities and differences in the skills, theory and value constituents across the agencies and identities of professional workers in health, social care, legal and educational settings in child protection work
- how the range of professional values and different models such as social and medical models which underpin the separate professions involved in child protection work can influence interprofessional working
- how different professional backgrounds and expectations of each others' professional roles can affect the key area of effective communication between professionals and agencies in child protection work
- how care versus control debates as key elements of child protection vary between the professions and agencies involved and affect interprofessional working
- the nature and effects of leadership and status perception of different professionals in the multidisciplinary setting of child protection work.

Definitions of multidisciplinary work in child protection

Since the late 1980s, literature, research and expert opinion have focused on a range of negative and positive determining factors impacting on inter-agency and multidisciplinary work in child protection. However, before considering the issues inherent to multidisciplinary work in this sector, it is useful to consider the various definitions of collaborative working as operationalised within and between specifically linked agencies involved in the child protection process. The terms 'interdisciplinary' and 'multidisciplinary' working appear to be used interchangeably in the literature. Wilson and Pirrie (2000) suggest that the key issues about definition relate to epistemology, professional boundaries and number of staff who work together. They argue that personal commitment, shared purpose and role clarity are the defining features. McGrath (1991) defines interprofessional working as collegiate practice based on confidence in the expertise of other professionals.

Issues in the multidisciplinary child protection environment: professional identities and roles

Social workers, educationalists, legal and health care professionals are trained using specific knowledge constructs, distinct professional values and principles and relevant skills. While it is obvious that there may be an overlap in the three core elements for all health and social care professionals, it is also clear that there are a number of fundamental differences in the skills, theory and value constituents. For example, as noted in Chapter 14 of this volume, there are differences in opinion which arise from application of the social and medical models in health and social care settings. The former often provides a more precise rationale for some of the problems which may present in the protection of children and young people, whereas the social model is frequently more complex and offers a multilayered view of the issues and possible resolution within a collaborative environment.

Concomitantly, the identities of professional workers in health, social care, legal and educational settings are influenced by a range of professional values, which underpin the separate professions. Both the incongruencies and similarities in values shared by the workers from different perspectives may act either as a conciliatory force or as a divisive catalyst within the multidisciplinary setting. For example, social workers practice under the auspices of person-centred and community empowerment values and strive to employ a partnership approach with children and families. Indeed they are trained to be fully aware of the ethical conflicts that may ensue as a result of the clashes between their statutory role and supportive function within the child protection process. However, ethical dilemmas engendered by the care/control debates in child protection social work may not be viewed as having the same level of importance by workers who have a judicial role or a primarily medical affiliation.

Differences in professional opinion and viewpoints are outlined in research on core groups in child protection, undertaken by Harlow and Shardlow (2006). Findings revealed that social workers perceived other professionals to be uncertain about referral thresholds: they may refer inappropriate cases unnecessarily, concerned about trivial matters, and would therefore make minor referrals which did not require further action. On the other hand, Hudson (2002) purports that distinct professional identities and differences in opinion are crucial to workers and that any attempt to blur the professional boundaries

Exercise 9.1

What might each professional need to take into account from their understanding of other's roles and goals in working with the families and children in interprofessional working?

How can they ensure they get to know, appreciate and take account of other professional cultures in child protection work?

may increase non-collaboration and engender defensiveness in the team. Alternatively, it is more beneficial to reduce the feeling of 'otherness' while utilising the diverse opinions and differential knowledge bases to enhance team working.

Professional roles

Inextricably linked to the concept of professional identity are the professional roles of the team members, their perceptions of these roles and how they evolve and develop within the collaborative setting. In an examination of roles within a multidisciplinary family support environment, Harlow and Shardlow (2006) underlined the importance of an increased understanding of professional roles in the multi-agency team. Findings also indicated a heightened awareness and reciprocal understanding of the roles of the different professionals involved in the team, specifically in relation to education and social work professionals. This was perceived to have been achieved via the dismantling of communication barriers and an understanding of 'others' expectations

Key learning points

Core issues for successful outcomes in multidisciplinary child protection work

A number of authors and researchers have identified a cluster of core issues which can lead to successful outcomes in multidisciplinary child protection work:

- professional identity
- co-location
- professional value base
- leadership
- team building
- agency policies
- agency processes.

These include professional identity and roles, co-location, similarities and differences in professional value bases, leadership, team building and agency policies and processes (Darlington *et al.*; 2005; Devaney, 2008; Frost and Robinson, 2007; Glennie, 2007; Harlow and Shardlow, 2006; Malin and Morrow, 2007; Packard *et al.*, 2006; Skinner and Bell, 2007).

and team members' professional roles and remit in working with children. Social workers also felt that multi-agency working engendered a reduction in partner agencies' negative perceptions of their role and service that they provided. They perceived this as helpful in making earlier referrals and providing a less stigmatising experience for families. Ultimately, this was viewed as having a positive impact on the attainment of more effective outcomes for children, young people and families (Harlow and Shardlow 2006).

Perception of status differentials

Issues of status perception were also highlighted in research which considered the position of professionals in the multidisciplinary setting in child protection work (Frost and Robinson, 2007). Social workers perceived health care professionals to have an elevated perception of their status and as roles were redefined, boundaries of expertise were questioned. Social workers were particularly disconcerted by the perception of differential role status as expressed by the 'tall hat' metaphor in the following comment: 'a lot of people with tall hats are overawed by their own status' (Frost and Robinson, 2007, p. 195).

This view is also corroborated by Geva *et al.* (2000), who underlined that power and status differentials among team members precipitated negative outcomes for service users, students and colleagues within the team. They highlighted that self-reflection and feedback from colleagues may assist professionals' awareness of each other and of how they present to clients and students in the work setting. Similarly, Frost and Robinson (2007) emphasised that the negative perceptions of role status may be offset by the positive elements of multidisciplinary working. The research participants in the study agreed that the collaborative approach served to consolidate a sense of professional identity, one which could be moulded and enhanced by expanding the team's knowledge of clients' needs and the needs of other agencies (Frost and Robinson, 2007). There was also an emphasis on the creative energy of the team environment as it embraced and forged the individual characteristics within the multi-agency teams. Any challenges presented could be addressed when the team culture supported and nurtured professional expertise, irrespective of profession role or perceived status (Frost and Robinson, 2007).

Leadership in multi-agency working

Leadership has been outlined as a crucial element of effective interagency working by a number of authors (Frost and Robinson, 2007; Mizrahi and Abramson, 2000), particularly in working with some of the role and value differences often experienced within the multidisciplinary environment. Frost and Robinson (2007) highlight leadership as key to successful outcomes in collaborative working. In Frost and Robinson's (2007) research on safeguarding children in multidisciplinary teams, they cited examples of effective managers who were able to work across organisational divides to promote the best interests of children. They also stated that managers must be able to address operational and identity issues in a skilful and sensitive manner.

Findings from a study by Mizrahi and Abramson (2000) indicated that perception of leadership in case collaboration between doctors and social workers was significantly different between both groups. Of the 100 participants in the study (50 from each profession), 68 per cent of social workers identified themselves as case *co-coordinators*, while only 12 per cent of doctors reported that they perceived the social worker as the case coordinator. Conversely, 55 per cent of the doctors perceived themselves as case coordinators, whilst only 3 per cent of the social workers agreed with this perception of the leadership role. The remaining 32 per cent of doctors and 23 per cent of social workers saw this as a collaborative leadership role.

Co-location

Alongside the sharing of information, skills, values, knowledge and opinions, multidisciplinary teams often share physical space and office space. There is evidence to suggest that co-location is beneficial to multidisciplinary teamworking because it facilitates the immediate sharing and analysis of informal and formal communications (Moran *et al.*, 2007). One of the major themes from research undertaken by Frost and Robinson (2007) focused on the impact of co-location and the consequences for information-sharing and confidentiality issues. A number of participants in the project highlighted major concerns around restricted access to health databases, differing opinions on the design of record keeping and varied perceptions of systems for recording case closures. Constructively, the problem was addressed within the office, via collaboration on new guidelines for recording and exchanging information relevant to case closures.

Barriers to effective multidisciplinary working

The literature on multidisciplinary working and child protection is notable because of the range of identified barriers which permeate the discussion. These are perceived as having a key role in hampering the implementation of sound multidisciplinary working. Among the many barriers to effective collaborative working, inadequate training, unrealistic expectations, poor communication and inadequate resources are reiterated throughout the literature (Darlington *et al.*, 2005; Devaney, 2008; Frost and Robinson, 2007; Glennie, 2007; Harlow and Shardlow, 2006; Malin and Morrow, 2007; Packard *et al.*, 2006; Skinner and Bell 2007).

Exercise 9.2

How can each professional involved in child protection work ensure that their role is understood by the others in the professional network so that assumptions about these do not negatively affect the well-being and protection of the child(ren) involved?

How can they ensure that they understand how others see their role in the assessment/intervention and review of the work to ensure the same thing?

Training

Effective multidisciplinary working is greatly undermined by a lack of tailored and targeted training, specifically the absence of high-quality training which defines the remit of collaborative practice and translates ideological representations of collaboration into practice in a pragmatic fashion. Darlington *et al.* (2005) analysed some of the factors which either enhance or hinder multidisciplinary practice between child-protection services and mental health services. An analysis of workers' perceptions of barriers to collaboration indicated that inadequate training was perceived as a major obstacle to effective joint working. The authors concluded that joint training should focus on the attainment of flexible boundaries, dispel interagency myths and challenge negative perceptions of others within multidisciplinary working.

There is also evidence to suggest a continuum of training which aims to develop an awareness and application of multidisciplinary working within child protection; this ranges from the informal 'how we might work together' initiatives to more structured and formalised training programmes. During the 1990s, there was a move towards more established and formal interagency training (Department of Health, 1991) and a drive towards established standards for interagency practice (Charles and Glennie, 2003; Shardlow *et al.*, 2004). It was anticipated that formal training in multidisciplinary working would encourage the formulation of shared understandings and communication between professionals, enhance sound decision-making based on information sharing and encourage increased understanding of the tasks, roles and responsibilities in shared practice (Department for Education and Skills, 2006).

Communication

As outlined above, a primary aim of multidisciplinary training is to work towards effective and consistent communication with and between agencies and agency workers. However, it is not always possible to communicate on a collaborative level because of differing communication styles or as a result of communication which remains at the level of basic information sharing. Devaney (2008) considered interprofessional working in child protection via research conducted with 28 experienced child welfare professionals. The findings underlined a recurring theme of the importance of communication between professionals and between professionals and families. Open and regular communication which incorporated an analysis of the issues in the family and a joint consideration of how to progress the work were highlighted as indicative of sound collaborative practice. On the other hand, effective communication between all professionals was not always achievable, particularly in relation to the involvement of GPs in the process. This limited communication with GPs in the child protection arena has also been highlighted by Lupton and colleagues (2000). The benefits of increased communication between agency workers were also cited by Polnay (2000) in a study of GP attendance at child protection case conferences. Over two-thirds of the 112 GPs questioned in the study would have attended the case conference if personally telephoned by the social worker.

Resources

Resource limitations are common and shared elements of the daily work by professionals involved in family and childcare services and particularly within the realms of child protection services. Research participants in Darlington and colleagues' (2005) study identified a lack of resources as the greatest barrier to effective multidisciplinary working. This finding is validated by other studies which have emphasised that lack of appropriate resources and time constraints detract from effective collaborative working in more complex cases. On a practical level, results from a study of interagency working in an early intervention team showed unequal distribution of resources within multi-agency sites, such as schools, where room allocation was often limited and prioritised to medical practitioners (Moran *et al.*, 2007). However, Darlington (2005) also cautions that while lack of resources may hamper the effort to achieve effective collaborative working, it is also clear that adequate resourcing will not automatically provide the panacea for all problems in the multidisciplinary working environment.

Case study

Janine Stewart is a 24-year-old single parent who has three children – Becky aged five, Kirsty aged four and Lee aged six months. As a care experienced young person, she has been known to Social Services for many years. Due to living in a family where her father was dependent on drugs and alcohol, she witnessed regular episodes of domestic violence and when her mother committed suicide when she was eight years old, Janine was initially fostered with her two siblings. However, in her teenage years, her foster parents found her challenging behaviour difficult to manage: she often stayed out till early morning, went missing on several occasions and there were concerns that she had been engaged in prostitution and shoplifting. She was transferred to a long-stay residential unit and remained there until she moved into a flat when she was 17. Janine's flat soon became a focal point for all-night parties and her neighbours regularly complained about her behaviour to the police and housing authority. Janine was employed in a local Tesco, enjoyed her work and was regarded as a reliable worker.

She got pregnant shortly after she met Kalim, aged 20, who had been a care experienced young person; he was employed as a car mechanic and in the early stages of their relationship was mutually supportive. However, when he lost his job shortly after Becky was born, the couple began to experience difficulties. The health visitor was concerned about Janine's mental health and encouraged her to seek medical treatment. Her GP diagnosed postnatal depression and referred Janine to the community mental health team for support. She attended a mother and toddler group and for a while things were stable.

However, the impact of unemployment led to regular rows between the couple and episodes of domestic violence. Janine moved into the Women's Aid hostel on several occasions but returned home after a couple of weeks. Concerns were expressed by staff in the hostel about Janine's lack of patience with the children (Kirsty was two years old) and her unrealistic expectations of the children's behaviour. When 'fingertip bruising' was observed on Kirsty's arms, Social Services were informed and child protection procedures were initiated. Both Becky and Kirsty were made subjects of child protection plans following a multidisciplinary meeting. As part of this, Janine and Kalim were willing to accept family support services and both engaged actively with parenting classes.

Family circumstances improved when Kalim was employed through a local garage and until recently there were no concerns expressed. Becky and Kirsty have been doing well at school nursery, and although Janine experienced postnatal depression after Lee's birth she has been supported by her health visitor and community psychiatric nurse.

The police have been contacted recently by Janine complaining about Kalim's aggressive behaviour towards her; he has threatened to throw her out of the house. He alleges she has been selling her prescription drugs and leaving the children unattended. When Social Workers contacted the nursery, teachers conveyed concerns about Kirsty's withdrawn behaviour and Becky's aggressive outbursts towards other children.

In a child protection planning meeting coordinated by Social Services, the professionals involved – GP, health visitor, community psychiatric nurse (CPN), teachers, police, domestic violence liaison officer, social worker and family support worker – begin to share concerns about the family's current functioning and the specific needs of the children. The health visitor expresses concern about Janine's mental health, she feels she is under a lot of stress and is concerned about the impact of this on her care of Lee. This view is shared by the CPN. The GP indicates he has seen Kalim recently and he is of the opinion that his aggressive behaviour results from his worries and frustration about being unemployed again. When the teachers outline their concerns about Kirsty's nursery school behaviour, the family support worker adds that she has suspicions that Kirsty is often scapegoated by Janine. The police confirm that they have received information from local informants that Janine is dealing in drugs but they have no evidence to arrest her. Opinions are voiced about the risks to which the children are exposed and the need for immediate action.

Case Study Questions

1. Identify the specific roles of the professionals involved in the above case study.
2. What is the purpose of the child protection meeting?
3. How would you begin to undertake an assessment of the family and the individual children's needs?
4. What contribution does each professional make to this assessment?

Positive outcomes in multidisciplinary child protection

Despite the apparent difficulties and complex issues inherent in multidisciplinary practice in child protection services and the resulting impact of the issues on successful outcomes for children and families, it is clear that positive results are precipitated by the collaborative approach. Moran *et al.* (2007) highlight that working within a multidisciplinary environment led to renewed commitment and enthusiasm for the job, fostered a creative approach and increased autonomy in practice. There was also an enhanced understanding of professional roles and modes of working and an increased confidence in relation to intervention thresholds, both of which enabled partner agencies to make more appropriate and quicker referrals.

Harr *et al.* (2008) outlines two models of good practice in interdisciplinary teamwork for the assessment and treatment of child abuse in a hospital setting. The multidisciplinary teams operate in two hospitals; in an established team in a Texas hospital and a newly formed multidisciplinary team within a Brazilian hospital. The Texan Referral and Evaluation of Abused Children (REACH) team members demonstrated a collaborative working model based on mutual trust and professional respect for the role of each worker. There was also evidence of clear and consistent communication, both in-house and with external agencies. Furthermore, the interests and needs of clients took precedence over professional status or individual gain in a dynamic process, which was reflected upon in a team-based approach.

Key learning points

What promotes good practice in child protection work:

- clear communication
- time taken to develop communication between members of team
- develop mutual trust and respect
- joint training initiatives
- clear procedural protocols.

Exercise 9.3

Consider the issues which provide arguments for close multiprofessional and interagency working, and the types of factors which might militate against this.

The Northern Ireland context

In Northern Ireland, as with the rest of the UK, government departments and concerned agencies and professionals have been challenged by current and what often seems like perennial public and media concerns about perceived local failings in the provision of child protection (safeguarding[1]) services, a cornerstone of any postmodern Western democracy (DHSSPS,[2] 2006; RQIA,[3] 2009; Toner, 2008). Historically, as a result of a local government deficit prior to the establishment of the Northern Ireland Assembly, Northern Ireland safeguarding legislation and policy tended to mirror, with some slight modifications, developments in England and Wales. For over three decades 'direct rule' government from Westminster meant that local politicians and child care professionals had little influence over child protection developments. Examples of this would be the primary Northern Ireland child care legislation, the Children (NI) Order 1995 that in essence is very similar to the Children Act 1989 in England and Wales, updated with the Children Act 2004.

Similarly, the interagency safeguarding aspirations contained in policies in England such as, *Working Together* (Department of Health, 1988), updated by *Working Together Under the Children Act* (Department of Health, 1991), and most recently by the *Working Together to Safeguard Children* (HM Government, 2010) policy, revised in relation to the Laming (2009) recommendations from the Baby P (Peter) inquiries in Haringey. All these English issues are also reflected in policy development in Northern Ireland and recognised as practice issues for professionals working in child protection. We can similarly chart the history of Northern Irish interagency child protection policy drivers, from *Co-operating to Protect Children* (DHSS,[4] 1989), through to the current *Co-operating to Safeguard Children'* (DHSSPS, 2003), which is due for revision soon as part of the DHSSPS 'Reform Implementation Strategy' (2008), following on from *Overview Report*[5] (DHSSPS, 2006).

In Northern Ireland one of the major recommendations of the 1989 policy guidance, *Co-operating to Protect Children,* was the establishment of local Area Child Protection Committees (ACPCs), in each of the previously established Health Boards, with lower-level Child Protection Panels being established in the Social Services Community Trusts (TCPPs). This *Co-operating to Protect Children* policy was Northern Ireland's first systematic attempt to regionalise and standardise the child protection policies, procedures and guidance available to all relevant professionals. It also clarified the roles of various professionals and agencies in handling individual child protection cases and suggested the importance of multidisciplinary training in safeguarding children (DHSSPS, 2003).

The ACPCs in Northern Ireland, as in other parts of the UK, were intended to bring together senior staff in social services, police, education, health and the non-government sector, in interagency forums, to plan and oversee the development and coordination of child protection services in their local area (Evans and Millar, 1993; Wright, 1999). These committees oversaw the development of the now familiar child protection case conference and the child protection register (DHSS, 1989) and was an attempt to develop a common ethos and understanding of what constituted child abuse, and how it could be best managed. The work of the ACPCs in Northern Ireland like England, are now overseen by a regional Safeguarding Board for Northern Ireland (SBNI), as part of the DHSSPS reform strategy. This section will discuss whether the interagency and interprofessional

---

[1]The terms 'child protection' and 'safeguarding' will be used interchangeably and describe the same concept.
[2]Department of Health, Social Services and Public Safety (DHSSPS), Northern Ireland.
[3]Regulation and Quality Improvement Authority (RQIA), Northern Ireland.
[4]Department of Health and Social Services (DHSS), now the DHSSPS (Northern Ireland).
[5]DHSSPS (2006), Our Children and Young People – Our Shared Responsibility: Inspection of Child Protection Services, Overview Report.

aspirations of the original ACPCs have yet to be realised, necessitating continual reforms and developments such as the Safeguarding Board in Northern Ireland and Professor Eileen Munro's review of child protection in England (2010/11).

As a DHSSPS report that reviewed the development of child protection services suggested 'Agencies and statutory bodies come from very different backgrounds and ways of working. It requires continual application to agree a common approach' (DHSSPS, 2003, p. 162).

One significant policy advancement in Northern Ireland was the emergence of the Regional Policy and Procedures[6] (ACPC, 2004), which streamlined a wealth of different ACPC policies and procedures that had been developed by each individual ACPC since 1991. One of the stated aims of the Regional Policy and Procedures (2004) was the concept of 'shared responsibility', which was understood to mean that 'effective child protection is firmly based on co-operation between staff and agencies and shared decision-making' (ACPC 1.15).

The roles and responsibilities of the main agencies and professionals are set out in detail in chapter 3 of this document (ACPC, 2004, 3.1–3.131). The professional interfaces include social work, nursing, allied health professionals, medical staff, education staff and the police.

If the Department's mantra 'Child Protection is Everyone's Business' (DHSSPS, 2003) and the partnership aspirations of the Children (NI) Order 1995 were to be realised, then a climate and structure that encouraged and supported interprofessional respect, ethos and collective responsibility was required. The question must be asked if policy initiatives and legislation alone can deliver an improvement in interagency working to safeguard and protect vulnerable children in Northern Ireland. Unfortunately, it would appear that this is not the case as Northern Ireland continued to have child abuse deaths and subsequent case management reviews that criticised the level of interagency effectiveness.

The local challenges and opportunities

There are of course some localised structural and cultural differences in how child protection services have developed and are delivered in all the UK countries. However, proximity to each other and the role played by professional bodies (many UK-wide) such as the professional Royal Colleges (for example Nursing, General Practice, Psychiatry and Psychology) does provide some opportunity for standardised professional practice in the UK. The collaborative nature of other regulatory agencies such as the Social Care Councils encourage inter-country collaboration and the sharing of best practice, including the often stark lessons from child death inquiries throughout the UK.

Northern Ireland is unique as it is the only home country that shares a land border with another European country, the Republic of Ireland. This presents both challenges, such as alleged child abusers fleeing over the border to the other jurisdiction, and opportunities for cooperation, as evident in the North–South Ministerial Council (NSMC) meetings, when new procedures for cross-border, sex-offender management, vetting and information sharing were agreed as part of a North–South Safeguarding Agenda (2008).

It can be seen, therefore, that Northern Ireland's position on the child protection compass means it must look south, as well as east, for inspiration and information on the best way to enhance interagency and interprofessional practice. Northern Ireland, or as some citizens prefer to call it the 'north of Ireland', is a small country with a population of 1.7 million citizens (NISRA[7]). It has particular child protection challenges for public services and statutory agencies, following on from the legacy of the 'troubles', and over three decades of political upheaval and civil unrest that claimed more than 3,500 lives. Two examples of this would be that the Police Service of Northern Ireland could still not investigate child abuse in some areas

---

[6]Regional child protection policies – endorsed by all four Northern Ireland Area Child Protection Committees.
[7]Northern Ireland Statistics and Research Agency (NISRA).

without stringent security measures in place for home visits and historically child witnesses are often video interviewed, under Achieving Best Evidence (1999) and Joint Protocol procedures (2004), in fortified police stations rather than in normal offices. In delivering and locating child protection services, there is still often local duplication of many public services, e.g. health centres and schools, to meet the needs of a still fairly religiously segregated society. One community would not travel into an area perceived to belong to the 'other side' – religiously and politically. Nevertheless, public support for the protection of children in Northern Ireland is strong and the public, political representatives and the media have high expectations and are not slow to condemn agencies when they are perceived as having failed to protect vulnerable children, (Toner, 2008; O'Neill, 2008; The Overview Report, DHSSPS, 2006).

Unlike other parts of the UK, Northern Ireland has had for many years a perceived advantage in having an integrated department of Health and Social Services, and it now includes public safety, thus the DHSSPS. However, any DHSSPS departmental initiatives to encourage good interagency safeguarding practice have also had to deal with the fact that on the ground a whole range of health and social care professionals and services can be competing for budgets, status and role demarcation. There may be separate executive accountably for the management of their part of the child protection system and it can still be perceived as being the primary (or sole) responsibility of the social services part of the organisation. Also the separate Department of Education, Northern Ireland (DENI), for example, may have different priorities than the Department of Health, Social Services and Public Health when it comes to allocating teachers' time to service the child protection system, and even within the DHSSPS GPs can only be advised to attend child protection case conferences concerning their patients, and as a result attendance is limited. Co-operating to Safeguard Children (Department of Health and Social Services, 2003) asserts that:

> Safeguarding children depends upon effective information sharing, collaboration and understanding between families, agencies and professionals. Constructive relationships between individual workers and agencies

needs to be supported by senior management in each agency (CtSC 1.15).

In looking east and the sustained child protection crisis that emerged in England in 2009, despite Lord Laming's Report (2003) and recommendations after Victoria Climbié's death in Haringey, although all of Lord Laming's reports (2003, 2009) only apply to England, most home countries, including the DHSSPS in Northern Ireland, have used many of the recommendations as a template to audit their own child protection services and learn any lessons that could improve interagency and interprofessional safeguarding practice (DHSSPS, 2008; RQIA, 2009).

An interagency 'health check' of child protection services

The challenge for all professionals directly or indirectly responsible for the delivery of safeguarding services in Northern Ireland is to deliver strategic and higher levels of interagency collaboration (Hallet and Birchall, 1992; Miller and McNicholl, 2003). In some countries this involves the merging of previously separate organisational and professional systems. It could be asserted that the Northern Ireland structures and policy initiatives have not yet achieved the levels of integration envisaged by some commentators (Horwarth and Morrison, 2007).

In Northern Ireland, the conclusions of the most recent child death/child abuse inquiries (The Overview Report, DHSSPS, 2006; McElhill Inquiry 2008; O'Neill Inquiry 2008; Toner, 2008) have echoed the findings from previous UK inquiries (Laming 2009) and those in the Republic of Ireland (Murphy Report 2009). The cumulative effect of over 30 years of child abuse inquiries/serious case reviews has been to produce the same recommendations and further detailed procedures and guidance. They all recommend more accountability (usually within agency) strengthened managerial control, additional training and the assertion that (often very busy) professionals need to communicate more effectively with each other (Department of Health, 2003; Munro, 2005; Reder and Duncan, 2003).

The Overview Report (DHSSPS, 2006) was a multidisciplinary, interagency inspection of child protection services in Northern Ireland covering all five health and social care trust areas. It found that despite some examples of good interagency practice, there was a failure on the part of some organisations to adequately discharge their statutory responsibilities to protect vulnerable children. The outcome of the report was the development of a 'reform implementation strategy' led by the DHSSPS, including the development of a single assessment framework (UNOCINI[8]) for assessing risks and needs that was to be adopted by all agencies and professionals working with children and families and coordinated by social services.

The DHSSPS (2006) report also concluded that 'ownership of ACPC's and Trust CPP's and their effectiveness in discharging their corporate role was limited. Consequently, arrangements for interagency communication and effective engagement ... needs to be significantly strengthened' (DHSSPS, 2006, 1.15).

The Toner Report (DHSSPS, 2008) into the McElhill fire tragedy that claimed seven lives, including all five children and the subsequent inquest (Omagh 2009), confirmed that Mr McElhill, a convicted sex offender, had deliberately started the fire. The ramifications of this particular tragedy have yet to be fully realised but the report (Toner, 2008) was

Exercise 9.4

On a scale of 1–5 (in terms of difficulty), consider how you and your profession could achieve the following recommendations:

- Establish a common language for use across all agencies to help those agencies to identify who they are concerned about.

  1 easy 2 3 4 5 very difficult

- The seeking or refusal of parental permission must not restrict the initial information-gathering and sharing.

  1 easy 2 3 4 5 very difficult

- When communication with a child is necessary for the purposes of safeguarding and promoting that child's welfare, and the first language of that child is not English, an interpreter must be used.

  1 easy 2 3 4 5 very difficult

- The child has been spoken to alone.

  1 easy 2 3 4 5 very difficult

Laming (2003) Climbié Report, recommendations 13, 18, 36 and 40.

critical in respect of the working interface and professional accountability of staff in the Western Health and Social Care Trust and most agencies involved, including the police, probation service and medical and mental health services. It commented that

> Robust governance arrangements are essential in building public credibility and are underpinned by the need to have in place systems to ensure compliance with clinical and social care governance standards as outlined in the DHSSPS guidelines.
>
> (Toner, 2008, 1.11)

The O'Neill Inquiry in the EHSSB[9] and WHSSB[10] reviewed the safeguarding practices of a range of agencies involved with Mrs O'Neill, who had mental health issues and her daughter (Lauren aged nine years) who sadly was a victim when her mother decided to end both their lives in 2005. The subsequent report was also very critical of the services involved: mental health hospital and community services; primary health care; social services and a

A closer look

The findings of the Overview Report (DHSSPS, 2006) included the following recommendations:

- the need for a review of structures, leadership and accountability in child protection
- clear regional thresholds for access to services
- consistent interpretation and implementation of policy and procedures and associated protocols
- a uniform approach to assessment of need and risk analysis.

(DHSSPS, 2006, 1.18)

---

[8]Understanding the Needs of Children in Northern Ireland (UNOCINI).
[9]Eastern Health and Social Services Board (EHSSB), replaced in 2008 by the new Belfast Health and Social Care Trust.
[10]Western Health and Social Services Board (EHSSB), replaced in 2008 by the new Western Health and Social Care Trust.

private counselling service. The O'Neill report (2008) highlighted a lack of understanding of roles and responsibilities in relation to child protection, poor communication among all professionals, between mental health and child care services and between professionals and the other family members.

Once again the best practice as outlined in the current DHSSPS guidance (2003 and 2006) appeared to be *not working* in practice, which is concerning in its own right. But this also raised the spectre, as mentioned by commentators such as Munro (2005), Horwarth and Morrison (2007), Parton (2006), Hayes and Spratt (2008), that perhaps the policies and procedures are *unworkable* within the currently configured interagency structures that deliver child protection services in Northern Ireland. This view could also be construed from some of Munro's (2011) conclusions in her final review report into the child protection system in England. Indeed, any more policy or legislative changes, in themselves, will not provide a safer child protection system, unless better interagency and interprofessional child protection practice is prioritised and developed throughout the UK.

Conclusion

This chapter has outlined the key professional issues related to interdisciplinary working in child protection. While elements of effective working are identified, the reader is encouraged to consider how **processes and procedures are framed by jurisdictional contexts** and more importantly how interagency structures militated against effective practices to safeguard children and young people. The chapter considers how such factors as professional roles, identities and **perceptions about differential status can impact on professional communication,** ultimately affecting effective multidisciplinary working. The case study defines some of these issues and conveys the tensions experienced in such work. In highlighting the positive outcomes associated with multidisciplinary practice in child protection, the reader is reminded of the benefits and how potential challenges can be addressed. Utilising one UK jurisdiction to illustrate

contemporary structures and practices, we have explored how current practice has emerged against a backdrop of policy and significant legislative reforms. More recently critical reviews of practice have reinforced perceptions of deficits in interagency working, raising questions about the effectiveness of current practice within present structures. Ultimately it is argued that **the professional challenge lies in prioritising interagency working in child protection** instead of developing additional policy or legislative frameworks to safeguard children and young people.

Further reading

Stafford A, Vincent S and Parton N (eds) (2010) *Child Protection Reform across the UK*, Edinburgh: Dunedin Academic Press.

Heenan, D. and Birrell, D. (2011) *Social Work in Northern Ireland,* Bristol: The Policy Press.

Useful websites

www.scie.org.uk
Social Care Institute for Excellence

www.ncb.org.uk
National Childrens Bureau

www.clicp.ed.ac.uk
The University of Edinburgh/NSPCC Centre for UK-wide Learning in Child Protection

References

Charles, M. and Glennie, S. (eds) (2003) *Promoting Quality, Standards for Interagency Training to Safeguard Children,* 2nd edn, London: NSPCC.

Darlington, Y., Feeney, J. A. and Rixon, K. (2005) Interagency collaboration between child protection and mental health services: practices, attitudes and barriers. *Child Abuse and Neglect* 29 (10), 1085–98.

Department for Education and Skills (2006) *Working Together to Safeguard Children, A Guide to Inter-agency Working to Safeguard and Promote the Welfare of Children,* London: The Stationery Office.

Department of Health (1989) *Co-operating to Protect Children,* Belfast: DHSS.

Department of Health (1991) *Working Together Under the Children Act 1989: A Guide to Arrangements for*

Inter-Agency Cooperation for the Protection of Children from Abuse, London: HMSO.

Department of Health and Social Security and the Welsh Office (1988) *Working Together: a Guide to Arrangements for Inter-Agency Co-operation for the Protection of Children from Abuse,* London: HMSO.

Department of Health and Social Services (2003a) *A Better Future: 50 Years of Child Care in Northern Ireland, 1950–2000,* Belfast: DHSS.

Department of Health and Social Services (2003b) *Co-operating to Safeguard Children,* Belfast, DHSSPS.

Department of Health, Social Services and Public Safety (2006) *Our Children and Young People – Our Shared Responsibility,* Overview Report, Belfast: DHSSPS.

Department of Health, Social Services and Public Safety (2008), *Development Strategy for Personal Social Services Staff in Children's Services: Guidance for Northern Ireland Health and Social Care Trusts,* Belfast: DHSSPS.

Devaney, J. (2008) Interprofessional working in child protection with families with long-term and complex needs, *Child Abuse Review* 17(4), 242–61.

Evans, M. and Miller, C. (1993) *Partnership in Child Protection,* London: National Institute for Social Work.

Frost, N. and Robinson, M. (2007) Joining up children's services: safeguarding children in multidisciplinary teams, *Child Abuse Review* 16 (3), 184–99.

Geva, E., Barsky, A. E. and Westernoff, F. (2000) Developing a framework for interprofessional and diversity informed practice, in E. Geva, A. E. Barsky and F. Westernoff. (eds) *Interprofessional Practice with Diverse Populations: Cases in Point* (pp. 1–28), Westport, CN: Greenwood.

Glennie, S. (2007) Developing inter professional relationships: tapping the potential of inter-agency training, *Child Abuse Review* 16, 171–83.

Hallet, C. and Birchall, E. (1992) *Coordination in Child Protection,* London: HMSO.

Harlow, E. and Shardlow, S. M. (2006) Safeguarding Children: challenges to the effective operation of core groups, *Child and Family Social Work* 11 (1), 65–72.

Harr, C., Fairchild, S. and Souza, L. (2008) International Models of Hospital Interdisciplinary Teams for the Identification, Assessment, and Treatment of Child Abuse, *Social Work in Health Care* 46 (4), 1-16.

Hayes, D. and Spratt, T. (2009) Child Welfare Interventions: Patterns of Social Work Practice, *British Journal of Social Work* 39(8), 1575–1579.

HM Government (2010) *Working Together to Safeguard Children: A Guide to Inter-Agency Working to Safeguard and Promote the Welfare of Children,* London: HM Government.

Horwarth, J. and Morrison, T. (2007) Collaboration, integration and change in children's services: Critical issues and key ingredients, *Child Abuse and Neglect* 31, 55–69.

Hudson, B. (2002) Interprofessionality in health and social care: the Achilles' heel of partnership? *Journal of InterProfessional Care* 16 (1), 7–18.

Laming, H. (2003) *The Victoria Climbié Inquiry: Report of an Inquiry by Lord Laming,* CM5730, Norwich: HMSO.

Laming, H. (2009) *The Protection of Children in England: A Progress Report,* London: Department for Children, Schools and Families.

Lupton, C., Khan, P. and North, N. (2000) The role of the general practitioner in child protection, *British Journal of General Practice* 50, 977–81.

Malin, N. and Morrow, G. (2007) Models of inter professional working within a Sure Start 'trailblazer' programme, *Journal of Inter professional Care* 21 (4), 445–57.

McGrath, M. (1991) *Multidisciplinary Teamwork,* Aldershot: Avebury.

Miller, C. and McNicholl, A. (2003) *Integrating Children's Services: Issues and Practice,* London: Office of Public Management.

Mizrahi, T. and Abramson, J. S. (2000) Social work and physician collaboration: perspectives on a shared case, *Social Work in Health Care* 31 (3), 1–24.

Moran, P., Jacobs, C., Bunn, A. and Bifulco, A. (2007) Multi-agency working: implications for an early-intervention social work team, *Child and Family Social Work* 12, 143–151.

Munro, E. (2005) A systems approach to investigating child abuse deaths, *British Journal of Social Work* 35, 531–46.

Munro, E. (2011), *The Munro Review of Child Protection: Final Report, A Child-Centred System,* London, Department of Education.

Murphy, Y. (2009) Report by Commission of Investigation into Catholic Archdiocese of Dublin, Dublin: Department of Justice and Equality.

North–South Safeguarding Agenda (2008), *Developing New Child Protection Safeguarding Structures in Northern Ireland,* Belfast: Northern Ireland Assembly Briefing Note 43/10.

O'Neill Report (2008), *Report of the Independent Inquiry Panel to the Western and Eastern Health and Social Services Boards, May 2007 – Madeline and Lauren O'Neil,* Western Health and Social Care Board and Eastern Health and Social Care Board, Belfast: DHSSPS.

Packard, T., Jones, L. and Nahrestedt, K. (2006) Using the image exchange to enhance interdisciplinary team building in child welfare, *Child and Adolescent Social Work Journal* 23 (1), 86–106.

Parton, N. (2006) *Safeguarding Childhood: Early Intervention and Surveillance in a Late Modern Society*, Basingstoke: Palgrave MacMillan.

Polnay, J. C. (2000) General practitioners and child protection case conference Participation, *Child Abuse Review*, 9, 108–23.

Reder, P. and Duncan, S. (2003) Understanding Communications in Child Protection Networks, *Child Abuse Review* 12, 82–100.

RQIA (2009) *Child Protection Review Reports, Stages 1-3,* Belfast: Regulation and Quality Improvement Authority.

Shardlow, S., Davis, C., Johnson, M., Long, T., Murphy, M. and Race, D. (2004) *Education and Training for Inter-agency Working: New Standards,* Manchester: Salford Centre for Social Work Research, University of Salford.

Skinner, K. and Bell, L. (2007) Changing structures: necessary but not sufficient, *Child Abuse Review* 16, 209–22.

Toner, H. (2008) *Independent Review Report of Agency Involvement with Mr Arthur McElhill, Ms Lorraine McGovern and Their Children*, 2008, WHSSB and EHSSC, Belfast: DHSSPS.

Wilson, V. and Pirrie, A. (2000) *Multidisciplinary Teamworking: Beyond the Barriers? A Review of the Issues,* SCRE Research Reports 96, Edinburgh: SCRE.

Wright, F. (1999) Consensus and conflict in the multidisciplinary child protection process: a review of the selected literature, *Child Care in Practice: Northern Ireland Journal of Multi-Disciplinary Practice*, 5(2), 161–70.

Chapter 10
Children in need, looked-after children and interprofessional working

Nick Frost

Chapter summary

This chapter will argue that there has been a step change in interprofessional working with children in need and looked-after children since the passage of the Children Act, 2004, which led to the development of children's trusts arrangements across England. This step change has involved moving perceptions of work with these groups of children and young people from being seen as largely the responsibility of Social Services Departments (as they were) towards a more collective and shared approach.

Learning objectives

This chapter will cover:

- how supporting children in need is a crucial element of children's services: local authorities are required under S.17 of Children Act 1989 to provide family support services
- how effective family support can prevent family problems becoming worse – it should be able to reduce the incidence of child abuse and of children becoming looked after
- how your professional practice can contribute to this process.

Exercise 10.1

- Who works in family support?
- Which professionals do you think might be a member of 'the team around the child'?
- Who else might be involved in family support?

What is family support?

In order to fully address interprofessional practice in family support we first have to clarify our use of terminology and exactly what the meaning of the term 'children in need' is.

'Children in need' are defined by Section 17 of the Children Act 1989. The Act places a 'general duty' on the local authority as follows:

(a) to safeguard and promote the welfare of children within their area who are in need; and

(b) so far as is consistent with that duty, to promote the upbringing of such children by their families,

(c) by providing a range and level of services appropriate to those children's needs

This duty is central to understanding family support, and effectively acted as a key stimulus in developing family support practice in England. The duty is proactive, whereas previous legislation tended to be reactive, and crucially identifies a group of children as being 'in need'. However, the way that children in need are actually identified is complex and difficult to put into practice. According to Section 17(10) of the 1989 Act a child in need can be identified as follows:

(a) he is unlikely to achieve or maintain, or to have the opportunity of achieving or maintaining, a reasonable standard of health or development without the provision for him of services by a local authority under this Part;

(b) his health or development is likely to be significantly impaired, or further impaired, without the provision for him of such services; or

(c) he is disabled

There are many problems with this definition. It is far from clear which children fall into this group and which do not. Also, the term 'children in need' is redolent of charity and also suggests that somehow a group of children exist who do not have 'needs'.

For these reasons in this chapter we will use the term 'family support' to analyse work around Section 17, rather than the phrase children in need. Family support suggests a positive approach, is a term in daily use and allows us to examine practice across an extensive range of settings and organisations who have embraced the term.

Family support practice

Family support is now a widespread practice existing across many settings – including schools, children's centres, health and voluntary sector organisations – both in England and internationally (see Dolan, Canavan and Pinkerton, 2006).

What is the current state of play in terms of practice in relation to family support? It can be argued that family support practice is in retreat in its 'traditional' social care setting. Social workers in local authority settings are under increasing pressure, from Ofsted in particular, to focus on safeguarding and child protection (Frost and Parton, 2009). While family support practice can be found in local authority settings it tends to be with families that are already recognised as having child protection issues. The threshold for being allocated a social worker has increased and such workers are unlikely to work with families requiring only 'assistance, support and advice'. In times of financial retrenchment there is a danger that family support will suffer when scare resources focus more and more on child protection.

While family support has declined in local authority social care settings it has developed and extended as an area of practice elsewhere. Since 1989 the practice of family support has become a broad one, with many locations and with many professionals practising in the field. Arguably family support is a practice in search of a definition and a home. It is 'de-centred' practice both in terms of where it is carried out and in terms of defining what it actually is (Canavan, Dolan and Pinkerton, 2000).

Family support is also a practice that involves many activities and levels of practice. The idea of seeing family support existing at different levels has its roots in the work of Parker (1980) and Hardiker and colleagues (1991) around the related concept of 'prevention'. Parker argued that preventive practice took place at three levels:

1. *Primary* providing general support to a wide range of families without stigma

2. *Secondary* a more targeted approach to families with identified particular needs

3. *Tertiary* targeted at avoiding children spending extended periods separated from their families (see Parker, 1980, p. 45).

Thus we can see that family support is both complex and many-layered.

More recently Penn and Gough argued that family support is

> one of those phrases that is used so often it has almost lost its meaning: or rather it encompasses so may meanings that it is difficult to disentangle them. The term is used loosely to cover many kinds of intervention with many different kinds of target groups.
>
> (2002, p. 17)

This lack of precision, perhaps paradoxically, exists alongside the expansion of family support as a practice:

> family support has become a major strategic orientation in services for children and families. It now occupies a significant place within the array of care and welfare interventions. It has global currency.
>
> (Dolan, Canavan and Pinkerton, 2006, p. 11)

Gilligan (2000) develops the idea of family support existing at different levels and argues that this diverse and uncertain deployment of the term can be best seen as existing in three forms:

1. *Developmental family support* building universal services locally to support all children and families

2. *Compensatory family support* seeking to support disadvantaged families through special provision

3. *Protective family support* which seeks to strengthen the coping and resilience of individual families (2000, p. 15).

Developmental family support can be seen as universal services that can be used without stigma by wide sections of the population – they might include school-based services, such as breakfast clubs, and services such as national helplines.

Compensatory family support is more explicitly targeted than developmental family support. These services may exist specifically in poorer areas in order to challenge the impact of social inequities, and might include home visiting, respite care and centre-based

activities such as parenting classes. In England Sure Start, a major family support project that existed between 1998 and 2007 in local areas represents a good example of such practice (Glass, 1999).

Protective family support exists to address high levels of need. Gilligan describes it as

> to promote the child's safety and development and prevent the child leaving the family by reducing stressors in the child's and family's life, promoting competence in the child, connecting the child and family members to relevant supports and resources and promoting morale and competence in parents.
>
> (2000, p. 14)

This type of family support would tend to work with individual families, most often identified by a referring agency as in need of services.

How is family support practice underpinned by interprofessional practice? Firstly, family support tends to be a holistic form of practice – seeing children and families as requiring support across the traditional organisational divides – social care, education, health, day care and so on. For family support practice to be effective it needs to address all these issues – and therefore, by definition, cannot be a single profession activity. Secondly, family support practice needs to relate to families in all their diverse forms – diversity relating to ethnicity, sexuality and family structure, for example.

In England the process of family support is increasingly driven by the Common Assessment Framework (CAF) – a form of interprofessional assessment that works in partnership with families, with focus on strengths and practical help and assistance for the family. Where a CAF has been undertaken a lead professional (LP) will be allocated. The current author undertook a local evaluation of the work of LPs where they were also allocated a budget to support their work, thus becoming Budget-holding Lead Professionals (BHLPs). A summary of this work is provided below to indicate how family support is profoundly a multidisciplinary process. The evaluation involved an in-depth analysis of six CAFs, where parents and relevant professionals were interviewed, and a documentary analysis of 25 case summaries.

Thus the CAF process emerges as a form of family support, facilitated by the existence of a budget and

A closer look

Identifying and responding to need – using the CAF

Twenty-five written case summaries produced by BHLPs were analysed and this process demonstrated that poverty and lack of access to goods and services underpinned all the situations. Poverty seemed to be central to many families where the parent/carer lacks the resources to address their situation. The other primary challenge was the range of health issues that affected the families in a number of ways. Concerns about poverty and health were closely followed by educational needs in the form of school uniforms for children, or transport costs for children to attend schools or day care.

It can be seen that this sample of families faced a range of issues that cross traditional organisational divides, and therefore required an interprofessional approach.

The range of interventions provided by professionals were extensive – there is not a 'typical' CAF, nor a 'typical' deployment of the budget. This reflects the flexibility and the responsiveness of the BHLP system. It is personalised in the sense that it responds personally and uniquely to the needs of the child and their family, based on careful assessment.

The CAF process enabled a range of organisations to coordinate and work together in a structured manner towards common agreed goals. A number of factors often needed to come together in order to effectively address the issues facing families:

- the CAF needed to be flexible and responsive to individual situations
- all the parents and carers interviewed greatly appreciated the outcome of the intervention

- all the parents and carers interviewed appreciated the speed and timeliness of the response
- the responses were solution-focused – a challenge was assessed and concretely responded to
- many of the assessed issues existed in a wider context of ongoing life challenges – in our six in-depth cases there were chaotic lifestyles, substance abuse, domestic violence, child protection concerns and housing problems
- the parents/carers and BHLPs were equally appreciative of the availability of the budget, the service provided and the outcomes
- parent/carers tended to provide a narrative around their particular concrete challenge, while the BHLPs tended to place this in a wider context of more persistent challenges
- there were no negative comments from the parent/carers about the BHLP, who were perceived as listening, approachable and responsive.

The interprofessional approach to intervention was facilitated by the CAF process and enhanced the delivery of outcomes for families. The BHLP process emerges strongly and powerfully from the data as an excellent example of solution-focused, strength-based, partnership working. It seems to deliver concrete outcomes for parent and carers, albeit in a wider context of complex and demanding lifestyles. The BHLPs themselves are empowered by a process that delivers real change and makes a concrete difference to those they work with. According to the case summaries gathered by the BHLPs the interventions from the various professionals have significantly increased the health and well-being of all the families concerned, as classified using the five outcomes.

fundamentally interprofessional in the approach that is taken.

Working with children in care

Having examined the practice of family support we now move on to work with 'looked-after children'. As with children in need, this group of children and young

Key learning points

- Children in care require effective interprofessional working if they are to be enabled to reach their full potential.
- Children in care require stability in high-quality placements and opportunities to participate fully in decisions about their lives.
- How your professional practice can contribute to this process.

Case study

Family support

This case study examines how a family support intervention can work positively to address family challenges.

Family structure

Father 28, child 7(female), child 5 (male), child 4 (male).

Reason for referral

The local social work team recommended in an action plan at a child protection conference that referral should be made as the father had become primary carer for three children and they had identified support needs for the family at home.

Family history

This was a White English family where the parents had separated. The three children were removed from mother's care and moved in with father due to fears of potential neglect. All three children are subject to a child protection plan following domestic violence between parents and issues relating to the mother's drinking and neglect. The children were made subject to a plan under the categories of emotional abuse and neglect; however, since residing with dad the neglect issue has been addressed.

Family support needs

- the family are currently living with father at grandmother's house in a two-bedroom property, which is consequently overcrowded
- anger management issues for father
- parenting support for father
- benefits/financial advice
- supported family to access family group conference service

Actions by family support advisor to date

- housing application submitted
- liaised with housing on behalf of family to ensure assessment was undertaken and the family were re-housed as a matter of priority
- family re-housed in three-bedroom property and supported to obtain furniture etc. through local charities and so on
- supported to complete community care grant to obtain furniture etc.
- support in accessing benefits, including school dinners, child tax credits
- initiated joint visit with facilitator of anger management sessions
- encouraged and supported to attend anger management
- supervised contact with mum and children at Anytown Tea Time Club
- provided information and encouraged dad to access dad's support through dad's group
- discussed one-to-one parenting with dad to identify any parenting needs
- supported family to access Family Group Conference service to address issues around contact with mum and arguments between both parents. It was decided not to hold any further reviews but family agreed it would be useful to reconvene if the children were no longer subject to a plan in future
- IFS continues to work closely with social care and school – attending all review meetings

---

Exercise 10.2

- Who works with children in care?
- What professional and non-professional roles are necessary?
- Who else is part of the team around the child?

---

people are also defined by the Children Act, 1989 and include children accommodated under Section 20 of the Act, where a court order is not required:

> Every local authority shall provide accommodation for any child in need within their area who appears to them to require accommodation.

Children can also be placed in care following court proceedings under Section 33 of the Act:

> Where a care order is made with respect to a child it shall be the duty of the local authority designated by the order to receive the child into their care and keep him in their care while the order remains in force.

While looked-after children is the legally correct phrase for thinking about this group of children and young people, there is an alternative phrase which, as with family support, is in everyday use: 'children in care'. In this chapter we will utilise this latter phrase.

In England at any given time there are approximately 60,000 children in care, with the majority of them being placed with foster carers (Frost and Parton, 2009). It should be recalled that due to children coming in and out of care in a given year many more than 60,000 will come into contact with the care system.

It is argued here that children in care have in recent years become increasingly subject to interprofessional support and intervention. Arguably, prior to the Children Act 1989, children in care were seen as the major, or even the sole, concern of social workers. The strengthening of the role of the local authority (as opposed to the Social Services Department) within the 1989 Act and the introduction of the concept of looked-after children helped to emphasise the fact the child in care was a shared corporate responsibility, highlighted by the use of the phrase 'corporate parent' to outline the overall responsibility of the local authority (see Stein,

2009, p. 13). The process was also strengthened by the introduction of the Looked-after Children assessment forms, often called LAC forms, which contained a strong emphasis on the holistic child – where many factors including health, education and leisure were explored.

The Children Act 2004, and the subsequent development Children's Trust arrangements, embedded the interprofessional working with children in care. This was often institutionalised through the establishment of multi-agency panels to develop and steer practice and policy development with children in care. This policy shift was given an increased emphasis by the Care Matters process, which is worthy of some detailed attention in this context.

Care Matters is a policy initiative focused on children in care and, as the name suggests, a specialist element of the 'Every Child Matters' policy stream. The Care Matters approach contains interprofessional work at its heart. It sees the young person as a whole and therefore requires a holistic professional approach. The approach is underpinned by four key themes:

> DCSF's Placement Stability Development Project found that improvement strategies which address all four factors – 'An improved front door', 'Strong management grip', 'Improved choice' and 'Improved support' are likely to be most effective.
>
> (Department for Children, Schools and Families, 2008a, 2.16)

The Green Paper, 'Care matters: transforming the lives of children and young people in care', was published in October, 2006, and represented the start of a major policy initiative from the New Labour government. A period of consultation followed, and in the spring of 2007 the White Paper, 'Care matters: time for change', was published. The Children and Young Persons Act, reflecting by and large the content of the White Paper, received the Royal Assent in 2008. This was followed by a concrete action plan, *Care Matters: Time to deliver for children in care*.

The *Care Matters* process presents a radical vision – offering a way forward for a group of children, many of whom have suffered a catalogue of abuse and disadvantage, which historically has often been supplemented, rather than resolved, by the care system (see the Utting

Reports of 1991 and 1997). The Green Paper argued this point as follows:

'The State has a unique responsibility for children in care. It has taken on the task of parenting some of society's most vulnerable children and in doing so it must become everything a good parent should be

(Department of Health, 2006, 1.1)

The White Paper makes a related point:

A good corporate parent must offer everything that a good parent would provide and more, addressing both the difficulties which the children experience and the challenges of parenting within a complex system of services.

(2007, 1.20)

These are important statements which finally represent a break with the Poor Law idea that care should be 'less eligible' (that is not as desirable as living in the community). The Care Matters process normalises being in care in the sense that the standard should be that of the 'good parent'.

This rhetoric is brought together by a pledge to children in care to ensure that they receive a reasonable level of care (see White Paper, 2007, 1.25). The pledge is aimed at providing a guarantee of the standard of care offered by the local authority and its partners.

The Care Matters process then seems to be a genuine attempt to modernise the care system and to rescue it from the legacy of poor outcomes with which it is often, and perhaps unjustly, associated (Stein, 2006).

In order to emphasise the interprofessional nature of Care Matters we will focus on one aspect of process – the central place of education.

Educational issues for children in care have featured frequently in recent legislation including in the Children Acts of 1989 and 2004, and the Children (Leaving Care) Act, 2000. Despite this focus educational outcomes for children in care have been poor, while improving slightly in recent years.

The Care Matters documentation devotes considerable space to education which is arguably the dominant theme of the reform process. In summary the White Paper proposes the following in relation to school age children:

- high-quality early years education for children in care

- a requirement to ensure that care planning decisions do not disrupt education and that moves in years 10 and 11 should only be in exceptional circumstances
- Ofsted review of the position of children in care in 2008/9
- children in care should only be excluded from school as a last resort
- alternative provision for excluded children in care from day one
- improvements in National Minimum Standards for foster and residential care relating to education
- a strengthened role for the designated teacher
- a virtual school head for children in care in each local authority
- personal education plans for children in care
- funding to pay for extra help for children in care not reaching their targets
- specified extended services for children in care
- improved home-school agreements
- an improvement in services for children with special educational needs.

(Department for Education and Skills, 2007, 4.10–4.56)

This brief summary hardly does justice to the width and depth of the Care Matters proposals relating to the education of children in care. In addition there are a range of proposals relating to further and higher education. This seems to be an attempt to address poor educational outcomes for the care population, as education is often identified as a route out of poverty and poor outcomes for children in care.

In an official review of recent research on children in care, Stein argues the centrality of interprofessional working as follows:

Several of the studies contained within the Overview point to the importance of integrated working. The *Reunification* study showed that both multi-agency assessment and monitoring was associated with better outcomes for children and young people, in respect of stability after returning home...Interprofessional working was identified in the *Educating Difficult Adolescents* study as an important dimension of the *Quality of Care Index,* and as facilitating effective participation and advocacy work.

(Stein, 2009, p. 126)

A closer look

Another study summarised by Stein identifies seven enablers of inter-agency collaboration:

- understanding and respecting roles and responsibilities of other services
- good communication, regular contact and meetings
- common priorities and trust
- joint training
- knowing what services are available and who to contact
- clear guidelines and procedures for working together
- low staff turnover. (2009, p. 126)

We can see then, that at least at central government level, there has been a strong emphasis on interprofessional working with children in care. We have focused here on educational issues, and it should be noted that if space allowed a similar case could be made around health, accommodation and leisure concerns.

How can these worthy intentions be put into practice? In 2008 the government published an action plan to guide the local implementation of the Care Matters process, which contains a strong emphasis on interprofessional working. It argues that

Local partners should ensure that they:

- are able to undertake high quality assessments to support good decision-making about when to admit children in care;
- ensure the provision of specialist intensive multi-agency family support services where care is not the right option; and
- provide intensive and responsive rehabilitation and support where care is a short term option.

(Department for Children, Schools and Families, 2008a 2.5)

Again the emphasis on education can be perceived:

The local authority will also have to ensure that a child or young person's education is not disrupted as a result of care planning decisions, especially at Key Stage 4. Stability is fundamental to ensuring a good education for all children and children in care experience too many changes of school places'

(2008a, 2.13)

The holistic, interprofessional approach is also reflected in policy approaches to children in care:

Case study

This case study demonstrates how professionals need to work together to address the holistic needs of children and young people.

Fiona is 16 and has been living with her foster carers for 3 years. She is subject to a care order – she was neglected by her mother who had a severe alcohol problem.

Fiona receives support from many professionals. She has some mild learning difficulties and has support in school from a learning mentor. She has a social worker who she gets on well with and whom she meets regularly.

Fiona has recently met with a Pathway Planning Advisor who is helping her to think about independent living and when she would be able to move on to her own flat – which Fiona is very keen on. She is also in touch with the looked-after children health team; they have been talking to Fiona about her sexual health.

Fiona has recently re-established contact with her mother and is helping care for her mother, particularly at weekends. Fiona is also in contact with a young carers support group.

Fiona attends her own review meetings, where the school, social worker, foster carers, Pathway Planning and health professionals get together to help Fiona plan for the future.

The professionals who work with Fiona try to communicate with each other and actively involve Fiona in all decisions about her future. The aim is to support Fiona to make a successful transition to adulthood.

As well as thinking about how they can improve the support offered by social workers, local partners should consider the range of services in place for foster and residential carers to help them to support children in care. There should be a broad package of high quality education health and leisure services on offer to ensure the wide range of children's needs are being met.

(2.15)

Thus we can see that policy and practice with children in care has become increasing interprofessional in the approach taken.

Interprofessional work in family support and with children in care

It has been argued here that professional work in the fields of family support and children in care was largely seen as part of social work practice dominated by professional social workers, often based in local authority social services departments. The dominant role of social workers has been displaced in different ways, in family support it has been almost entirely displaced and is now largely undertaken by a wide range of workers – family support workers, parent support workers, outreach workers – often located in health or education settings and/or employed by the voluntary sector. In terms of children in care, social work remains the dominant profession, but with education, health, youth work and other professionals playing an enhanced role. In both fields, therefore, interprofessional work is central.

A future for interprofessional working in family support and with children in care

In this chapter we have argued that in the fields of family support and work with children and young people in care we have a seen a fundamental shift towards enhanced interprofessional working.

It has been argued that in order to address children and young people's needs in the round, a holistic interprofessional approach is required. In retrospect it seems strange that we used to see children has having needs that fell in separate boxes that were responded to by separate, silo-based organisations. While we do not yet have sufficient rigorous research evidence to demonstrate that the outcomes for these groups of children and young people have improved dramatically, the research we have reported suggests a positive direction that should be sustained and developed if we are to improve the lives of these vulnerable groups of children and young people.

A skill-base for interprofessional practice in work with vulnerable children and young people

We have a considerable body of knowledge about what service users expect from professionals. The research here is remarkably consistent. Here we draw on Cree and Davis (2007) who spoke to 59 service users, with experience of a wide range of services, and from research undertaken as a backdrop to the Government's work on Care Matters (DCSF, 2008a).

Cree and Davis summarise service users' expectations as follows:

> responsiveness, building relationships, being person-centred, providing emotional and practical support, being holistic, balancing rights, risks and protection, being evidence-based, future-orientated and there for the long term
>
> (Cree and Davis, 2007, p. 149)

In a different context young people in care were asked about their views of social workers. They reflected as follows on their negative experiences:

> You get to know one then they leave.
> I have had around 30 social workers in 10 years.
> I thought you were meant to get a working relationship with social workers, but it's like I don't even know her.

And on what they wanted from a social worker as follows:

> The qualities my ideal social worker would have are: to be friendly and compassionate, to listen to what I

want and what ways I can go around things to get it, to always be there for me, not to nag at me when I don't know what to do for my future.

(Department for Children, Schools and Families, 2008b, p. 9)

The views of service users can be used as a basis for developing a positive practice. We also know what helps to ensure effective interprofessional practice (the remainder of this chapter draws on Anning *et al.*, 2006). Reflecting on this knowledge we can perhaps suggest the professional skill sets that are required to take practice in this field forward.

Shared planning, procedures and systems

Effective interprofessional teamwork requires shared procedures that have been developed with the participation of all professionals involved. However, procedures need to be more than pieces of paper and need to be enacted and owned by front-line staff. Reflective practice is an interactive process through which informed, thinking professionals interpret and enact procedures in the best interest of children and young people. Procedures and protocols must be regularly reviewed and consulted around and, when necessary, changed and reformed to reflect changes in practice. This process forms part of a learning loop where policy structures practice, but where practice should, in turn, inform and reform policy.

Leadership vision

A key variable in implementing effective practice in interprofessional work is the leadership offered by senior staff. Effective leadership involves individuals who can work in the ever-changing world of interprofessional practice and characterised by the skills of motivating staff, providing a vision and supporting reflective practice.

Role clarity and a sense of purpose

One challenge of responsive interprofessional working is that roles can become blurred and complex. Effective interprofessional working should not imply that people lose a sense of purpose and clarity about their professional roles. Each worker should have a clear role and a definite sense of purpose of how they can contribute to the overall purposes of the team or the plan for each child.

Addressing barriers related to status/hierarchies

Interprofessional work is difficult. One reason for this is the legacy of status and hierarchical barriers. It is important that when diverse professionals come together, they respect each others skill set and then they may find that the differences are not as great as they imagined. One advantage of an interprofessional team interacting on a day-to-day basis when they are co-located (the sharing of office and other space by professionals) is that this can help break down some professional prejudices and ease the practicalities of communication.

Agreed strategic objectives and shared core aims

Staff in interprofessional settings need to have a clear sense of shared objectives and core aims. The exact nature of this will be dependent on the specific setting and purpose of the team, but all teams delivering child and family services have a shared rationale within the broad framework provided by the Children Acts of 1989 and 2004, and the 'five outcomes'. The five outcomes provide a springboard for a shared sense of common purpose across children's services. The Children's Workforce Development Council (CWDC) have also developed a Common Core of competences which can help to drive a strong sense of working together (see www.cwdcouncil.org.uk).

Effective communication between team members and partner agencies

Most interprofessional teams have to relate to a range of agencies who may fund, second, host or manage the team. Whatever these structures and funding streams they need to be clear and transparent to providers and users of the service.

Co-location of service deliverers

The idea of co-location is encouraged in the Green Paper, Every Child Matters (Department for Education and Skills, 2003), and the subsequent stream of official guidance. The idea of co-location has become a reality in many services – within children's centres, youth offending and family support teams providing prime examples. There is evidence to suggest that co-location enhances communication, learning and understanding of roles. It is important to note that co-location assists, but does not guarantee, effective joint working.

Acknowledging professional diversity

Interprofessional teams represent differing professions with diverse roles. We have seen that a wide range of professionals have a role to play both in relation to family support and children in care. While interprofessional working attempts to improve coordination between these groups, it should not attempt to ignore differences. Team members need to be encouraged to celebrate their differences, and also perceive that they are held together by a shared vision and sense of purpose (Ancona *et al.*, 2007).

Awareness of impact of change on service users

Effective interprofessional practice crucially revolves around effective partnership with service users. Practitioners should be acutely aware of the impact of interprofessional practice on service users. Evidence is beginning to emerge that suggests that interprofessional practice can have a positive impact on service users (see *Children and Society*: Special Issue, 2009).

Joint client-focused activities and professional development

The most effective interprofessional working emerges from actual practice. Professionals should be encouraged to work together across professional boundaries – and then to reflect on this through tools such as case discussions, joint training and group supervision. These methods provide powerful opportunities for developing a shared approach to practice.

A strengths-based approach

Effective practice in the field of family support and with children in care can be effectively underpinned by a strengths-based approach. This means that professionals recognise and aim to build on the strengths and positives of children, young people and their families. Effective interprofessional work needs to be underpinned by shared values and a shared approach (Fleischer *et al.*, 2006).

Conclusion

This chapter has provided an outline of how professionals can work together in the fields of family support and children in care. It has been argued that by working together professionals can improve outcomes for children and young people within their families and when and if they come into care.

The primary points are that:

- professionals can work together to provide effective family support for children and young people who live together with their family
- tools such as the Common Assessment Framework can assist such processes
- children in care have needs which can be successfully addressed through multi-professional practice
- we have research evidence which identifies the challenges facing professionals working together and how these can be addressed.

We can conclude, then, that if we place children and young people at the heart of the process, it is possible to construct a 'team around' the child/young person which is capable of delivering an effective service with the child's interests at the centre of every aspect of the intervention. Indeed, adopting this kind of approach actually facilitates good interprofessional working.

Further reading

Family support

Dolan, P., Canavan, J., Pinkerton, J. (2006) (eds) *Family Support as Reflective Practice*. London: Jessica Kingsley Publishers. A fascinating collection of papers, with an international flavour. The editors are enthusiastic in proposing a 'reflective practice' approach to planning and delivering family support.

Penn, H. and Gough, D. (2002) The price of a loaf of bread: some conceptions of family support. *Children and Society* 16(1), 17–32. A useful and accessible paper which draws on a local authority case study to develop some wider ideas about family support.

Children in care

Stein, M. (2009) *Quality Matters in Children's Services*, London: Jessica Kingsley Publishers. A very good summary of a wide range of government-funded case studies relevant to working with children in care. Written in an accessible fashion, the book points to the importance of interprofessional working in this field.

Department for Children, Schools and Families (2008) *Care Matters: Time to Deliver for Children in Care*. London: DCSF. Care Matters is a crucial change programme for children in care – this is a progressive and interprofessional approach to working with children in care.

References

Ancona, D., Malone, T. W., Orlikowski, W. J. and Senge, P. M. (2007) In praise of the incomplete leader. *Harvard Business Review*, February, 94–99.

Anning, A., Cottrell, D., Frost, N., Green, J. and Robinson, M. (2006) *Developing Multi-professional Working for Integrated Children's Services*, London: OUP.

Canavan. J., Dolan, P. and Pinkerton, J. (2000) *Family Support: Direction from Diversity*, London: Jessica Kingsley Publishers.

Children Act (1989) www.opsi.gov.uk/acts/acts/acts1989.

Children and Society (2009) Special issue: The outcomes of integrated working, Chichester: John Wiley & Sons, Ltd.

Cree, V. and Davis, A. (2007) *Social Work: Voices from the Inside*, London: Routledge.

Department for Children, Schools and Families (2008a) *Care Matters: Time to Deliver for Children in Care*, London, DCSF.

Department for Children, Schools and Families (2008b) *Piloting the Social Work Practice Model: A Prospectus*, London: DCSF.

Department for Education and Skills (2006) *Care Matters: Transforming the Lives of Children and Young People in Care*. London: DfES.

Department for Education and Skills (2007*) Care Matters: Time for Change*, London: DfES.

Department for Education and Skills (2003) *Every Child Matters*, London: DfES.

Dolan, P., Canavan, J. and Pinkerton, J. (eds) (2006) *Family Support as Reflective Practice*, London: Jessica Kingsley Publishers.

Gilligan, R. (2000) Family support: issues and prospects, in J. Canavan, P. Dolan, and J. Pinkerton, (eds) *Family Support: Diversion From Diversity*, London: Jessica Kingsley Publishers.

Fleischer, J., Warner, J., McCulty, C. J. and Marks, M. (2006) Youth advocacy, in P. Dolan, J. Canavan, and J. Pinkerton (eds) *Family Support as Reflective Practice*, London: Jessica Kingsley Publishers.

Frost, N., Lloyd, A. and Jeffrey, L. (2003) *The RHP Companion to Family Support*, Lyme Regis: Russell House Publishing.

Frost, N. and Parton, N. (2009) *Understanding Children's Social Care*, London: Sage.

Glass, N. (1999) Sure start; the Development of an Early Intervention Programme for Young Children in the United Kingdom. *Children and Society* 13, 257–64.

Hardiker, P., Exton, K. and Barker, M. (1991) *Policies and Practices in Preventive Child Care*, Aldershot: Avebury.

Parker, R. (1980) *Caring for Separated Children*, London: MacMIllan.

Penn, H. and Gough, D. (2002) The price of a loaf of bread: some conceptions of family support. *Children and Society* 16(1), 17–32.

Stein, M. (2006) A wrong turn? *Guardian*, 6 January.

Stein, M. (2009) *Quality Matters in Children's Services*, London: Jessica Kingsley Publishers.

Utting, Sir W. (1997) *People Like Us: The Report of the Review of the Safeguards for Children Living Away from Home*, London: HMSO.

Utting, W. (1991) *Children in Public Care: A Review of Residential Child Care*, London: HMSO.

Chapter 11
Older people

Michelle Cornes

Chapter summary

In the UK, the concept of personalisation is at the forefront of the health and social care policy agenda (HM Government, 2007). Personalisation emphasises the importance of professionals working together to tailor public services according to need and to open up opportunities for greater flexibility and choice. It is important to begin from the premise that there is a strong fit between the concepts of personalisation and interprofessional practice and that one will not be achieved without the other:

> Interprofessional working is not about fudging the boundaries between the professions and trying to create a generic care worker. It is instead about developing professionals who are confident in their own core skills and expertise, who are fully aware and confident in the skills of fellow health and care professionals, and who conduct their own practice in an non-hierarchical and collegiate way with other members of the working team, so as to continuously improve the health of their communities and to meet the real care needs of individual patients and clients.
>
> (McGrath, 1991 quoted in CAIPE, 2007, p. 8)

At a strategic level, personalisation poses new challenges for collaborative practice because it requires local partnerships to work together to produce a broader range of services for people to choose from. A key principle of personalisation is social inclusion in which support is as much about enabling service users and carers to access universal services (such as transport, leisure and life-long learning) as well as more traditional care services such as domiciliary, residential and nursing home care (Department of Health, 2006). The Department of Health (DH) (2008, p. 5) makes the point that:

> Importantly the ability to make choices about how people live their lives should not be restricted to those who live in their own homes. It is about better support, more tailored to individual choices and preferences in all care settings.

At the level of front-line practice, personalisation should mean more power and resources being shared with people at the front line – service users, carers and front-line workers – so

▶

143

they are empowered to 'co-produce' their own solutions to the difficulties they are best placed to know about (Carr, 2008).

In making this vision a reality for older people and their carers, a key challenge will be extending the principles of personalisation into the sphere of integrated care and support planning where the social and medical models of disability rub side by side. In exploring what progress has been made toward achieving this policy goal for older people, this chapter focuses on integrated work across agencies and different professionals in one particularly challenging practice area (delayed hospital discharge) and two contrasting policy solutions for encouraging integrated work across agencies and different professionals (the reimbursement process and intermediate care).

Learning objectives

This chapter will cover:

- the range and nature of collaborative interprofessional working arrangements necessary to provide an effective and person-focused set of services for older people
- how personalisation approaches are key to producing a broader range of services for people to access, and how these might be considered jointly by different agencies and professionals
- how the key principles of *social inclusion, personalisation, self-directed support* and *co-production* pose new challenges for local collaborative practices in assessment, support and rehabilitation processes; and how these must include an assessment of the individual and their carers' wishes and ambitions, and the contributions each can make in achieving these as part of interprofessional working and local interagency policies and arrangements
- the importance and operation of assessment tools and frameworks, including Single Assessment Processes (SAPs) and Comprehensive Geriatric Assessments when assessments, treatment or care decisions are made, and the place of proposals for a Common Assessment Framework in the future for interprofessional and interagency working.

Integrated care and support planning

Increasing frailty and ill health will mean that for some older people promoting independence, well-being and choice will require access to a range of different services and professionals including doctors, nurses, physiotherapists, occupational therapists, speech and language therapists, podiatrists, pharmacists, dentists, nutritionists, continence advisors, optometrists, audiologists and social workers. According to Swift (2005), the activities of any one discipline may at best be wasted or at worst harmful if they are not related to an assessment and planned programme of care. However, a common understanding of coordinated care is often

assumed when, in reality, the concept is neither clearly defined nor completely understood (Ehrlich *et al.*, 2009).

In England and Wales, the statutory framework which underpins interagency and interprofessional working for older people and other vulnerable adults is outlined in Section 47 of the NHS and Community Care Act 1990. Under this section of the Act, if during an assessment it appears that the person may have health or housing needs, the local authority must invite the NHS or housing authority (if different from the assessing authority) to participate in the assessment. There is however no statutory obligation on the NHS or the housing authority to cooperate (Mandelstam, 2005).

The early guidance which accompanied the 1990 Act introduced to the UK the concept of Assessment and Care Management (Social Services Inspectorate/ Scottish Office Social Work Services Group 1991a, b). The central task of the care management process is to coordinate a holistic assessment of need (a community care assessment) which draws together a range of 'specialist' medical and non-medical assessments. Thereafter the task becomes one of coordinating the different professional inputs and services into an overarching (integrated) care plan; delivering a 'seamless service' in which the boundaries between primary health care, secondary health care and social care are invisible to the service user and their carers (Department of Health, 1990, s.1:8/1:9).

In England, the guidance on community care assessment was revised in 2001 with the introduction of the Single Assessment Process (SAP) (Department of Health, 2001a, 2002a). This aimed to improve assessment practice specifically as it relates to older people. Ormiston (2002) points out that it may be helpful to think of 'unified' rather than 'single assessment', as SAP is intended solely to ensure that relevant information about a person is brought together whenever treatment or care decisions are made, thereby streamlining the process and reducing duplication for service users. More recently, proposals have been tabled for a Common Assessment Framework (CAF) (Department of Health, 2009a). This will have generic application across all care groups and is principally targeted at finding IT solutions to the problem of sharing information across agencies. Significantly, the guidance on SAP and CAF do not depart radically from the earlier guidance on community care assessment and care management. Indeed, when launching SAP it was acknowledged that local authorities had been striving to implement the stages of single assessment for some ten years and that the onus was now on health to adopt a similar approach (Department of Health, 2002a). SAP did however introduce four new distinct assessment types (contact, overview, in-depth and Comprehensive Geriatric Assessment). Comprehensive geriatric assessment (which is a practice relevant across the UK) is defined by the British Geriatrics Society (2010) as a multidimensional and usually interdisciplinary diagnostic process comprising a number of specified domains (see A closer look below). Circumstances which will warrant a comprehensive geriatric assessment and therefore an interprofessional response include:

- an older person admitted acutely to hospital who is likely to develop specialist medical care needs, based on a case-finding approach in a general ward
- transfers of care for rehabilitation/re-enablement
- a frail patient prior to surgery or experiencing two or more geriatric syndromes of falls, delirium, incontinence or immobility
- a person receiving intermediate care or other community-based rehabilitation.

(British Geriatrics Society, 2010, p. 1)

Abendstern *et al.* (2008) point out that the greater participation of older people in the assessment process may conflict with the role of assessment as a professional tool. Indeed, the first key challenge for personalisation is that the circumstances that will warrant a

A closer look

Components of comprehensive geriatric assessment (British Geriatrics Society, 2010, p. 1)

Domains	Items to be assessed
Medical	Comorbid conditions and disease severity
	Medication review
	Nutritional status
	Problem list
Mental health	Cognition
	Mood and anxiety
	Fears
Functional capacity	Basic activities of daily living
	Gait and balance
	Activity/exercise status
	Instrumental activities of daily living
Social circumstances	Informal support available from family and friends
	Social network such as visitors or daytime activities
	Eligibility for being offered care resources
Use or potential use of telehealth technology	Transport facilities
	Accessibility to local resources

comprehensive geriatric assessment are also circumstances when older people by virtue of their frailty or illness may not be in a position to take control of, or even participate in, the assessment and care planning process. According to Lymbery (2010), the policy rhetoric which surrounds personalisation does not engage sufficiently with the complexity of managing the balance between the enhancement of individuals independence against the reality that – for many – dependence, vulnerability and the need for protection are dominant features of their lives. The law and policy guidance surrounding what to do in such circumstance is complex. Under the 1990 NHS Community Care Act it is permissible under emergency circumstances to arrange services without assessment, given that an assessment should be carried out as soon as is practicable (s.47 [5,6]). In terms of cognitive impairment, the Mental Capacity Act (2005) has enshrined in law the notion of 'presumption of capacity' and a requirement to provide appropriate support to enable people to participate in decision making about their care. This might include so-called advance care planning and the completion of a statement of the person's wishes and preferences about their future care (Department of Health, 2007). However, pressure on services at key transition points may make these legislative guidelines difficult to translate into practice and can cause considerable tension between different professional groups such as social workers and hospital discharge coordinators (nurses). For example, until the advent of so-called interim care or intermediate care, pressure to free-up hospital beds meant that a common problem was older people being moved straight from hospital into permanent residential or nursing care without affording them with enough time for rehabilitation or proper decision making with regard to the choice of suitable care home (Cornes et al., 2008).

To achieve optimum outcomes for older people and the efficient use of services overall, assessment must include expert medical and nursing input to ensure the accurate diagnosis and assessment of potential for rehabilitation. In the context of community care, rehabilitation is defined in its broadest sense as an enabling process in which societies, communities, agencies and professionals meet the social, psychological, physical and economic needs of the person through knowledge, skill, respect, understanding and agreement. Importantly, it has long been recognised that personalisation and 'co-production' are important components of the rehabilitation process given that it must include an assessment of where the individual and their carers are, where they wish to be and the contributions each must make to achieving their ambitions and meeting their needs (Baker et al., 1997).

When planning for recovery and/or rehabilitation it is likely that a plethora of specialist assessment tools and outcome measures will be used (Hastings, 2005). For example, for nutritional status this might be weight or recent weight change. For gait and balance it might be speed of walking six metres or ability to stand unaided for a minute. For cognition it would be a tool validated for older people such as the Mini Mental State Examination (British Geriatrics Society, 2010). It is crucially important that there is a consistent approach between the different professional groups as to how this information will be coordinated. In the earlier guidance on assessment and care management, local authorities were identified as 'lead agents' for the organisation and delivery of interdisciplinary community care with social workers acting as 'care managers'.[1] More recent guidance has largely eroded the lead role of the local authority social worker and it is now acknowledged that the lead worker might be a single person or possibly a multidisciplinary team of professionals who convene to coordinate the individuals care and support needs (Department of Health, 2009a). The care manager may also be the older person themselves:[2]

The Community Care Direct Payments Act 1996 enabled local authorities to make cash payments to service users in lieu of directly provided services. While

---

[1] In the UK, the term 'case' management was rejected in favour of 'care' management to highlight that it was the care and not the person being managed (Social Services Inspectorate/Scottish Office Social Work Services Group (1991b).
[2] Compared to other service-user groups, the take-up of direct payments has been traditionally low among older people (Leece and Leece, 2006).

direct payments can be used to purchase services from the voluntary and private sector, many people choose to use the money to employ their own personal assistants, essentially becoming their own care managers.

(Glasby and Duffy, 2007, p. 2)

In social care, 'self-directed support' is a key concept within the personalisation policy agenda (Carr, 2008). However, in health, while there is considerable interest in self-care it is suggested that particularly for people with long-term conditions and a range of complex health and social care needs, having someone to lead on the care planning process and to coordinate services can have a hugely positive impact for the person and their carer (Department of Health, 2009b). Significantly, within the CAF guidance (Department of Health, 2009a), the concept of the 'lead worker' relates to the 'professional care worker':

> Personalisation happens in the interaction between a health professional and patient . . . The key thing [the patient wants] is a reliable, known point of contact with the system, who knows about their life circumstances as well as their condition. This key liaison must know about local support services and proactively keep up with the patient even by telephone or email.
>
> (Sarner, 2010, p. 12)

It is the role of the lead worker to collate the summary findings from all the different specialist assessments into an overarching, single care plan that is owned by the person but can be accessed by those providing direct care/services or other relevant people as agreed by the individual (e.g. their carer) (Department of Health, 2009b). The expectation is that everyone with a both a long-term health condition and social care needs will have an integrated and personalised care (support) plan if they want one (Department of Health, 2006). The care planning process should:

- promote choice and control, putting the individual, their need and choices at the centre of the process
- be anticipatory and proactive with contingency (or emergency planning) to manage crises episodes
- facilitate joint working, ensuring that people receive coordinated care packages, reducing fragmentation between services

- provide information and support for self-care
- focus on goals and outcomes that people want to achieve, including carers.

(Department of Health, 2009b, p. 11).

To guide the process of integrating the different specialist components into an overarching care (support) plan, it is helpful if the different professional contributors agree to work within a shared 'outcomes framework'. Outcomes refer to the impacts or end results of services on a person's life. Outcomes-focused services therefore aim to achieve the aspirations, goals and priorities identified by service users, in contrast to services whose contents or forms of delivery are standardised or determined solely by those who deliver them. One framework developed specifically for use with older people is shown in the table in the next 'A closer look: Outcomes Framework (based on a review of the research evidence on the outcomes valued by older people)' overleaf (Glendinning *et al.*, 2006). Although this framework was designed for use in social care it is potentially very useful for guiding interprofessional practice because it facilitates teamworking around common goals and, very importantly, renders technical or clinical information into everyday language which is accessible to all stakeholders including older people and their carers. Importantly, Glendinning *et al.* (2006) alert us to the distinction which needs to be made between 'change

Key learning points

Triggers to indicate the need for a comprehensive geriatric assessment

Circumstances which will warrant a comprehensive geriatric assessment and therefore an interprofessional response include:

- an older person admitted acutely to hospital who is likely to develop specialist medical care needs, based on a case finding approach in a general ward
- transfers of care for rehabilitation/re-enablement.
- a frail patient prior to surgery or experiencing two or more geriatric syndromes of falls, delirium, incontinence or immobility
- a person receiving intermediate care or other community-based rehabilitation.

(British Geriatrics Society, 2010, p. 1)

A closer look

Outcomes framework (based on a review of the research evidence on the outcomes valued by older people)

Outcomes involving change	Improvements in physical symptoms
	Improvements in physical functioning and mobility
	Improvements in morale
Outcomes involving maintenance and prevention	Meeting basic physical needs
	Ensuring personal safety and security
	Having a clean and tidy home environment
	Keeping alert and active
	Having social contact and company, including opportunities to contribute as well as receive help
	Having control over daily routines
Service process outcomes	These refer to the ways that services are accessed and delivered and include:
	Feeling valued and respected
	Being treated as an individual
	Having a say and control over services
	Value for money
	A 'good fit' with other sources of support
	Compatibility with, and respect for, cultural and religious preferences

Source: based on Glendinning *et al.* (2006)

outcomes' and 'maintenance outcomes'. This is to ensure that older people who may have only limited rehabilitative potential are also enabled to make choices and to receive personalised care and support.

Barriers to delivering good practice

Despite growing recognition of the importance of adopting a personalised and integrated way of working, the approach is still not widespread enough and barriers persist (Department of Health, 2009b). In a review of the international literature on care coordination, Ehrlich *et al.* (2009) conclude that although

Key learning points

Summary of integrated care and support planning:

- The central task of integrated care and support planning is to coordinate a holistic assessment of need which draws together a range of specialist medical and non-medical assessments. Different professional inputs and services should be integrated into an overarching care plan which is personalised and individually tailored; delivering a seamless service in which the boundaries between different services are invisible to the service user and their carers.
- To achieve optimum outcomes for older people and the efficient use of services overall, assessment must include accurate diagnosis and assessment of potential for rehabilitation.
- It is important to ensure that older people and their carers are actively engaged in these processes and supported to act as care managers if that is their wish, for example through the use of individual budgets and direct payments.

complex systems are capable of being flexible for those who must navigate them over a protracted period of time, they are usually experienced as being fragmented, confusing and overwhelming.

At the root of the problem is the compartmentalisation of health and social care services. In many countries, regulation of health care is by either a national health system (as in the UK and Nordic countries) or a social insurance system administered by central government (as in Germany and the Netherlands), whereas social care is overseen by local or regional government (Billings and Leichsenring, 2005; Jacobs *et al.*, 2009). According to Ware *et al.* (2003), separate budgets for health and social care can undermine joint working. As Wistow (1990) points out, while local authorities were identified as lead agents for community care they were only ever responsible for the social care element of it, with health authorities remaining responsible for all those elements which they provide. In terms of what this means for front line 'joint working' practices it has been observed that

Social services assess needs for home care, day care, residential and nursing care while community nurses assess needs for the health services they provide.

When practitioners identify a need for a service which is perceived as being outside of their area or domain, the collaborative process is one of 'handing over the stick' or 'passing the baton' and ensuring that the older person is 'referred on' for further assessment by another agency.

(Cornes and Clough, 2001a, p. 64)

Worth (1998) has pointed to the considerable mutual suspicion that can exist between health and social care professionals about the adequacy of each others' assessments and the culture of seeing for oneself. The practice of 'gatekeeping' can become rife in times of resource constraints when the aim is to assess people out of support rather than to provide it (Beresford, 2009). According to Walker (1994) the community care system quickly became discredited by competition in some areas between health and social services to avoid supporting the most costly frail older people.

While some measures have been introduced to address these structural issues,[3] it is significant that the health and social care funding divide will be taken forward in terms of the implementation of personalisation with separate direct payments for health[4] and social care:

[Direct payments for health] will mirror the principles and arrangements underlying social care direct payments. This should promote the integration of care, and greatly benefit those individuals who receive direct payment in both systems or move from one system to the other.

(Department of Health, 2009c, p. 6)

This is at odds with the user perspective, given that we know service users do not distinguish between health and social care needs but see both as part of overall support and personal care needs (Glasby and Duffy, 2007).

In terms of the potential for collision between different professional cultures and the medical and social models of disability, it was noted earlier that while social care promotes the principle of self-directed support, long-term (health) condition management advocates the role of the professional care manager. It has since been noted that progress on personalisation has been patchy and hesitant and that progress has been particularly limited in relation to service users with complex needs (Commission for Social Care Inspection (CSCI), 2009).

Cornes and Clough (2004) argue that another very practical reason for the continuation of silo delivery of support from multiple agencies is that in social work as elsewhere, case loads are such that there is often very little time left to undertake the

Key learning points

Summary of barriers to delivering good interprofessional practice:

- Both in the UK and elsewhere delivering integrated support and care planning for older people is particularly challenging. This is often attributed to the compartmentalisation of health and social care.
- Assessment is often linked to gatekeeping which can make collegiate working between different professionals difficult in times of resource constraints.
- Heavy case loads often make it difficult for front-line health and social care practitioners to find the time to undertake the practical tasks of care coordination (e.g. setting up and attending case conferences and multidisciplinary meetings).
- For service users and carers, the above factors make accessing the care system confusing and difficult. The experience is usually one of fragmented provision rather than seamless services.

---

[3]Some measures have been introduced to overcome these structural barriers. In England, the 'flexibilities' contained in Section 31 of the Health Act 1999 have put in place the legal frameworks for 'pooled budgets' and 'care trusts'. Care trusts are a new type of primary care organisation that can commission both health and social care services, while the rationale for pooled budgets is that resources contributed to the pool by partner organisations will lose their distinctive health and social care identity (Glasby and Peck, 2004). However, only a small number of care trusts have been set up to date.

[4]Primary Care Trusts are already able to offer personal health budgets that do not involve giving the money directly to individuals. The Health Act (which received Royal Assent on 12 November 2009) extends these options by allowing selected primary care trust sites to pilot direct payments. http://www.dhcarenetworks.org.uk/_library/Resources/Personalhealthbudgets/PHB_newsletter_Dec_09_tagged.pdf, accessed 15 March 2010.

practical tasks of care coordination (e.g. setting up and attending case conferences and multidisciplinary meetings).

Other studies report similar findings, suggesting that few local authorities have been able to operate intensive-care management schemes for older people thereby translating into practice the interdisciplinary care management approach described in the policy frameworks above (Jacobs *et al.*, 2009). Kharicha *et al.* (2004) conclude that the underlying assumption that a greater degree of integration provides benefits to older people and their carers is a perspective that at times obscures the issue of resource availability, especially in the form of practical community services such as district nursing and home help.

Hospital discharge

One area where the tensions between health and social services often manifest is in the hospital discharge process. Delayed discharge from hospital has been identified as a problem in the UK since the birth of the welfare state (Schimmel, 1964). It is largely a problem associated with the care of older people who have ongoing need for support (Henwood, 2006). For older people staying in hospital for longer than necessary poses particular risks: hospital-acquired infections, falls, loss of mobility, social isolation, depression and loss of independence (Booth and Mead, 2007). A review of the evidence (Jacobs *et al.*, 2009) suggests that the most common cause of delayed discharge is organisational issues, including many involving coordination with social services (for example, where a person is waiting for completion of an assessment or a place in a care home). A recent report in Health Service Journal (Smulian, 2009) suggests that some 33 per cent of beds might be 'inappropriately occupied' both in terms of delayed discharge and admission to hospital for 'social' rather than 'medical' reasons. To address these issues, two key policy measures have been implemented in England, the reimbursement process and intermediate

care, both of which have since been acknowledged as being effective in reducing the rate of delayed discharge (Godfrey *et al.*, 2008). In the remainder of this chapter, we explore the impact of each of these very different policies for personalisation and joint working.

The reimbursement process

In 2002, the Department of Health announced its intention to tackle so-called bed blocking by introducing a system of reimbursement or 'cross-charging' similar to those introduced in Scandinavia (Department of Health, 2002b). What is distinctive about this approach is that it sets out very clear (statutory) guidelines for joint working around hospital discharge and, in a nutshell, enables the hospital acute trust to impose penalties on social services if they fail to comply (see box below). According to the Department of Health (2003) the reimbursement process is fundamentally about supporting best practice in interagency working around discharge planning as regards clear and timely communication with colleagues and patients.

The reimbursement process was enshrined in the Community Care (Delayed Discharges etc.) Act of 2003 and was implemented in England with effect from 5 January 2004. In England, social services can be held liable to charges of £100 per day (£120 in London) if a patient is found to be occupying an NHS acute hospital bed for the sole reason that they are waiting for a community care assessment or the delivery of community care services. As Booth and Mead (2007) point out, 'the intention is not that social services should make payments to the NHS, but that they should avoid doing so by providing services to their residents more rapidly'.

In a study of the impact of reimbursement (Godfrey *et al.*, 2008), it was noted that the main advantage of the Community Care (Delayed Discharge etc.) Act was that it did provide a robust framework as to what is expected of different parties in the hospital discharge process. Medical and nursing staff felt that the

A closer look

Summary of the reimbursement process

- NHS bodies have a statutory duty to notify social services of a patient's likely need for community care services (referred to as an 'assessment notification' or Section 2 notification). Section 2 notifications should only be made after patients' eligibility for continuing NHS care has been assessed. Where possible, assessment notifications should include an estimated date of discharge.

- There is a defined timescale – a minimum interval of two days for social services to complete the individual assessment and provide appropriate social care services.

- A second notification (Discharge Notification or Section 5 notification) follows completion of a multidisciplinary assessment and gives notice of the proposed day on which discharge will take place (minimum 24 hours notice).

- A reimbursement charge is paid by social services to the acute trust if the fact of social services not having met their obligations – that is to assess the patient (and carer if appropriate) and provide social care services within the set time – is the sole reason for the delay in discharge from hospital. If any element of the delay is related to NHS areas of responsibility then reimbursement does not apply.

- NHS bodies have to make both notifications to social services if a claim for reimbursement is to be triggered. The charge applies from 11 a.m. on the day after the proposed discharge date identified by the NHS in the discharge notification, or three days after social services have been given an assessment notification of a patient's likely need for community care services, which ever is later. If services are not in place after 11 a.m., the full daily charge will apply from that day onward.

Section 2 notifications had contributed to speedier response times from social work colleagues as regards arrangements for community care assessment. However, it was reported that the Section 5 had become a potent symbol of systemic tensions in the discharge process. On the wards, Section 5s were not issued in keeping with the guidance as a routine way of alerting the multidisciplinary team as to the proposed date of discharge. Instead Sections 5s were issued sparingly by health staff and were only 'put on' certain cases to alert social services that this particular patient was now a priority for discharge planning. According to one health professional in the study, 'We find that Section 5s prompt social workers a little bit . . . if you don't do a Section 5 patients can just languish a little bit'. On the wards, the effect of the Section 5 was to shift responsibility for delays down to individual social workers. Social workers argued that Section 5s were often 'used as a bat to beat us with' and felt unfairly singled out in the context of the wider multidisciplinary team. For example, if a delay was due to a wait for an occupational therapy assessment then the occupational therapists would not be subject to the same pressure and treatment as the social worker. Where it was perceived that a Section 5 had been issued unreasonably then the temptation was for social services to 'start playing things by the book', for example, returning a form because it had not been filled in correctly. Reimbursement was said to fuel this kind of low-level negativity and to have taken a lot of the goodwill out of the system.

In speeding up the system to deliver appropriate and timely discharge, there was little evidence of personalisation. One patient interviewed for the study described the ward as being like a 'sausage machine' with older people being processed through the wards in quick succession. A carer interviewed for the study described a process of negotiation and attrition when it came to making arrangements for her father to be discharged from hospital into a nursing home:

[Ward staff] are under pressure to have the bed for others to come in. I think if you are not strong, you might have ended up anywhere . . . because they are desperate to move them on. We were told that he has been in the bed too long. But on the other side, it was unhelpful for dad to stay there. He wasn't so well in hospital. If things are in place, they should move.

(Young and Stevenson, 2006, p. 340)

Intermediate care

Introduced in England as part of the National Service Framework for Older People (Department of Health, 2001a), intermediate care, like reimbursement, also has its roots in the desire to tackle delayed discharge from hospital. However, it can also work to prevent inappropriate admissions to hospital by providing access to rapid response health and social care in times of acute illness or crises. While reimbursement concentrates on speeding-up patient flow through the hospital, intermediate care works to actively bridge the transition from hospital to home by providing short-term access (usually for between two and six weeks) to rehabilitation and re-enablement (see Figure 11.1). This can be provided either in the person's own home or in a

designated care home. Jacobs *et al.* (2009) note that the focus on rehabilitation in older people's services has now largely been subsumed by the intermediate care agenda in the UK.

Intermediate care delivers its objectives of prevention of admission and speedier discharge through cross-professional working, with a single assessment framework, single professional records and shared protocols (Department of Health, 2009d). The essence of good practice in intermediate care is that people are seen as a whole, not just in terms of cognitive and physical abilities but as individuals in a social setting. It is this that defines its multidisciplinarity, which may be expressed through either multidisciplinary teams or new partnerships between services (Godfrey *et al.*, 2005). In many areas, 'co-location' is a common feature of intermediate care with different professionals (social workers, community nurses, occupational therapists and physiotherapists) and other groups of workers (health care assistants, support workers and social care workers) coming together to share the same building or office space. Volunteers have also been integrated into intermediate care teams with some success (Cornes, Weinstein and Manthorpe, 2006).

Although there is great diversity in provision, the evidence suggests that those intermediate care ser-

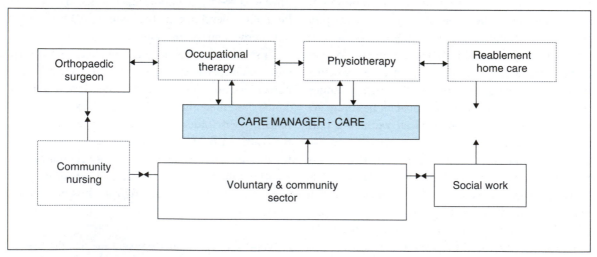

Figure 11.1 Care planning for intermediate care

vices which bring together strong interprofessional teams and devolved resources are working very effectively when it comes to delivering personalised support and the outcomes valued by older people (Glendinning *et al.*, 2006). Significantly, it has also been observed empirically that interdisciplinary working is more developed in intermediate care than that which exists in mainstream services (Godfrey *et al.*, 2005). However, this poses a significant problem in that once the intermediate care service is withdrawn, mainstream care services do not always continue to work in the same way, which can leave some older people feeling abandoned (Glendinning *et al.*, 2006, Manthorpe *et al.*, 2006). A key criticism of intermediate care is that it is time-limited when many older people may require ongoing support (Young *et al.*, 2005). According to Young and Stevenson (2006, p. 340) the challenge remains as to how to make the 'good practice' evident in intermediate care applicable across the wider system of care:

> It is useful to consider the underlying principles of intermediate care: multi-agency working; comprehensive shared assessments and person-centred care based on an enabling (rehabilitation approach). There is no fundamental reason why these good practice principles should be confined to intermediate care services. Rather the policy of intermediate care could be viewed as a stepping stone, a practical mechanism, to introduce these important concepts as acceptable and routine new ways of supporting older people.

Case study

Referral and allocation

Mrs Brown has fallen and fractured her hip. On admission, ward staff refer Mrs Brown to the Hospital Social Work Department and to the coordinator of the Hospital Intermediate Care Team (ICT). Following surgery, monitoring of Mrs Brown's progress on the ward suggests that the ICT coordinator is best positioned to lead on the SAP and to act as care manager.

Single assessment

The findings of the assessment are that Mrs Brown has excellent rehabilitative potential and that her needs could best be met by an intermediate package of care provided in her own home for a period of six weeks.

Care planning for intermediate care

The intermediate care plan involves the coordination of many different professionals and agencies, including professionals and care staff not directly employed or seconded to the hospital ICT. All are working towards the overarching goal that Mrs Brown will be fully independent within the next six weeks.

Prior to discharging Mrs Brown from hospital, a home visit is carried out as part of the SAP. It is noted that Mrs Brown is in danger of falling again because her carpets are uneven. The care manager telephones the local Handy Van scheme which now has procedures in place which means people meeting the eligibility criteria for intermediate care get priority. The Handy Van makes a visit within 24 hours of the phone call from the care manager – thus permitting plans for early discharge to stay on track. The occupational therapist also provides a range of aids and adaptations such as a board to help Mrs Brown get in and out of the bath.

On Mrs Brown's return home from hospital, the house is warm and some basic food supplies have been provided by the local Age UK Home from Hospital Scheme. A volunteer sits with Mrs Brown to make sure

▶

she has settled in as she was feeling very anxious about returning home alone. Later that afternoon, the community nurse visits to check the wound is healing and to make sure Mrs Brown is not in any pain following her hip operation. The nurse phones the physiotherapist to confirm that Mrs Brown is home and feeling well enough for a visit tomorrow.

The following morning, the intermediate care team physiotherapist works with Mrs Brown to agree a series of rehabilitation goals. Mrs Brown's main goal is that she will be fit enough to walk to the local shops unaided within six weeks. An exercise plan is agreed and the goals written up and shared with the rest of the intermediate care team. Mrs Brown tells the physiotherapist that before her fall she had experienced some dizziness. Arrangements are made for Mrs Brown to have a full check-up with her GPs and for a visit to the falls clinic which looks at a wide range of issues.

The social worker has arranged for the reablement home carers to come in to help prepare meals and to help Mrs Brown get washed and dressed in the morning. The re-enablement carers encourage Mrs Brown to do things for herself and to practice the exercises that have been left for her by the team physiotherapist. The carers accompany Mrs Brown the first few times she goes outside, gradually increasing the distance walked until Mrs Brown achieves her goal of walking to the local shops. At the end of the six-week period of intermediate care, Mrs Brown is walking well but it is still lacking in confidence and feeling depressed. She is worried what she will do when the carers no longer visit. To ease the transition back to full independence, the social worker arranges for an Age UK volunteer to continue to visit everyday for a further three weeks. The Age UK volunteer encourages Mrs Brown to join the local Over 50s exercise class and to pursue her dream of learning to speak a foreign language.

Outcomes	Action required and by whom	Date for review
To ensure Mrs Brown's confidence improves as regards being home alone.	Home care team to visit once a day to check that Mrs Brown is looking after herself properly (eating well, taking her medication and managing her personal care).	Four weeks.

Exercise 11.1

Read the case study. Mrs Brown is about to be discharged from the intermediate care team but unfortunately things have not gone to plan and she has not regained as much independence as was anticipated. Further problems have come to light with regard Mrs Brown's mental health as she seems to becoming increasingly forgetful. The intermediate care team has referred the case to you (you are a social worker based in the local older people's social work team in the community) and you have decided to convene a case conference.

1. **Draw up an invitation list. Who should be invited to the case conference?** (Refer to the section on integrated care and support planning and consider which professionals you think it would be useful to speak to face-to-face. What level of assessment would you opt for? Which assessments would you like to see copies off? Do you envisage any difficulties in accessing this information? Would you invite Mrs Brown to the case conference? What would be the advantages and disadvantages of doing so?)

2. **Prepare an agenda for the case conference.** (In the case conference think about which areas you would need to cover, e.g. what has happened to date; issues that have been identified in the various assessments; discussion and agreement of any shared

outcomes and the plans for delivering these. What scenarios do you think might lead to conflict arising between the different professionals in attendance? How could this be managed? You and your colleagues have a very high case load, how do you think this would impact on the above activities?)

3. **Summarise the outcome of the case conference by completing an integrated care plan.** Refer to the 'A closer look' boxes on pages 145 and 148 to create a checklist of the range of issues you might need to consider. It is important that you document

not only your own input, but also that of the other agencies and professionals involved.

4. **As the social worker:** consider who the other professionals are and their roles in this process, and the problems and possibilities in organising support through these.

5. **If you are a professional from one the groups who would provide areas of support:** consider what your attitudes and approach would be to collaborating and being involved in assessments and any plans made. What are the problems and possibilities for you in working through these processes?

Key learning points

Summary of policy measures aimed at improving joint working around hospital discharge for older people:

- Two key policy measures have been implemented in England – the reimbursement process and intermediate care – both of which have helped reduce the rate of delayed discharge from hospital.
- The main advantage of the reimbursement process is that it provides a robust framework as to what is expected of different parties in the hospital discharge process. However, the framework is very complex and the threat of fines has not improved relationships between health and social services.
- Intermediate care works to actively bridge the transition from hospital to home by providing short-term access (usually for between two and six weeks) to rehabilitation and re-enablement. Research suggests that this is a service which provides the outcomes valued by older people. However, the time-limited nature of the service means that older people can be left feeling abandoned when the service is withdrawn.

Conclusion

Conceptually, coordinated care cannot exist unless different professional groups agree to work within a shared framework. In this chapter, we have explored the evolution of one such framework which originated under the auspices of the 1990 NHS Community Care

Act. However, **different funding streams for health and social care bring with them different channels or veins of assessment and care management (gateways)** which often compete with one another rather than promote collaborative joined-up working. The policy of reimbursement is particularly interesting in that it effectively compelled sign-up to a common framework for multidisciplinary working around hospital discharge by introducing new laws and the threat of fines for non-compliance on one of the parties. While reimbursement has been associated with a reduction in the number of delayed discharges, it has proved unpopular and difficult to implement. Furthermore, the culture it has created does not sit well with either personalisation or the spirit of collegiate working which is so fundamental to interprofessional practice.

The evidence suggests that where things are working well is in the context of intermediate care which has been linked to both personalisation and better outcomes for older people. However, by conceptualising intermediate care as a short-term service, there is a sense in which this has added to the maze of multiple assessment and care management (Cornes and Clough, 2001b) rather than working to **challenge the baton-passing culture which often passes for interprofessional practice** within the current care system. The challenge remains then as to how to move what are essentially pockets of good practice into the mainstream of service delivery. Beresford (2009) concludes that this is essentially a question of more adequate resourcing and that **if social care is to be fully accessible to all service users and better integrated with health, then the two require consistent funding arrangements,** which reinforce their overlaps and interrelations rather than encourage their separateness and isolation. However, the issue of further evolving and ensuring system-wide commitment to a common framework for interprofessional and integrated working should not be underestimated. As policy on personalisation develops further apace it will be important to get beneath the rhetoric and to start to answer important questions such as: **when is professional case management preferable to self-directed support and when is care provision by a care worker preferable to self-care?**

Useful websites

www.dh.gov.uk

Department of Health

www.scie.org.uk

Social Care Institute of Excellence

www.ageuk.org.uk

Age UK

www.caipe.org.uk

Centre for Advancement of Interprofessional Education

References

Abendstern, M., Clarkson, P., Challis, D., Hughes, J. and Sutcliffe, C. (2008) Implementing the Single Assessment Process for older people in England: lessons from the literature, *Research, Policy and Planning* 26 (10), 15–31.

Baker, M., Fardell, J. *et al.* (1997) *Disability and Rehabilitation: Survey of Education Needs of Health and Social Service Professionals,* London: Disability and rehabilitation Open Learning Project.

Beresford, P. (2009) Social care, personalisation and service users, *Research, Policy and Planning* 27 (2), 15–31.

Billings, J. and Leichsenring, K. (eds) (2005) *Integrating Health and Social Care Services for Older Persons: Evidence from Nine European Countries*, Farnham: Ashgate.

Booth, A. and Mead, T. (2007) *Delayed Transfer of Care. Health Management Specialist Library: Management Briefing,* http://www.library.nhs.uk/healthmanagment, accessed 3 August 2007.

British Geriatrics Society (2010) *Comprehensive Assessment for the Older Frail Patient – Best Practice Guide* (3.5, January), http://www.bgs.org.uk/index.php?option=com_content&view=article&id=195:gpgcgassessment&catid=12:goodpractice&Itemid=39, accessed 15 March 2010.

CAIPE (2007) *Creating an Interprofessional Workforce: An Education and Training Framework for Health and Social Care in England*, London: CAIPE, http://www.caipe.org.uk/silo/files/cipw-fw-doc.pdf, accessed 25 January 2010.

Carr, S. (2008) *Personalisation: A Rough Guide*, London: Social Care Institute of Excellence.

Commission for Social Care Inspection (CSCI) (2009) *Cutting the Cake Fairly: CSCI Review of Eligibility Criteria for Social Care*, London: CSCI.

Cornes, M. and Clough, R. (2001a) *Assessment in Community Care: Disputed Territory*, Lancaster: Lancaster University.

Cornes, M. and Clough, R. (2001b) The continuum of care older people's experiences of intermediate care, *Education and Ageing* 16 (2), 179–202.

Cornes, M. and Clough, R. (2004) Inside multidisciplinary practice: implications for single assessment, *Journal of Integrated Care* 12 (2), 3–13.

Cornes, M., Manthorpe, J., Donaghy, E., Godfrey, M., Hubbard, G. and Townsend, J. (2008) Delayed discharge from hospital: supporting older people to exercise choice, *Working with Older People* 12 (1), 16–20.

Cornes, M., Weinstein, P. and Manthorpe, J. (2006) *The Evaporation Effect: Final Evaluation of the Help the Aged Intermediate Care Programme for Older People*, London: Help the Aged.

Department of Health (1990) *Community Care in the Next Decade and Beyond,* London: HMSO.

Department of Health (2001a) *The National Service Framework for Older People*, London: Department of Health.

Department of Health (2002a) *The Single Assessment Process for Older People,* Circular HSC 2002/001: LAC (2002)1, London: Department of Health.

Department of Health (2002b) *Consultation on Proposals to Introduce a System of Reimbursement around Hospital Discharge*, London: Department of Health.

Department of Health (2003) *The Community Care (Delayed Discharges, etc.) Act 2003: Guidance for Implementation.* HSC 2003/009: LAC (2003)21, London: Department of Health.

Department of Health (2006) *Our Health, Our Care, Our Say: A New Direction for Community Services*, London: Department of Health.

Department of Health (2007) *Advance Care Planning: A Guide for Health and Social Care Staff,* London: Department of Health.

Department of Health (2008) Local authority circular LAC (DH)(2008)1: *Transforming Social Care,* London: Department of Health.

Department of Health (2009a) *Integrated Care and Support Planning (ICSP) High Level Process,* London: Department of Health.

Department of Health (2009b) *Supporting People with Long Term Conditions: Commissioning Personalised Care Planning – A Guide for Commissioners,* London: Department of Health.

Department of Health (2009c) *Guidance on Direct Payments: For Community Care, Services for Carers and Children's Services,* London: Department of Health (updated 2010)

Department of Health (2009d) *Intermediate Care – Halfway Home. Updated Guidance for the NHS and Local Authorities,* London: Department of Health.

Ehrlich, C., Kendall, E., Muenchberger, H. and Armstrong, K. (2009) Coordinated care: what does that really mean? *Health and Social Care in the Community* 17 (6), 619–27.

Glasby, J. and Duffy, S. (2007) *Our Health, Our Care, Our Say – What Could the NHS Learn from Individual Budgets and Direct Payments?* Birmingham: University of Birmingham (Joint Health Services Management Centre and In Control Discussion Paper).

Glasby, J. and Peck, E. (eds) (2004) *Care Trusts: Partnership Working in Action,* Oxford: Radcliffe Medical Press.

Glendinning, C., Clarke, S., Hare, P., Kotchetkove, I., Maddison, J. and Newbronner, L. (2006) *Outcomes-focused Services for Older People,* London: SCIE.

Godfrey, M., Keen, J., Townsend, J., Moore, J., Ware, P., Hardy, B., West, R., Weatherly, H. and Henderson, K. (2005) *An Evaluation of Intermediate Care for Older People,* Leeds: Leeds University.

Godfrey, M., Townsend, J., Cornes, M., Donaghy, E., Hubbard, G. and Manthorpe, J. (2008) *Reimbursement in Practice: The Last Piece of the Jigsaw? A Comparative Study of Delayed Hospital Discharge in England and Scotland,* Stirling: Stirling University.

Hastings, M. (2005) The process and outcome of rehabilitation, in A. Squire, and M. Hastings, (eds) *Rehabilitation of the Older Person: A Handbook for the Interdisciplinary Team,* Cheltenham: Chapman and Hall.

Henwood, M. (2006) Effective partnership working: a case study of hospital discharge, *Health and Social Care in the Community* 14 (5), 400–407.

HM Government (1990) NHS and Community Care Act, London: HMSO.

HM Government (2003) Community Care (Delayed Discharges etc) Act, London: Department of Health.

HM Government (2005) Mental Capacity Act, London: Department of Health.

HM Government (2007) *Putting People First: A Shared Vision and Commitment to the Transformation of Adult Social Care,* London: HM Government.

Jacobs, S., Xie, Chengqiu., Reilly, S., Hughes, J. and Challis, D. (2009) Modernising social care services for older people: scoping the United Kingdom evidence base, *Ageing and Society* 29, 497–538.

Kharichi, K., Levin, E., Illiffe, S. and Davey, B. (2004) Social work, general practice and evidenced-base policy in the collaborative care of older people: current problems and future possibilities, *Health and Social Care in the Community* 12 (2), 134–41.

Leece, D. and Leece, J. (2006) Direct payments: creating a two-tiered system in social care? *British Journal of Social Work* 36 (8), 1379–93.

Lymbery, M. (2010) A new vision for adult social care: continuities and change in the care of older people, *Critical Social Policy* 30 (1), 5–26.

Mandelstam, M. (2005) *Community Care Practice and the Law,* London: Jessica Kingsley Publishers.

Manthorpe, J., Cornes, M., Watson, R. and Andrews, J. (2006) *Intermediate Care and Older People: Building a Case for Continuous Care,* London: Help the Aged.

Ormiston, H. (2002) The single assessment process, *Managing Community Care* 10 (2), 38–43.

Sarner, M. (2010) Burnham gets personal with tailored care drive, *Health Service Journal* 7 January, 12–13.

Schimmel, E. M. (1964) The hazards of hospitalization, *Annals of Internal Medicine* 60, 100–110.

Social Services Inspectorate/Scottish Office Social Work Services Group (1991a) *Care Management and Assessment: Practitioners' Guide,* London: HMSO.

Social Services Inspectorate/Scottish Office Social Work Services Group (1991b) *Care Management and Assessment: Managers' Guide,* London: HMSO.

Smulian, M. (2009) Total place: pooling power, *Health Service Journal,* 17 December, 30–31.

Swift, C. (2005) Disease and disability in older people – the effectiveness of specialist interdisciplinary health-care services, in A. Squire and M. Hastings (eds) *Rehabilitation of the Older Person: A Handbook for the Interdisciplinary Team,* Cheltenham: Chapman and Hall.

Walker, A. (1994) *Half a Century of Promises. The Failure to Realise Community Care for Older People,* London: Counsel and Care.

Ware, T., Matosevic, T., Hardy, B., Knapp, M., Kendall, J., and Forder, J. (2003) Commissioning care services for older people in England: the view from care managers, users and carers, *Ageing and Society* 23 (4), 411–428.

Wirth, A. (1998) Community care assessment of older people: identifying the contribution of community nurses and social workers, *Health and Social Care in the Community* 6 (5), 382–386

Wistow, G. (1990) *Community Care Planning: A Review of Past Experiences and Future Imperatives,* London: Department of Health.

Young, J., Robinson, M., Chell, S., Sanderson, D., Chaplin, S., Burns, E. and Fear, J. (2005) A prospective study of frail older people before the introduction of an intermediate care service, *Health and Social Care in the Community* 13 (4), 307–312.

Young, J. and Stevenson. J. (2006) Intermediate care in England: where next? *Age and Ageing* 35, 339–341.

Chapter 12
End-of-life care

Suzy Croft

Chapter summary

The focus of this chapter is interprofessional working in palliative care settings. It provides a particular focus from the perspective of social work as a means to examine key issues for good practice in interprofessional working, and how this relates to such issues for other professions. It also sets out how the role of one profession – social work – with its wide-ranging and holistic nature, might not be fully appreciated by the other professions which have perhaps clearer and more closely focused boundaries than social work. Arising from this, issues of information-sharing, roles of the different professions in relation to assessments, and managing interventions and decision making in interprofessional working in this area are considered.

   The role of social workers, and some other key professionals, in palliative care settings has until very recently had little attention paid to it in the professional literature (Beresford *et al.*, 2008; Reith and Payne, 2009). The focus here is on issues arising from specialist palliative care social work, and the other groups working in this area; i.e. professional work concerned with end-of-life issues. This addresses two groups of service users. These are people with life-limiting illnesses and conditions and those facing or who have experienced bereavement. It is an area of social work where issues of interagency and interprofessional practice are at the heart of day-to-day work and where social work and social workers have long had to grapple with many of the problems and barriers that continue to operate in the way of effective coordination and collaboration between agencies and professions; this consideration then gives wider, more generalised lessons for other areas of interprofessional working, as explored at the end of this chapter.

Learning objectives

This chapter will cover:

- key issues in understanding interprofessional working in palliative care settings, in terms of what the aims of the services are, what is intended from them and then how these aims can be implemented in practice
- the roles of professionals and agencies involved in palliative and end-of-life care. Interprofessional issues are examined, both positive and where they throw up challenges in,

▶

159

for example, the effects of applying different assumptions from social and medical models, and suggestions are examined as to how these might be resolved

■ an analysis of how improvements in interagency and interprofessional collaboration can be brought about in services through developing holistic and person-centred support and practice

■ how the promise of moving beyond professional and agency preoccupations and boundaries to work in line with the rights and needs of service users might be realised.

The relevance of specialist palliative care social work

Specialist palliative care social work includes a body of practitioners experienced in working in the multidisciplinary teams and integrated settings increasingly required of social work, and operates in a wide range of both statutory and non-statutory agencies. While the focus of specialist palliative care social work is on end-of-life care and bereavement, it can also involve child protection work, work with families and children, disabled people, mental health and other adult service users. Specialist palliative care social work, like palliative care more generally, has highlighted its holistic approach, seeking to address psychological, personal, social and spiritual issues (Sheldon, 1997). As Lloyd observed in 1997, specialist palliative care social work is

> not immune to the broad changes in the delivery of health and social care which increasingly characterize postmodern societies. In Britain, the survival of such practice faces a considerable challenge in the face of the changes ushered in by the National Health Service and Community Care Act (NHSCCA), 1990.
>
> (Lloyd, 1997, p. 175)

Like other forms of social work it has also had to learn to 'operate in conditions of cultural and religious pluralism' (Lloyd, 1997, p. 176). The continuing issues this raises are highlighted by Gunaratnam (2006a, b). At the same time, specialist palliative care social work is perhaps one of the most universalist areas of modern mainstream social work. Staff in such settings can expect to encounter service users with a wide range of social, economic, class, employment and cultural backgrounds and increasingly, particularly in metropolitan areas, are working with

groups facing particular barriers and exclusions, including refugees and asylum seekers. Palliative care work is also being faced with new challenges, with increasing public discussion about death and dying and pressure for change in legislation relating to euthanasia, assisted dying and bioethical interventions. These now raise new issues about quality of life and rights to death which relate to the role of social work, and the other professions involved.

Specialist palliative care social work can also be seen as a branch of social work that has stayed most true to traditional understandings of social work roles and responsibilities (Monroe, 1998; Oliviere et al., 1998). But specialist palliative care social work also highlights broader tensions experienced in social work which have international relevance and significance and significance for interagency and interprofessional working. The issues relate to types of approaches in social work that service users may value and find helpful, even where social control may be involved, and approaches to social work that may be externally imposed by policy-makers and political and ideological considerations, as well as through some interpretations of professionalisation.

What we do know from empirical research is that palliative care service users generally highly value specialist palliative care social work. A UK-wide in-depth qualitative research study explored their views of such social work practice (Beresford et al., 2007). This included the two groups of service users already described who can access palliative care and palliative care social work; people with life-limiting illnesses and conditions and people facing bereavement. Both groups generally found such social work very helpful, highlighting the value they attached to their relationship with the social worker, their personal skills and qualities, flexibility, commitment and ability to offer both practical and personal support. In some cases

A closer look

What service users value in their relationships with professionals

Evidence from one study (Beresford *et al.*, 2007) suggests that service users highly valued their contact with palliative care social workers. They highlighted the crucial importance that the *relationship* with the social worker played in their experience of social work and identified the following key points:

- the quality of the relationship between service user and social worker
- the personal qualities of the social worker
- The nature and process of the work with them.

Over and over again the service users emphasised that they felt the social worker had built a relationship of trust and mutual respect with them. They valued:

- the informality, flexibility and respectful approach of the social worker. Service users felt they were able to work out their own agenda in partnership with the social worker. They had permission to talk about any issue of importance with no sense of hurry.
- the fact that the social worker was available not just to the service user but also to their families and partners.
- the social workers were reliable and delivered promised action. If they did not know the answers they said so and showed a willingness to find out.

It may therefore be helpful for all professionals working in palliative care to recognise the importance of:

- taking time to build up a relationship with service users/patients
- understanding the need to go at the service user's own pace
- Understanding the importance of following through on promised action.

they contrasted this with their experience of other professions involved (Beresford *et al.*, 2007). Such social work may therefore offer a helpful starting point for exploring positive practice in human services, given the evidence we have from service users about such a cooperative and holistic relationship-based, person-focused approach.

Palliative care: a holistic approach and collaborative working

Many professions and agencies are involved in palliative and end-of-life care. The hospice team, for example, may include a doctor, clinical nurse specialist in the community, occupational therapist, physiotherapist, lymphoedema therapist, day centre staff, nurses and health care assistants, dietician, chaplaincy and social worker. Other outside professions and occupations are also frequently involved, including a district nurse, psychologist, surgeon, bereavement counsellor, hospital consultant, human resources, school, housing and benefits agency staff.

The sensitivity to the importance of multi-agency and multidisciplinary working in palliative care grew out of the emphasis placed on an holistic approach pioneered in the modern hospice movement by Dame Cicely Saunders (Saunders *et al.*, 1995). However, it is not necessarily easy to retain such a holistic focus and there are growing signs that this is the case.

A wide range of pressures can currently be identified as operating against such a holistic approach, to the detriment of specialist palliative care social work,

Exercise 12.1

Note down your own list of pressures you can see working against a holistic approach in palliative/end-of-life care services.

Note down the potential positive benefits for service users of good collaborative interprofessional working in palliative/end-of-life care services.

and other professionals' work in this field. I would suggest that these include:

- Medical dominance in health care. This has been reinforced as palliative care has more recently been reintegrated as part of the medical mainstream (Sheldon, 1997).
- Inadequate funding – funding for palliative care, as with other longer-term non-curative conditions, has not matched that for acute services. Social work is at particular risk because it is not seen as a core medical service. Some hospices, for example, have never had social workers and some have lost them with cuts.
- The NICE Guidelines for palliative care services do not include social workers as a core member of the end-of-life care team; although we know that they are much valued by service users. It is also questionable whether the End-of-Life Care Strategy pays adequate attention to social and social care issues that are addressed by social workers.

The importance of the social

There is an irony in current moves to remedicalise palliative care, because the social needs which social workers are particularly adept at dealing with seem to be gaining significance in this field. For example:

- Medical and other developments mean people are likely to live longer with life-limiting, inherited and more complex conditions and social needs are therefore likely to become more central.
- Palliative care is being seen as helpful for a widening range of conditions. It is no longer only the province of people with cancer, but also can include people with end stage cardiothoracic conditions, including chronic obstructive pulmonary disease, HIV/AIDS, multiple sclerosis, motor neurone disease and so on.
- An increasing emphasis is being placed in palliative care on addressing equality and diversity issues better, particularly in relation to ethnicity, class and culture in providing end-of-life care.

- It is becoming less clear when people are actually 'dying', with resulting concerns currently about people being moved on to nursing and residential homes where end-of-life care is inadequately developed and social support important.

What were once acute medical conditions creating short-term medical needs are thus now being converted with medical and other advances, as well as some social changes into longer-term chronic needs and particularly into social needs. The social needs to be met will be many and varied, and these need to be appreciated and provided for by the different professionals involved, with social work coordinating and providing the personalised holistic approaches so valued by service users within the team.

People will need help adjusting to physical and psychological changes, which may be longer-lasting or permanent.

- They will need help with material issues like employment, income, benefits, housing and so on.
- In a public service system that prioritises choice and the active citizen, patient and service user, they are likely to need help in gaining those skills and capacities for these to be equally available.
- People will need help both at the end of life and facing bereavement in dealing with what may be increasingly complex and longer-term relationship issues.

What this highlights in palliative and end-of-life care is the importance of the social and holistic understanding for such practice. This emphasises the need for both such a social understanding across professions and social work itself in interagency and interprofessional palliative care practice. In social

Key learning points

- Specialist palliative care social work is evidenced to be highly valued by service users.
- Social workers are not officially included in the core palliative care team.
- Some palliative care services, particularly children's hospices, do not have social work staff.

work and social care, interest has recently grown in personalisation, or more person-centred support (Carr with Dittrich, 2008). This places an emphasis on tailoring services, support and practice to the rights and needs of the individual. This could help offer the kind of unifying focus for practice that is likely to enhance collaboration across agencies and professions.

However, different agencies and professions have different starting points for practice and collaboration, which can create barriers for both.

Generally the multidisciplinary team within a palliative care setting will consist of the following roles:

- clinical nurse specialists (sometimes known as Macmillan nurses) with a specialist background in palliative care
- social workers who may also offer bereavement support
- occupational therapist
- physiotherapist
- palliative care consultant.

Some teams may also include access to other roles such as dietician, lymphoedema therapist, volunteer coordinator and complementary therapist.

The general aim of the team is to help people cope with the effects that illness may be having on their life and the lives of their families, friends and partners.

The medical members of the team will have as their focus the assessment and management of people's pain and symptom control and on the needs that may arise as a result of these problems, looking at how these can be managed in the most effective way to improve quality of life. For example the clinical nurse specialist and/or doctor may focus on how to control pain, nausea, constipation and confusion. The physiotherapist may concentrate on maintaining reasonable mobility and the occupational therapist will be looking at suitable aids and adaptations to help maintain independence at home.

This work may also include referral to other services including arranging for hospice@home, respite care, hospice admission, volunteer support, day service and referrals to external agencies for support.

However, all members of the team would expect to be able to offer emotional support to patients in their contact with them. This will be especially true of the clinical nurse specialists, working in the community, who will also be able to offer some basic advice and help on welfare benefits.

In this respect the role of the clinical nurse specialist and that of the social worker may well overlap, but where teams work well together the clinical nurse specialist will be able to refer on to the social worker when it is felt a patient and/or family need much more in-depth help with emotional, social, practical and psychological support, continuing on into bereavement after the death of the patient. Palliative care social workers are usually skilled in counselling and family work. The combination of skills offered by the social worker makes a unique contribution to the psychological and social aspects of the multi-professional team caring for patients, their families and carers.

Often the clinical nurse specialist and the social worker in the team will work jointly together. So while the nurse may concentrate on the patient's problems with pain and medication and in addition offer emotional support to that patient, the social worker may, for example, be sorting out welfare benefits, applying for re-housing, supporting other family members including young children and so on.

In this way the team is able to offer a holistic service to the patient.

Case studies

The different cultures, traditions, status, power, histories and ways of doing things of different occupational groups have significant implications both for how they work as a team and the helpful consistency (or otherwise) when they work together. We can see this through three case study examples focusing on:

- breaking bad news
- team meetings
- management styles.

Case study 1

Breaking bad news

Hospital doctors place a big emphasis on further possibilities and further treatments for patients to hold their illness. For example, for people with inoperable cancer, there is often a reluctance to say 'this is the best it will be; this is your good time, to enjoy if you can'. For people whose business is saving lives, it can be difficult to be honest that people have an inoperable, incurable condition and that they will die. As one Macmillan nurse said, 'Mr Johnson's good time will be lost because he was put on a chemotherapy [research] trial that made him very ill'. He had to come off it. It predictably achieved nothing, but lost him time when he could have had reasonable quality of life. The Macmillan nurses and social workers seem more open to saying to a patient or service user that it isn't essential or necessarily the best thing to have more treatment, but to consider instead concentrating on what you can enjoy now. Because of their different orientation it can be possible for them to be more open and honest – if, of course, they judge that a person will be able to deal with it – to tell them that such treatment is very unlikely to have any beneficial effect.

Case study 2

Team meetings

The best team meetings at one palliative care centre are the day centre meetings. There is much less of a focus on people's medical issues and the meetings are not mainly led by medical members of the team – doctors or nurses – but much more by day centre staff who are not necessarily nurses. Much more emphasis seems to be placed on the contribution of all members of the team. The aim of the meetings is to discuss new referrals, admissions to day care, to do three-monthly reviews of people coming to day care and to discuss whether people should be discharged. The primary purpose is offering the sort of service we should be offering to the patient – are we working with them in the way we should be? People don't primarily come to the day centre for medical reasons, the emphasis is more on their social and psychological needs. These meetings are attended by the physiotherapist, occupational therapist, social worker, day centre coordinator, nurse and doctor. Meetings seem to work well to enable shared understanding and collaboration. For example, an older Irishman who comes with prostate cancer that is not particularly active. The doctor wants to discharge him as he feels the patient doesn't have particular palliative care needs and 'we shouldn't encourage dependency'. Other members of the team, however, point out that far from encouraging dependency his attendance fosters independence and his ability to live at home successfully. This is agreed.

Key learning points

Barriers to interprofessional working

Interprofessional working may sometimes be stressful for all involved. The key barriers to effective working can be:

- where the needs of patients and families are not the clear primary focus of a team and the demands of managers or other external forces have got in the way
- team members are not clear and confident about their own roles
- team members are not clear about the roles of other colleagues
- a hierarchy of importance exists within the team. So, typically, the doctor's voice is more respected than that of the nurse and the social worker and so on
- there are not clear structures for decision making, for example multi-disciplinary team meetings where the voice of all professionals is listened to and valued but real decisions are taken outside of the meeting
- there has been no support and training offered around interprofessional working. We are not always born knowing how to do this!

Case study 3

Management styles

The social work team at one hospice includes four qualified social workers, two part-time. The team leader's management style is based on open communication and discussion, working to be supportive, with regular formal team meetings with an agenda and notes. There are also frequent informal discussions in-between times. Members of the team also receive clinical supervision from the team leader on a regular basis about service users they have concerns about. The aim is to have a team which has a clear identity and sees itself as a unit in the hospice with its own ethos as well as sharing the overall hospice ethos, with agreed goals and values.

The hospice management style, recently imported with the acquisition of managers from the National Health Service, is much more formal. There are monthly heads of department meetings, with a set agenda which is worked through. They are currently considering using a pro forma to shape discussion. The plan is that each professional discipline within the hospice will report back at these meetings how they are meeting developmental targets set by the managers.

Significantly it is becoming clear that where nurses, occupational therapists and others are having problems, they tend to discuss them with other professionals rather than at these meetings. The managers therefore do not hear directly about them. The meetings do not serve as a forum for discussion, but rather as information exchanges, almost entirely providing information upwards to the managers, rather than a two-way exchange. Decisions do not seem to be made at these meetings, but elsewhere. The meetings are not seen as supportive and management meetings have lately been significantly increasing in both time and number. In order to have effective interprofessional working, such informal developments need to be actively discouraged, and proper protocols and guidance developed for and within teams to ensure the best coordination and information sharing in assessments and interventions for service users.

Insights for good practice, collaboration and joint working

Some of the insights that the experience of specialist palliative care social work can offer to our knowledge about interprofessional working have more to do with how it is different, than how it may be the same to other human service practice. Indeed it is often different in nature to other forms of social work as well as to the practice of other professions.

Exercise 12.2

Note down your own list of what the features of an effective teamworking approach in palliative/end-of-life care services would be.

Note down the potential positive benefits for service users of good teamworking in palliative/end-of-life care services.

Issues around assessment

Since the 1980s, the idea of assessment has become increasingly central in human services. With finite resources and a growing policy and organisational sense of the need to monitor and concentrate them where they are most needed, determining need for services and support has increasingly come to be seen as a priority. There has been a growing concern to develop methods of assessment that are 'efficient' and quantifiable, as well as being in line with 'performance targets'. Since the 1990s, there has also been a growing belief in the importance of involving the service user or patient in the process of assessment, so that their views and preferences can be incorporated.

This seems to have resulted in the increasing technicisation of assessment, making it more procedural and electronically based. Where services and support are discretionary, assessment processes have become even more tightly structured and potentially excluding. In social care, for example, which has been both needs- and means-tested, there are pre-assessment processes which may be telephone-based, operated through unqualified staff based in call centres, using scripted texts. In both social care and the benefits system, electronic and phone-based interviews and questionnaires have increasingly come to be used as a route to access support. Assessment is increasingly associated with the completion of substantial forms and in-depth bureaucratic interviews.

The development of the role of care manager in social care from the 1990s has been strongly associated with such an approach to assessment. The role of the social worker is framed in terms of managing a 'case' by making an assessment and then identifying an appropriate 'care package' and organising other professionals' input and services (Postle, 2002). This model, however, has not yet become the dominant one in specialist palliative care social work. Service users report that palliative care social workers do not carry out assessments in a formalised way. In the research study already cited, no service users referred to forms or checklists. Instead they painted a picture of the emphasis being placed on building the relationship between the specialist palliative care social worker and the service user. Assessment took place as an imperceptible part of that process.

Service users reported feelings of being at ease with the specialist palliative care social worker from the beginning, and thus being able to talk about issues that were important to them. They also felt that the specialist palliative care social worker had really listened to them. They were able to determine their own agenda and having feelings of control over what happened. They reported that the social worker was able to quickly pick up on cues as to what type of help was appropriate even when the service user was overwhelmed and not necessarily able to articulate what they wanted (Beresford *et al.*, 2007).

Professional boundaries

The role of social worker is not one that is well understood by the public or indeed by other professionals. Other professions seem to be much better understood by the public, as mentioned previously. Indeed, social workers have sometimes been criticised for not being clear enough about their role themselves. Certainly it is a role that is continually subjected to re-examination and redefinition. Professionals need to be prepared to be clearer with themselves and others in order to present these with clarity to service users and colleague professionals in order to ensure effective interprofessional working. Understanding and being clear about the social work role and that of other professionals is essential in a multidisciplinary team where there may seem to be overlaps in role and activity. Then it is crucial that the social worker and indeed any other professional be clear what they specifically have to offer from their professional position, and how to relate to those others' roles to provide the best assessments and services to the service user.

For example, nurses may feel that they offer patients emotional as well as clinical support and are not clear what social workers can provide that is more or different. They may wonder why social workers need to be involved. This can be a problem for social workers in palliative care. However, it can help for them to make clear that their scope and remit is wider than the patient. While the nurse may not have the brief or time, the social worker certainly is expected to address the wider needs of the family, the extended family and friends.

Joint working can be a helpful way of sharing understanding about expertise, helping to foster understanding of different professional boundaries as well as breaking down unhelpful assumptions about boundaries. This is readily instanced.

The social worker visits a patient at home who has been reluctant to admit to medical staff the severe physical pain he has, but having built up a good and broader relationship with the social worker, the patient is then more prepared to open up about it. Another patient can't see why he needs a Macmillan clinical nurse specialist in the community. His GP and hospital consultant both want him to. He saw her once and kept her at arm's length. His social worker, however, who doesn't have a treatment responsibility, is able to explain to him impartially more about it. A problem had cropped up for him and he had gone to casualty and waited in triage there till three in the morning. The social worker can keep a watching brief and be there for him in an ongoing way. She can help him see how the Macmillan nurse can offer a more helpful alternative, without him feeling she has a vested interest in doing so.

If a patient feels overwhelmed with many different issues and problems, then joint visits make it possible for each professional to take on different appropriate chunks from the first visit onwards. For example, a social worker and a Macmillan nurse made a joint visit to a woman overwhelmed by her own distress. Such visits can be really hard on your own because it is difficult to get clarity about what the main issues and difficulties are when someone is so distressed. Together, different perspectives and with combined understanding across the different professional disciplines mean that it is possible to work with the person to sort out with them what they see as the real problems, and to work out together how to help with them.

Sharing of information

What is key about information and information-sharing is who it is for. Recent problems highlighted in relation to IT systems operating in social work with children and families have highlighted the problems when information systems are seen primarily as serving managerial and bureaucratic ends, diverting practitioners from their practice and reducing their contact with service user. Key to good information-sharing is that it is primarily geared to helping service users. As one specialist palliative care social worker said in this vein

Good practice in information sharing? You write down what you have been doing with a patient or a family for everyone to see on the 'clinical record' – the patient's electronic notes. These are also available to the patient. So in the context of death and dying you need to be thoughtful about how you record and how you share information. Information on the clinical record is there readily to be shared. That's crucial. A big emphasis is placed on this in this hospice.

Information sharing seems to be done best by the professions with most direct contact with patients. It tends to be less well done by some of the medical staff because they still seem sometimes to be more of a law unto themselves and are not so good at communicating. It can create problems if you don't know what a doctor has told a patient and you can't find the doctor to ask. Doctors also may be less likely to read the notes. So a situation can arise where they might ask one social worker to see someone who has already been seen by another social worker. When you have good multi-professional meetings then you also share through the discussions about patients. We work with weekly meetings where there's the chance to discuss what information each professional has about the patient. Then there's an opportunity to develop a real discussion. Can I say that some of the best ones are when doctors are not there or can be kept in order! They might be challenged. You have to be assertive. But not all nurses seem so well equipped to do so by their training. At an inpatient meeting there could be twenty people. At a community team meeting, eight. The smaller numbers tend to work better. People take it in turn to chair, which is good. In bigger meetings nurses tend to feel intimidated. There's no training about running, being in or chairing meetings. That needs to happen much more.

(Personal Communication, 2010)

Different interventions

Specialist palliative care social work highlights not only the variety of practice interventions that different professions can offer, but also the very wide range of its own interventions. These seem to be more diverse than those from medical professionals. Interventions by palliative care social workers can be very fluid and arise for a wide range of reasons. As a result they can, for example, include offering emotional and psychological support, help with housing and benefits, talking to children in families and supporting another family member, as well as providing help with debt and offering advocacy and support to access other services.

This is illustrated by work with one service user. Mr B. is an asylum seeker with advanced cancer. He was sleeping with his wife on the floor of a family friend's home when the Macmillan nurse first visited.

She realised the value of a social work visit. Initial social work interventions included getting money from different charities for him as he was living on vouchers and didn't even have money for basic food, visiting him with an interpreter to get a proper history of what had happened and to check his understanding of his situation and then getting the local authority social services department to take responsibility for him, something which they had tried to avoid. Then the social worker liaised with his solicitor and gathered medical evidence to write letters of support for his application to remain in Britain. This was successful.

After he had been granted 'leave to remain' in this country, she helped him apply for housing and acted on his behalf in the bidding process used by the local authority to get a flat for those who had the appropriate number of points. She then helped him to apply for the benefits to which he was entitled. This included ESA (employment and support allowance which has replace incapacity benefit), Disability Living Allowance, housing and council tax benefit and carer's allowance for his wife. When he moved in to his new home, she spent a day setting up utility payments, informing relevant health and welfare agencies and helping him to establish a telephone land line. Mr B. said 'What would I do without a social worker? What would have happened if I didn't have one?'

The Macmillan nurse has had an ongoing involvement in this case and the two professionals liaise with each other to support Mr B. When the Macmillan nurse read the social worker's notes that mentioned that he seemed to have begun behaving strangely, she arranged his admission to the hospice for support and assessment. There it emerged that the cancer had spread to his brain.

Working towards person-centred practice

A recent national research and development project initiated by the Joseph Rowntree Foundation explored such person-centred support through the perspectives of service users, carers, face-to-face practitioners and managers (Glynn *et al.*, 2008). There was a strong

A closer look

The key components of person-centred support

Glynn and colleagues saw the key components of person-centred support as:

- putting the person at the centre, rather than fitting them into services
- treating service users as individuals
- ensuring choice and control for service users
- setting goals with them for support
- emphasising the importance of the relationship between service users and practitioners
- listening to service users and acting on what they say
- providing up-to-date, accessible information about appropriate services
- flexibility
- a positive approach, which highlighted what service users might be able to do, not what they couldn't do (Glynn *et al.*, 2008).

consensus about the definition of person-centred support between these different stakeholders. A wide range of different occupations and professions were represented in this project, including residential workers, housing and support workers, development workers, as well as people working with a wide range of groups, including people with dementia, lone parents, people at the end of life, people with learning difficulties, young people and so on. The resulting definition of person-centred support was strongly value-based, rather than emphasising techniques or procedures.

This provides a helpful unifying framework for practice across human service professions and agencies. It highlights the possibility of a form of practice which starts not from the priorities of the agency, is service-driven, or starts from the concerns and preconceptions of particular worker roles, but with the rights, concerns and potential of the service user. It points to helpful components for both the process, purpose and outcomes of practice. It provides a basis for developing practice that is person-centred – where the focus is on offering person-centred support rather than on the competing histories and traditions of different

Exercise 12.3

What barriers can you see working to prevent workers and agencies work in more person-centred ways? Think about your own experience, whether as a user of mainstream or human services or from working within them. What can get in the way?

agencies. Clearly different professions, services and agencies will have different contributions to make – something different to offer – but these can be guided by a consistent set of values and objectives, led by the rights and needs of service users. They can flourish under the umbrella principles of being *person*-centred.

Building on the person-centred approach set out at the beginning of this chapter, it is important to recall that in the *Standards We Expect* project as set out in Glynn *et al.* (2008), service users, workers, carers and managers identified a long list of barriers in the way of person-centred support and practice. These were big and small. Many related to problems in existing and traditional professional practice. They ranged from problems of resources to people working in outmoded and unhelpful ways because of past approaches to providing services and support. Such barriers included:

- people thinking they know what you want
- inflexibility – doing things the way they always have done
- lack of information for service users
- inadequate funding and resources
- charging policies that debar people from help
- inadequate staff time and unhelpful staff attitudes
- over-emphasis on risk and regulation
- poor communication
- failure to address culture and language issues
- institutionalisation
- negative experiences of user involvement
- measuring 'performance' in unhelpful ways
- being excluded by eligibility criteria
- family carers not equipped to support people's independence
- geographic inequalities
- lack of accessible transport
- ageism (Glynn *et al.*, 2008).

Addressing these issues is key to the provision of effective and holistic services to service users, and it would be therefore be valuable to use in auditing the practices of teams from these perspectives.

Overcoming barriers in the way of person-centred practice

Participants in this study had ideas for how to overcome the barriers that prevented people working in person-centred ways. Some spoke about changes that had improved their own services and practices, others referred to changes they thought were important for the future. Underpinning people's ideas was a clear belief that it represented a principled and value-based approach to support, rather than a set of mechanistic tools or techniques.

The three key stakeholders – service users, face-to-face practitioners and managers – all highlighted as key to overcoming barriers to person-centred practice:

- developing trust with and about service users, encouraging positive risk-taking, rather than being risk-averse
- pursuing a positive approach to service users that recognises and builds on their strengths rather than being preoccupied with their 'weaknesses'
- sharing good practice – supporting, rewarding and encouraging it
- promoting person-centred support
- providing training for person-centred support – which can strengthen the skills and capacity of both service users and practitioners
- improving communication – between practitioners and service users and between different practitioners
- developing effective user involvement and participation on both an individual and collective basis. (Glynn *et al.*, 2008)

Conclusion

Between them, the ideas listed above offer a basis for improving interagency and interprofessional collaboration through developing person-centred support and practice. This offers the promise of taking us **beyond professional and agency preoccupations and boundaries to work in line with the rights and needs of service users.** This raises issues for practice at both micro and macro levels, in relation to organisational as well as personal issues. As recent research on person-centred support or personalisation highlights, the key stakeholders who need to be involved for this to work and to be developed successfully are service users, carers and face-to-face practitioners (Beresford *et al.*, 2011). The latter includes those coming from the range of different occupational and professional positions that relate to the provision of social support. Thus **practice issues in palliative care, if they are to be truly person-centred, must always be holistic** in their orientation, involving and including these key perspectives. **Practice issues in palliative care and indeed all care and support must not only cut across professional boundaries and identities but also truly involve service users on equal terms**.

Further reading

Beresford, P., Fleming, J., Glynn, M., Bewley, C., Croft, S., Branfield, F. and Postle, K. (2011) *Supporting People: Towards a Person-centred Approach*, Bristol: The Policy Press.

Beresford, P., Adshead, L. and Croft, S. (2007) *Palliative Care, Social Work and Service Users: Making Life Possible*, London: Jessica Kingsley Publishers.

Altilio, T. and Otis-Green, S. (eds) (2011) *Oxford Textbook of Palliative Social Work*, New York: Oxford University Press.

Conway, S. (ed.) (2011) *Governing Death and Loss: Empowerment, Involvement and Participation*, Oxford: Oxford University Press.

Useful websites

Email: info@helpthehospices.org.uk

Help the Hospices

www.helpthehospices.org.uk/hospiceinformation

Hospice Information Service

Email: Enquiries@ncpc.org.uk

The National Council For Palliative Care

Email: susie.norton@stwh.co.uk

The Association of Palliative Care Social Workers

www.ncpc.org.uk

Dying Matters (Contact via The National Council for Palliative Care)

www.collegeofsocialwork.org

The College of Social Work

References

Beresford, P. Adshead, L. and Croft, S. (2007) *Palliative Care, Social Work and Service Users: Making Life Possible*, London: Jessica Kingsley Publishers.

Beresford, P. Croft, S. and Adshead, L. (2008) 'We don't see her as a social worker': a service user case study of the importance of the social worker's relationship and humanity, *British Journal of Social Work* 38 (7), 1388–407.

Beresford, P. Fleming, J. Glynn, M. Bewley, C. Croft, S. Branfield, F. and Postle, K (2011) *Supporting People: Towards a Person-Centred Approach*, Bristol, The Policy Press.

Carr, S. with Dittrich, R. (2008) *Personalisation: A Rough Guide*, Adult Services Report 20, London: Social Care Institute for Excellence.

Glynn, M., Beresford, P. *et al.* (2008) *Person-centred Support: What Service Users and Practitioners Say*, York: Joseph Rowntree Foundation/York Publishing.

Gunaratnam, Y. (2006a) A sweeter palliative, *Community Care*, 28 September–4 October, 36–7.

Gunaratnam, Y. (2006b) *Ethnicity, Older People and Palliative Care*, London: National Council for Palliative Care and Policy Research Institute on Ageing and Ethnicity.

Lloyd, M. (1997) Dying and bereavement: spirituality and social work in a market economy of welfare, *British Journal of Social Work* 27, 175-90.

Monroe, B. (1998) Social work in palliative care, in D. Doyle, G. Hanks and N. MacDonald (eds) *The Oxford Handbook of Palliative Medicine*, 2nd edn, Oxford: Oxford University Press.

Oliviere, D., Hargreaves, R. and Monroe, B. (eds) (1998) *Good Practices in Palliative Care*, Aldershot: Ashgate.

Postle, K. (2002) Working 'between the idea and the reality': ambiguities and tensions in care managers' work, *British Journal of Social Work* 32 (3), 335–51.

Reith, M. and Payne, M. (2009) *Social Work in End-of-Life and Palliative Care*, Bristol: The Policy Press.

Saunders, C., Baines, M., Dunlop, R. (1995) *Living with Dying*, 3rd ed., Oxford: Oxford University Press.

Sheldon, F. (1997) *Psychosocial Palliative Care: Good Practice in the Care of the Dying and Bereaved*, Cheltenham: Stanley Thornes.

Chapter 13
Rehabilitation and disabled people

Glenis Donaldson and Bob Sapey

Chapter summary

In this chapter we explore interprofessional working with people with disabilities from different perspectives – the professional perspectives that have informed much practice within social work, nursing, occupational therapy and physiotherapy; and the perspective of disabled people as the recipients of services. The challenge for professionals who work with people with disabilities is to listen to the experience of their service users and to find ways of incorporating what is learned into their practice. In order to do this, this chapter draws extensively on a study of disabled peoples' experiences of wheelchair use (Sapey *et al.*, 2005) and of physiotherapy (Donaldson, 2009). Both of these studies analysed their data from a social model of disability perspective as this was the best approach to valuing the experiences of disabled people. As the example above illustrates, disabled peoples' own expertise may lead to more convincing and sustainable solutions than that of the professional expert. While using the work of physiotherapists as an exemplar of issues involved in interprofessional working in this area, the chapter examines the roles and functions of the different professionals involved in work with people with disabilities, and how between them an effective service can be provided to people in need of services from a rehabilitation model, which we believe is the model which should guide interprofessional working with rehabilitation patients,[1] for reasons we will set out in the chapter. We argue that the full inclusion of the service user or patient is key to effective nature of interprofessional working with people with disabilities.

Learning objectives

This chapter will cover:

- the implications of social and medical models of disability, and key approaches to interprofessional work to meet their needs

▶

---

[1] It is important that disabled people are not assumed to be patients, but in the context of discussing disablement as it is theorised by health professionals, it is helpful to use the term patient as this describes how the service user is most commonly perceived.

- how contemporary rehabilitation discourses can promote autonomy and functional independence for people with disabilities, and how the role of professionals who work with them is to facilitate this individually and interprofessionally

- how professionals must not view key issues for people with disabilities as entirely to do with the body, but also personal and social implications, within coordinated services delivered by the variety of professionals involved, all of whom accept this basic premise

- how all professionals who work for people with disabilities need to provide services from the perspective of aiding service users develop creative solutions that are socially appropriate

- how professionals need to work in their own personal practice and through the other agencies/professionals in developing a whole-person response to the needs of people with disabilities.

Case study

Linda, who had sustained a spinal cord injury and has little use of her upper and lower limbs, talked about some of the assumptions that are made about people with physical impairments.

> A lot of people look at you and think that you can't walk, but for me not walking was the easiest bit to get over; it's all the underlying issues that are the problem. I don't really want people I don't consider to be close, to know the intimate details of the problem.

She described how the loss of bladder function and frequent urine infections have caused her much frustration and been very limiting.

> I'm incontinent, so with being incontinent I didn't want to have an indwelling bag; I was encouraged to do intermittent catheterisation. But I can't do it myself, the inserting of the catheter's not the problem, it's actually getting off the chair and getting undressed. I find the problem to be, because I'm small and my hands aren't strong, that I haven't got a long enough lever to grip round the toilet and pull myself across . . . Before I go anywhere I need to know if there's a toilet and if there isn't going to be one then I've got to make plans as to what I'm going to do, whether I'm going onto an indwelling bag for the day or try intermittent catheterisation. It restricts how long I can stay at the restaurant or the pub.

She was critical of rehabilitation therapists who tended to focus on her functional ability in an attempt to improve what they saw as the problem.

> Then you'd get the physio and they'd be saying this is what I want you to do, 'I want to you to lift your leg up and move it over here'. They'd explain, but no matter how hard they explained or demonstrated, I could never get it because there is no way on earth you can move your leg if you can't move it. They were giving me these sandbags to raise the level of the floor so that I could actually push up. Then I'd get back in the chair and I'm supposed to be doing it all on my own and I've got one physio pushing me up and the other lifting me in and they said 'oh well done'. My husband just sat there laughing saying 'this is not practical, she has not done anything'.

Linda felt that the therapists could not see her as an individual or understand the issues from her perspective; rather they were working to a different understanding of disablement gained through their occupational education and training, and they expected Linda to fit in with.

> I think individually they don't see it properly. It's like everything thing else, everything is global, everything is standard.

Linda was eventually able to take greater control of her situation by claiming direct payments and using the income to employ her own personal assistants. When she had control of the purse strings she was able to direct her personal assistants to assist her in ways that she found would best resolve the problems associated with her incontinence. It would not make any difference to Linda as to which member of the rehabilitation team was working with her – physiotherapist, occupational therapist, nurse or social worker – the issues she faced would not change. It may well be that the pressures to collaborate within interprofessional teams are such that the professionals become inclined to share the dominant biomedical understanding of disablement, thereby adding to the likelihood of the social context of needs being ignored.

Key issues here for Linda, and for those professionals who provide services for her, are:

■ Linda's impairment issues were viewed by professionals as entirely to do with her body, but for Linda they had personal and social implications.

■ By taking control of her own care through direct payments, Linda was able to be creative and to find solutions that were socially appropriate for her.

(Donaldson, 2009)

Exercise 13.1

Consider how you would approach your work with Linda personally, and through the other agencies/professionals, in developing a whole-person response to her needs.

Perspectives of rehabilitation work with people with disabilities

Rehabilitation interventions should be tailored to improve disabled people's lives rather than their bodies.
(Williams and Woods, 1988, p. 129)

Although Williams and Woods may have recognised aspects of Linda's experience, most contemporary rehabilitation discourse promotes autonomy and functional independence. These are understood by therapists to be 'unproblematic and universally desirable goals' for the 'patient' (Fine and Glendenning, 2005, p. 602). As such both concepts are considered by rehabilitation professionals to be key outcomes of rehabilitation (Desrosiers *et al.*, 2003) and within the rehabilitation literature the two terms are often closely associated. Proot *et al.* describe how during the process of rehabilitation the patient is

in a state of transition – from an individual who needs support to enhance autonomy and independence to one who gains autonomy and independence and needs less support.

(2000, p. 267)

The role of the different professionals should be to actively facilitate this process. Throughout much of the history of the physiotherapy profession, for example, the meaning of both of these concepts has been accepted by its members without question. However, in recent years both of these concepts have come under critical review. French, a physiotherapy academic, argues from a social model understanding of disability and uses experiential accounts of rehabilitation to question whether it was always in the best interest of disabled people to strive for functional independence. She suggests that narrow definitions of independence from health professionals can give rise to 'inefficiency and stress' (1994, p. 49) for patients. Whalley Hammell (2006), an occupational therapist and academic, argues from the same political stance and suggests that because there is a lack of an evidence base to support the assumption that independence is a universally valued goal, it must be ideological and reflect the dominant values of middle-class Western-orientated therapists. Social workers too have been encouraged to reject individualised approaches that pathologise and blame disabled people for the disadvantages they experience, rather they should adopt an approach in which disabled people are valued as citizens.

Other academics have argued that the notion of autonomy used in rehabilitation work with people with disabilities is individualised (Finkelstein, 2000; Swisher, 2002) and therefore lacks a social and

173

Key learning points

Approaching disabled people as valued citizens

- Disabled people should be seen as contributing members of society as both workers and valued customers.
- Disabled people should be recognised as empowered individuals.
- Disabled people should be seen as active citizens with all that implies in terms of rights and responsibilities.

(Oliver and Sapey, 2006, p. 41)

experiential basis. Disabled people (for example Barnes, 1991; Finkelstein, 2004) have often criticised professionals for giving them unrealistic goals and expecting them to accept services over which they have little control and which fail to help them gain equality of access to economic, social and political resources. They argue that disabled people are expected to accept standards of life that would be unacceptable to the therapists who ask this of them. There are broadly three responses from rehabilitation workers to these criticisms:

1. Entrenchment and defence of the biomedical model, including pathologising the criticisms of disabled people as arising from poor psychological adjustment to their disablement.
2. Development, refinement and strengthening of the biomedical model by attempting to include some aspects of the criticisms, most notably by the World Health Organization in the development of a bio-psychosocial model, but also in the organisational response of adult safeguarding to growth of ideas such as self-directed support.
3. Adoption of social model approaches to practice and a changed relationship between professionals and disabled people, such as is evident in Centres for Independent Living which have been developed by disabled people's organisations, and which employ therapists. This approach has become part of the government's personalisation policy and within social work has become a requirement of the General Social Care Council.

In the rehabilitation literature, functional independence is usually associated with an individual's ability to perform activities of daily living and mobility without assistance (van Vliet *et al.*, 2005). The role of the therapist is to teach the patient motor skills to enable the highest level of physical independence. Conversely, functional dependence is devalued and is described in negative terms as an individual attribute to be alleviated and/or minimised (Pomeroy, 2007). Therefore in physiotherapy, functional dependency has become a measure of physical need for professional intervention and functional independence is determined by the individual's physical attributes, judged against medically defined norms such as normal posture and gait. Importantly it is assumed that those identified as dependent are actively trying to seek to reverse this situation (French and Swain, 2004; Whalley Hammell, 2006). Some disabled researchers have for a long time argued that professionals' reasoning and actions are embedded in complex social, political, economic, cultural, intellectual and historical contexts and that their approach to practice is value-based (Abberley, 2004; Oliver, 1996). These academics argue that an ideology of normality pervades rehabilitation and allows therapists to wrongly assume that their professional valuing of functional independence is in fact a universal norm. Moreover, these norms are said to reflect dominant cultural values that are rarely challenged, 'a carnal hierarchy, where the non-disabled body is privileged and advantaged' (Hughes, 2004, p. 64)

Disability studies academics also argue that ideologies are inseparable from workings of power and ultimately serve the interests of the professional and not the person receiving rehabilitation. And they are sceptical of professional claims to impartiality in service provision. Those claims are based on the supposed scientific base of rehabilitation that has been adopted from medicine and has led to a focus on cure and body restoration.

The legitimacy and the scientific identity of rehabilitation professions has been closely linked to the discipline of medicine (Crotty, 1998) which has historically exerted collegiate control over the institutions responsible for the training of physiotherapists, nurses, speech and occupational therapists, while viewing social work's role as limited to aspects of a patient's life other than the body. The biomedical model of health, which evolved as a consequence of the scientific revolution in Europe in the seventeenth century, led to the analysis of living things as sets of mechanical parts; as machine rather than organic wholes (Hutchinson, 2004, p. 28). Descartes (1596–1650), one of several seventeenth-century philosophers whose mechanical conception of the human being was taken up by medical practitioners, was responsible for expounding the dualistic concept of the mind–body split (Descartes, 1989). This is based on the assumption that there is no significant interaction between mind and body; therefore, the two realms can be addressed by separate and distinct disciplines. The body became the subject of the natural sciences and the mind the topic of cultural sciences and humanities (Turner, 1992). Doyal (1991) argues that modern medicine continues to expound a mechanistic concept of health due to its primary concern with the body. A body could be considered to be healthy if it was in good working order like a properly functioning machine; conversely, a body was considered diseased if an impairment of its function could be found.

Within allied health professions the effect of illness and impairment are thought to have a devastating effect on independent living and to affect both the individual and their family and close associates (Laver Fawcett, 2007). The provision of appropriate therapy is one of the ways in which individual lifestyle and quality of life can be restored. Rehabilitative physiotherapy aims to maintain or restore actions that are considered to be critical to independence such as standing up, sitting down, walking, reaching, manipulation and balance (Carr and Shepherd, 2003; Whalley Hammell, 2004). These actions are considered to be fundamental to the performance of basic activities of daily living, for example, eating, drinking, washing, dressing, cooking, cleaning and travelling (Laver Fawcett, 2007). Just as psychologists have argued that people experiencing loss must pass through certain psychological processes to achieve recovery, many rehabilitation professions believe that their therapeutic activities are necessary and sufficient for the recovery of life skills.

For physiotherapists, a key group providing services, function can be reduced to simple components

that can be retrained. The process of physiotherapy rehabilitation therefore teaches the patient how to normalise deviation and adapt to their environment (Bobath, 1990; Carr and Shepherd, 1998). The assumption that normal function can be achieved underlies the use of neurological and biomechanical theories in neurological rehabilitation. This biological reductionism, the process of reducing any 'higher level or complex action into a lower level or simpler action' (Reed and Sanderson, 1999, p. 206), also reinforces the tendency to view people as patients, as an 'object to be manipulated' (Hutchinson, 2004, p. 29). There is a parallel to task-centred approaches to social work in which the ways of achieving ultimate goals are broken down into small steps which are felt to be more realistic and achievable. For the professionals the ultimate goal provides the motivation to achieve smaller goals; however, if these smaller goals are too remote that motivation may be lost.

The biomedical model assumes a top-down approach to health, where the role of the patient as the learner is to submit to the authority of the clinical expert whose dominance in the relationship is legitimised by the possession of scientific knowledge (French, 1994; French and Swain, 2004). In this context the role of the clinician is to both treat and educate, and 'patient compliance' is anticipated. However, encouraging compliance to long-term exercise as part of a rehabilitative regimen has proved challenging, and lack of patient motivation is one of the most commonly cited reasons for non-compliance in several studies (Campbell et al., 2001; Dishman and Ickes, 1981; Evenson and Fleury, 2007; Maclean et al., 2002; Sluijs et al., 1993).

Within rehabilitation professions, patient motivation tends to be defined as 'a behavioural tendency to persevere independent of situational reinforcements' (Dishman and Ickes, 1981, p. 423). Theoretical

Exercise 13.2

What can rehabilitation professionals learn from the points in the above sections on how they can talk to their service users/patients to ascertain from them their motivations, and not to impose their own assumptions?

frameworks and conceptual models, drawn mainly from the academic discipline of behavioural psychology, have been used to aid understanding of the intrinsic motivational factors that are associated with physical exercise compliance. Although some of these theories acknowledge the importance of cultural and social variables, very few have made an attempt to incorporate these in a meaningful way (Kaptein and Weinman, 2004). Furthermore, while it is recognised that motivation is an important issue in physical exercise compliance, no single model of motivation is universally accepted (Middleton, 2004). This is due to the lack of empirical evidence to verify the hypothesised relationship between motivation and proposed variables. Various models emphasising cognitive variables and processes have been used and these include the health belief model (Rosenstock, 1974) and the theory of planned behaviour (Ajzen, 1988). These models adopt a social–psychological approach to health behaviour that emphasises social cognitive factors, in particular the group of social cognitions that concern beliefs about the consequences of a given behaviour (de Wit and Strobe, 2004, p. 54). These give rise to an expectancy-value model, specifying the types of beliefs that should be used to predict a particular type of behaviour. This approach directs attention to the way in which patients conceptualise health threats and appraise factors that may inhibit or facilitate motivation and compliance. The use of these theoretical models, which incorporate a number of psychological explanatory variables, have arguably become accepted as key determinants of patient compliance and have now become firmly established as fact within the professional knowledge.

Key learning point

Donaldson (2009) has argued that therapists who draw exclusively on theories derived from health psychology to explain patient non-compliance run the risk of constructing non-compliance as pathological behaviour. Rather, what is needed is further inquiry into the patient's perspective and the use of a critical sociological knowledge about disability.

Disabled people suggest that social phenomena such as the institutional environment, the behaviour of the therapist and shared values can influence their compliance as well as cultural norms.

(Donaldson, 2009, p. 155)

However, the development of rehabilitation has been guided by the models of disability promoted by the World Health Organization. The model that dominated rehabilitation practice in the late twentieth century was the ICIDH (International Classification of Impairment, Disability and Handicap) (World Health Organization, 1980). The ICIDH originally developed a four-level hierarchy of function comprising disease, impairment, disability and handicap (see Figure 13.1). The four components of function were hierarchical. Functional limitations (disability) and social roles (handicap) are conceptualised in negative terms as the life-long personal and social consequences of disease and the resultant impairment.

Therapeutic services that followed this model targeted the medical needs of disabled people by focusing on issues of impairment. This model helped multidisciplinary team members such as physio and occupational therapists, speech therapists and psychologists identify their '*domain of concern*' (Laver Fawcett 2007, p. 235).

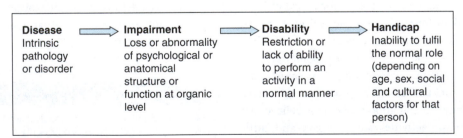

Figure 13.1 The hierarchy of the International Classification of Impairment, Disability and Handicap

Source: Based on information from World Health Organization (1980)

From a social model perspective the ICIDH came to epitomise the individualisation of the disadvantages disabled people faced, and Imrie (2004) argues that it has now been discredited for its medical foundation and for focusing on individual functional limitations as key determinant of disability. In 2001 the World Health Organization revised the ICIDH and proposed the International Classification of Functioning Disability and Health (ICF), which they argue had

> moved away from being a 'consequences of disease' classification to become a 'components of health' classification. 'Components of health' identifies the constituents of health, whereas 'consequences' focuses on the impacts of diseases or other health conditions that may follow as a result.
>
> (World Health Organization, 2001, p. 4)

In this model disability becomes a variation of human functioning caused by one or a combination of 'impairment, difficulties in executing activities, or problems the individual may experience in her involvement of life situations' (Imrie, 2004, p. 292). Importantly all these dimensions are considered to be co-equal and different facets of disablement. In most parts of the world this revised model has been embraced by rehabilitation professionals and some disabled academics (notably Shakespeare, 2006) have also suggested that this model can benefit disabled people. However, in the UK in particular the model has been criticised for its inclusion of the need for individual, psychological adjustment. In terms of interprofessional working this model is seductive because it appears to provide the compromise required to work together, but it may still be excluding of disabled people themselves (Figure 13.2).

For therapeutic practitioners the model sets the rehabilitation agenda in a social context while still recognising that disease has an important influence on a person's level of physical activity and social participation and on the process of rehabilitation (Wade and de Jong, 2000). The changes made mean that in the ICF, disability is a relational phenomenon whereby the functional limitations of impairment become disabling as a result of broader social and attitudinal relations. The ICF also differs from the ICIDH by stating that the presence of impairment does not necessarily indicate disease or that the individual should be regarded as sick. According to Bickenbach *et al.* (1999) the ICF embodies a biopsychosocial model of disablement that is a synthesis of social and medical understandings of disablement. The ICF framework conceives the determinants of functioning and health of individuals as a composite of physical, mental and social environments.

This model invites rehabilitation professionals to not only take a broader perspective of the causes of disablement, but also become involved in a wider range of aspects of their patients' lives. This would be good if the ICF were encouraging of a more qualitative approach to assessment which valued the experiential understandings of disabled people, but it remains essentially scientific in its construction and operation, which it is argued does not increase the likelihood that it will benefit disabled people any more than its predecessor, the ICIDH (Oliver and Sapey, 2006).

The adoption of a biopsychosocial approach is claimed to promote a holistic approach to rehabilitation, but the version of holism implicit within the model is one which does not sacrifice the advantages of the biomedical approach, so still works to the advantage of medical practitioner. Roberts (1994), a physiotherapy academic, examined medical claims of holistic practice based on the biopsychosocial model of health. Her work describes the theoretical approach of 'holism' (Smuts, 1952) as based on the belief that certain 'wholes are greater than their sum parts'. She explains that medicine has redefined holism in terms of the biopsychosocial model by dividing the body into three quite distinct but interrelated parts – a biological being, a social being and a psychological being – examining all three and then adding them together to make a whole. This, she argues ignores Smuts's premise that we need to look at the whole first to make any sense of the parts. Thus she concludes that, 'The biopsychosocial model is not holism by another name; it is an aberration of holism, which is attractive to (rehabilitative agents) physiotherapists, as it does not threaten the concept of the medical model' (Roberts, 1994, p. 365)

What this means is that the ICF fragments the function of an individual into physical, social and psychological divisions, allows the individual's functioning

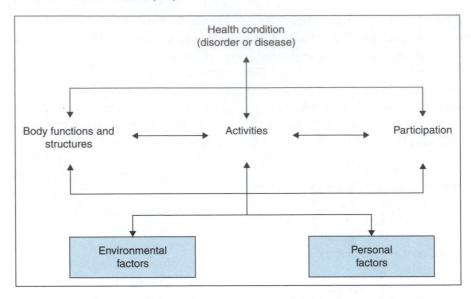

Figure 13.2 Interactions between the components of the International Classification of Functioning Disability and Health

Source: World Health Organization (2001, p. 18)

to be viewed as a medical issue and assumes that different types of intervention are appropriate at the different levels. This has encouraged health care professions to maintain specialised approaches to the problem of disablement and to make claims about the social advantages of their own particular intervention. Armstrong (1987) also notes that there is little evidence of the development or application of the biopsychosocial model outside biological and psychiatric sciences. This he argues implies a strengthening of biological and reductionist medicine while maintaining the subsidiary status of the social sciences. Thus the need for an alternative perspective on rehabilitation, one informed by disabled people, persists. In order to achieve this, different professionals need to grasp that interprofessional working must also include patients, although it may be that the term 'interprofessional' is itself a barrier as it implies a value of working with other professionals rather than patients. In mental health where some of these relationship issues have been discussed for some time, it has been argued that there is a need for a paradigm change in which professionals move from being experts to collaborators, while patients become citizens (Nelson *et al.*, 2001).

In the last few years the government have been pursuing a policy of personalisation of care through

Exercise 13.3

How can professionals ensure that they develop and maintain an individualised, person-centred planning approach at the heart of their own practice, and in advocating for this with other agencies/professionals providing services?

which they are attempting to give service users control of resources used to provide support with health and social care. They describe these changes as moving

> from the model of care, where an individual receives the care determined by a professional, to one that has person centred planning at its heart, with the individual firmly at the centre in identifying what is personally important to deliver his or her outcomes.
> (Department of Health 2008, p. 4)

Implications for practice

Professional approaches to rehabilitation have been influenced by medicine and in particular the World Health Organization's conceptualisations of disability and health. This has resulted in the development of therapies that aim to alleviate (cure) the effects of

A closer look

In 1976 the Union of Physically Impaired against Segregation proposed a relational model of disablement, which recognised that people with impairments were disadvantaged by the response of various institutions of society to their impairment. This became known as the social model of disability, but importantly the focus of intervention in this relational model was not the disabled person, but the social organisations that were causing their disablement.

> Disability is something imposed on top of our impairments, by the way we are unnecessarily isolated and excluded from full participation in society.
> ... it is absolutely vital that we get this question of the cause of disability quite straight, because on the answer depends the crucial matter of where we direct our main energies in the struggle for change. We shall clearly get nowhere if our efforts are chiefly directed not at the cause of our oppression, but instead at one of the symptoms.
> (UPIAS and Disability Alliance 1976, pp. 3–4)

This model does not provide simple or formulaic procedures for rehabilitation staff to follow, rather it requires them to re-examine the ways in which they use their skills and the ways in which they define their role. This might involve working collaboratively with a disabled person while acknowledging them as an expert, rather than aiming to be in an expert role. Holdsworth (1991) argued that in the context of social work, as the social model is redefining disability as a form of oppression, the aim of assessment should be geared to a person's need for empowerment.

impairment and to the dominance of individual explanations of disability.

Key learning points

Our studies suggest that there are several differences between the assumptions of professionals and the experience of disabled people.

- Professional approaches to functional independence can sometimes be socially impracticable.
- Functional independence is central to much rehabilitation practice, whereas interdependence is not shunned, but welcomed by disabled people.

- Therapists have assumed that patient compliance can be maintained if they address the individual's psychological traits. Disabled people suggest that social phenomena such as the institutional environment, the behaviour of the therapist and shared values can influence their compliance as well as cultural norms (Donaldson, 2009).
- Power relationships within rehabilitation settings may prevent disabled people from sharing their experiences with their therapists (French, 1994).

Exercise 13.4

What skills and approaches do professionals need to develop in order to foster appropriate levels of interdependence between providers and service users in and across services?

Conclusion

This chapter has examined how professionals can between them best provide holistic and comprehensive services to people with disabilities based on our knowledge of what service users require from the different agencies and professionals involved with them.

In order to develop effective interprofessional working in the area of rehabilitation, professionals should be educated and have an understanding of and **commitment to the social model of disability** and be encouraged to employ its reasoning to evaluate the holistic nature of their practice. When disability is examined in this framework the emphasis shifts away from the removal of problems associated with the impairment to the removal of barriers associated with the integration of the disabled person back into society. However, there are many aspects of the social model which seem to be incompatible with the medical approach to rehabilitation which dominates many occupational groups.

The social model requires rehabilitation professionals to re-evaluate their value system, which is often based on notions of normality. This process can be helped by giving greater consideration to the subjective nature of health and **the importance of disabled people's perceptions** of what constitutes the aims of their own rehabilitation. This knowledge should serve as a basis

A closer look

The patient-centred approach of an interprofessional team

Implications for practice

In a mapping exercise on a social work degree, one student drew two diagrams that described how she felt as a patient moving from child to adult services. As a child her consultant had not only treated her in a patient-centred way, but also took the responsibility to coordinate the interprofessional team (see Figure 13.3). In this situation she felt secure and the various professionals worked together in a coherent team.

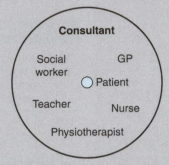

Figure 13.3 A patient-centred team

However, when she moved into adult services, the consultant decided that to empower her, she should be in charge of the team. The consultant withdrew from that role, but the team did not acknowledge the patient's authority and she did not know how to exercise such a professional role. As the professionals failed to respect the patient in this role the team began to disintegrate and the patient felt excluded (see Figure 13.4).

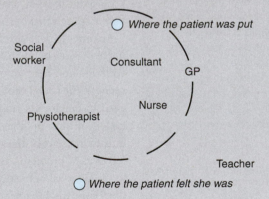

Figure 13.4 The 'patient-excluded' approach in interprofessional teams

Rehabilitation professionals need to be patient-centred, but they also need to ensure that they take responsibility for their own effective collaboration. The patient in this case needed to be valued for her position and experience, not put into a quasi-professional role.

of goal-setting and will involve greater collaboration between the individual therapists and disabled people towards agreeing the outcomes of therapy.

Individual budgets and self-directed support can enable disabled people to achieve autonomy and independence in their lives. If as Williams and Woods (1988) suggest, 'rehabilitation interventions should be tailored to improve disabled people's lives rather than their bodies', then it will be necessary for rehabilitation professionals to consider approaches that are not directed at the body and to make this part of their knowledge base. Donaldson (2009) found a consensus amongst disabled women that important aspects of their lives can be restricted if they lack access to the relevant information on which decisions can be made.

Most rehabilitation professionals set out to assist disabled people to improve their lives, but in the process of their education and employment they develop approaches to helping that are expert- rather than person-centred. The challenge of the social model of disability is not to say that rehabilitation professionals are not needed, rather that they should use their skills as a resource to **work collaboratively with disabled people to help them achieve their chosen outcomes**.

It may seem to those in a particular professional group that these recommendations would be more easily adopted by their colleagues in another group. For example physiotherapists and occupational therapists (see the relevant Chapters 19 and 21 respectively on the professions in this volume) may believe that dealing with social model issues is the domain of social work and that the best collaborative working practices will be achieved by each group maintaining their particular position. However, that view is from within an existing paradigm, whereas what is being demanded through a social model analysis is to reconceptualise disablement as a social problem, not an individual one. From this perspective the psychosocial concerns of the social worker are no more relevant than the biomedical concerns of the therapist, they all focus on the need for individual change. For Linda (see the Case study at the beginning of this chapter) her problem was not her incontinence but the restricted way in which her therapist viewed the potential solution. The eventual solution that worked for her was to take control of the budget for her care and to decide for herself how to meet her own needs. Her solution was outside of the range of techniques available to the physiotherapist and beyond the range of services offered by occupational therapists, incontinence nurses and social workers, emphasising the need for **a common value system** and agreed outcomes for service users to be developed amongst the different groups providing such services, based on a sound understanding of the issues which arise in the dynamics of the workings between such groups.

Further reading

Oliver, M., Sapey, B. and Thomas, P. (2012) *Social Work with Disabled People*, 4th edn, Basingstoke: Palgrave Macmillan.

Shakespeare, T. (2006) *Disability Rights and Wrongs*, Abingdon: Routledge.

Swain, J. and French, S. (2008) *Disability on Equal Terms*, London: Sage.

Thomas, C. (2007) *Sociologies of Disability and Illness: Contested Ideas in Disability Studies and Medical Sociology*, Basingstoke: Palgrave Macmillan.

Whalley Hammell, K. (2006) *Perspectives in Disability and Rehabilitation – Contesting Assumptions; Challenging Practices*, Edinburgh: Churchill Livingstone.

References

Abberley, P. (2004) 'A critique of professional support and intervention', in J. Swain, S. French, C. Barnes and C. Thomas (eds) *Disabling Barriers – Enabling Environments*, 2nd edn, London: Sage.

Ajzen, I. (1988) *Attitudes, Personality and Behaviour*, Buckingham: Open University Press.

Armstrong, D. (1987) Theoretical tensions in biopsychosocial medicine, *Social Science and Medicine* 25 (11), 1213–18.

Barnes, C. (1991) *Disabled People in Britain and Discrimination*, London: Hurst.

Bickenbach, J., Chatterji, S., Bradley, E. and Üstün, T. (1999) Models of disablement, universalisms and the International Classification of Impairments, Disability and Handicaps, *Social Science and Medicine* 48 (9), 1173–87.

Bobath, B. (1990) *Adult Hemiplegia: Evaluation and Treatment*, Oxford: Heinemann.

Campbell, R., Evans, M., Tucker, M., Quilty, B., Dieppe, P. and Donovan, J. (2001) Why don't patients do their exercises? Understanding non-compliance with physiotherapy in patients with osteoarthritis of the knee, *Journal of Epidemiology and Community Health* 55, 132–8.

Carr, J. and Shepherd, R. (2003) *Neurological Rehabilitation: Optimising Motor Performance*, Edinburgh: Butterworth Heinemann.

Crotty, M. (1998) *The Foundations of Social Research: Meanings and Perspectives in the Research Process*, London: Sage.

de Wit, J. and Strobe, W. (2004) 'Social cognition models of health behaviour', in A. Kaptein and J. Weinman (eds) *Health Psychology*, Oxford: Blackwell.

Department of Health (2008) *Local Authority Circular: Transforming Social Care*, LAC (DH) (2008) 1.

Descartes, R. (1989) *Selected Philosophical Writings*, translated by J. Cottingham, R. Stoothoff, and D. Murdoch, Cambridge: Cambridge University Press.

Desrosiers, J., Rochett, A., Noreau, L., Bravo, G., Hebert, R. and Boutin, C. (2003) Comparison of two functional independence scales with a participation measure in post-stroke rehabilitation, *Archives of Gerontology Geriatric* 37, 157–72.

Dishman, R. and Ickes, W. (1981) Self-motivation and adherence to therapeutic exercise, *Journal of Behavioural Medicine* 4, 421–38.

Donaldson, G. (2009) *What can physiotherapists learn from disabled people's experiences of rehabilitation using a social model perspective?* MPhil thesis submitted to Lancaster University.

Doyal, L. (1991) *The Political Economy of Health*, London: Pluto Press.

Evenson, K. R. and Fleury, J. (2007) Barriers to outpatient cardiac rehabilitation, *Archives of Physical Medicine and Rehabilitation* 20, 241–6.

Fine, M. and Glendenning, C. (2005) Dependence, independence or inter-dependence? Revisiting the concepts of care and dependency, *Ageing and Society* 25, 601–611.

Finkelstein, V. (2000) 'Professions allied to the community', in J. Swain, S. French, C. Barnes and C. Thomas (eds) *Disabling Barriers – Enabling Environments*, 2nd edn, London: Sage.

Finkelstein, V. (2004) 'Modernising services?', in J. Swain, S. French, C. Barnes and C. Thomas (eds) *Disabling Barriers – Enabling Environments*, 2nd edn, London: Sage.

French, S. (1994) *On Equal Terms: Working with Disabled People*, Oxford: Butterworth Heinemann.

French, S. and Swain, J. (2004) 'Whose tragedy? Towards a personal non-tragedy view of disability', in J. Swain, S. French, C. Barnes and C. Thomas (eds) *Disabling Barriers – Enabling Environments*, 2nd edn, London: Sage.

Holdsworth, L. (1991) *Empowerment Social Work with Physically Disabled People*, Norwich: Social Work Monographs, UEA.

Hughes, B. (2004) 'Disability and the body', in J. Swain, S. French, C. Barnes and C. Thomas (eds) *Disabling Barriers – Enabling Environments*, 2nd edn, London: Sage.

Hutchinson, J. S. (2004) 'Health, health education and physiotherapy practice', in S. French and J. Sim (eds) *Physiotherapy: A Psychosocial Approach*, 3rd edn, Edinburgh: Elsevier.

Imrie, R. (2004) Demystifying disability: a review of the ICF, *Sociology of Health and Illness* 26 (3), 287–305.

Kaptein, A. and Weinman, J. (2004) 'Health psychology: some introductory remarks', in A. Kaptein and J. Weinman (eds) *Health Psychology*, Malden, MA: Blackwell.

Laver Fawcett, A. (2007) *Principles of Assessment and Outcome Measurement for Occupational therapists and Physiotherapists: Theory, Skills and Application*, Chichester: Wiley & Sons.

Maclean, N., Phill, B., Pound, P., Wolfe, C. and Rudd, A. (2002) The concept of patient motivation, *Stroke* 33 (2), 444–8.

Middleton, A. (2004) Chronic low back pain: patient compliance with physiotherapy and advice and exercise, perceived barriers to motivation, *Physical Therapy* 9, 153–60.

Nelson, G., Lord, J. and Ochocka, J. (2001) *Shifting the Paradigm in Community Mental Health: Towards Empowerment and Community*, Toronto: University of Toronto Press.

Oliver, M. (1996) *Understanding Disability: From Theory to Practice*, Basingstoke: Palgrave.

Oliver, M. and Sapey, B. (2006) *Social Work with Disabled People*, 3rd edn, Basingstoke: Palgrave Macmillan.

Pomeroy, V. (2007) Facilitating independence, motivation and motor learning, *Physiotherapy* 93 (2), 87–8.

Reed, K. and Sanderson, S. (1999) *Concepts of Occupational Therapy*, 4th edn, Philadelphia, PA: Lippincott Williams and Wilkins.

Roberts, P. (1994) Theoretical models of physiotherapy, *Physiotherapy* 80 (6), 361–6.

Rosenstock, I. M. (1974) Historical origins of the health belief model, *Health Education Monographs* 2, 1–8.

Sapey, B., Stewart, J. and Donaldson, G. (2005) Increases in wheelchair use and perceptions of disablement, *Disability and Society* 20 (5), 485–505.

Shakespeare, T. (2006) *Disability Rights and Wrongs*, Oxford: Routledge.

Sluijs, E., van der Zee, J. and Kok, G. (1993) Difference between physical therapists in attention paid to patient education, *Physiotherapy Theory and Practice* 9, 103–17.

Smuts, J. (1952) *Jan Christian Smuts*, London: Cassell.

Swisher, L. (2002) A retrospective analysis of ethics knowledge in physical therapy (1970–2002), *Physical Therapy* 82, 692–706.

Turner, B. S. (1992) *Regulating Bodies: Essays in Medical Sociology*, London: Routledge.

UPIAS and Disability Alliance (1976) *Fundamental Principles of Disability*, London: Union of Physically Impaired Against Segregation and The Disability Alliance.

van Vliet, P., Lincoln, N. and Fox, A. (2005) Comparison of Bobath-based and movement science-based treatment for stroke: a randomised control trial. *Journal of Neurology, Neurosurgery and Psychiatry* 76, 503–508.

Wade, D. and de Jong, B. (2000) Recent advances in rehabilitation, *British Medical Journal* 320, 1385–8.

Whalley Hammell, K. (2004) 'The rehabilitation process', in M. Stokes (ed.) *Physical Management in Neurological Rehabilitation*, 2nd edn, Edinburgh: Elsevier Mosby.

Whalley Hammell, K. (2006) *Perspectives in Disability and Rehabilitation – Contesting Assumptions; Challenging Practices*, Edinburgh: Churchill Livingstone.

Williams, G and Wood, P. (1988) Coming to terms with chronic illness: the negotiation of autonomy in rheumatoid arthritis, *Disability & Rehabilitation* 10 (3), 128–33.

World Health Organization (1980) *International Classification of Impairments, Disabilities and Handicaps*, Geneva: WHO.

World Health Organization (2001) *International Classification of Functioning, Disability and Health*, Geneva: WHO.

Part Three

INTERPROFESSIONAL AND INTERAGENCY WORKING: SERVICE USERS, CARERS AND DIFFERENT PROFESSIONAL GROUPS

Chapter 14
Service-user issues:
Rights, needs and expectations

Peter Beresford

Chapter summary

Writing in the second decade of the twenty-first century, when concepts like user involvement, empowerment and co-production have become commonplace, it is easy to forget how recent a development this actually is. But it is important not to do this. Such involvement only became a requirement with legislation at the beginning of the 1990s. Social work, a pioneer in this field, had only started to seek the views of service users, let alone involve them, in 1970 (Mayer and Timms, 1970). There is at the most no more than 30 years, or a generation, of public service and professional engagement with the perspectives of service users. Yet those same services and professions have much longer histories and cultures, stretching back in some cases to at least the nineteenth century, if not before. Thus a discussion of interprofessional and interagency practice, which seeks to build seriously on service-user perspectives, as this book does, has two developments in complex relation to deal with. It must not only advance our understanding of interprofessional and interagency practice, it must also provide an adequate basis for understanding and engaging with service users, their organisations, aims and objectives, to do so. This chapter has a particular concern to help in taking forward this second task.

Learning objectives

This chapter will cover:

- the key issues entailed in involving service users' perspectives in effective interprofessional working
- the reasons why the service-user perspective should be central to all interprofessional working considerations and plans

▶

- attitudes, methods and approaches that can be used for the most effective incorporation of service-user interests
- barriers to integrated practice which fully includes service users
- how inequalities of power and status between agencies and professions, and the effects of social and medical models in interprofessional working, affect service-user involvement
- developing effective and inclusive service-user involvement in agencies and workforce.

Service users and their movements

Human services historically have tended to see the people who use them as individuals, family members or possibly members of broader groups and communities. But from the 1960s and 1970s, a wide range of such service users began to organise collectively and get together in their own organisations and movements. A number of reasons for this development can be identified. These include dissatisfaction with the services and support they were receiving, a new assertiveness linked with more liberatory political times and the emergence of broader movements, like the women's, black civil rights and the lesbian, gay, bisexual and transgender movement, as well as new political challenges to the welfare state coming from both the new political right and the radical left. Many different groups organised in this way, starting with the disabled people's movement and embracing people with learning difficulties, older people, mental health service users, people living with HIV/AIDS, young people who had been brought up in state care and so on (Beresford and Croft, 1993).

While it would be wrong to overstate the impact of these movements, it has been significant. It has led to major changes in ideas, culture, practice, policy, processes and legislation on a global scale. Groups that had previously often been hidden have gained a greater individual as well as political and cultural presence in societies. In countries like the UK, their viewpoints have begun to permeate the mainstream, just as they have made major steps along the long road to inclusion and equal rights (ODI, 2008). It is also an international development, finding various expressions in North America, Europe and the majority world (Aspis, 1997; Campbell and Oliver, 1996;

Charlton, 1998; Coleridge, 1993; Morris, 1996; Oliver, 1996, 1993; Priestley, 1999).

All these service-user movements have placed an emphasis on people's right to live on equal terms in mainstream society and to speak for themselves. They seek to challenge discrimination and to ensure appropriate and adequate support over which they are able to exert greater choice and control (Campbell, 1996; Campbell and Oliver, 1996; Carter and Beresford, 2000). Each of these movements has particular history, character, culture and traditions. However, they also seem to have some important things in common. All highlight the importance they attach to a number of features.

The response to these movements across the agencies and professions covered in this book has been uneven, some responding to them more effectively

Key learning points

Service-user movement views on what is important for them from agencies:

- service users speaking and acting for themselves
- working together to achieve change
- having more say over their lives and the support that they receive
- challenging stigma and discrimination
- having access to alternatives to prevailing medicalised interventions and understandings
- the value of user-controlled organisations, support and services
- a focus on people's human and civil rights and their citizenship; this has emerged later, but is increasingly evident of the survivors' movement
- being part of mainstream life and communities, able to take on responsibilities as well as securing entitlements.
  (Beresford, 1999; Beresford and Harding, 1993; Campbell, 1996; Campbell and Oliver, 1996)

than others. This can be expected to have an impact on both interprofessional working and how far approaches to such working reflect these developments effectively. This may relate to the different models underpinning these professions. Social work, for example, highlights a social model approach which takes account of the person in their broader context, while the medicalised individual model on which some other professions are still based is more likely to see the individual in isolation and focus on problems and pathologies within them (see below). Generally, those professions which draw on social models have tended to find it easier to address and include service-user perspectives.

Services versus lives

One of the themes running through service-user groups and movements is that people define themselves not in terms of services or practitioners, but rather in terms of their lives and their overall identity. Indeed, there is no agreed terminology for people in this field either accepted by service users and their organisations or providing a basis for agencies and professionals to adopt within their agencies, and for interagency working purposes. There are no existing words that adequately embrace all the groups and individuals who are included in these groups and movements. While 'service user' is the term most often used, many individuals dislike this term, because they feel it defines them passively and solely in relation to services they use, rather than taking account of their overall identity. This may include being a parent, a worker, a student, a volunteer, a partner and much more (Beresford, 2005). This desire to be framed in terms of your life, rather than the services that can impact on it, is epitomised by the name chosen by one national service-user organisation and network, *Shaping Our Lives*. This explicitly places an emphasis on people's lives rather than their services, framing them accordingly and highlighting the desire they have to shape their lives for themselves.

Thus service users understandably tend to take a holistic view of themselves and their situation. They do not frame themselves in terms of the particular services and professions that may interact with them and impact on their lives. This can make divisions that exist between such policies, services and professions, particularly difficult and unhelpful for service users. It means that they need to learn what their boundaries and different roles and cultures are, how to negotiate them and what to expect of them. It means life can become like 'pass the parcel', where one agency or practitioner passes the individual on to another and it is difficult to pin down where responsibility lies and how to secure the help and support that is needed.

The different professionals involved in delivering any one individual's services and support need to be alert to this important issue in service users' experience, and take it actively into account in planning their communication and work with that individual and with the other professionals that they are likely to liaise with in relation to that person.

Exercise 14.1

Check out the operation of any multi-professional team or agency you are familiar with:

- In agency or team literature or guidance, what models underpin practice – are they essentially individual or social models?
- What models underpin actual practice among team members – are they essentially individual or social models?
- If there are any discrepancies between these two, what might explain it?
- What if any meetings of the team/agency are service users and/or representatives of their organisations present?
- What part do they play in setting agency and professional agendas and how is this achieved?
- What issues for interprofessional working between the different professionals involved in the team might this raise?

Problems with traditional professional and service approaches

Working to move to more interprofessional and interagency approaches to practice also raises many complex issues from service users' perspectives. It is worth looking at some of these issues, if effective ways of overcoming them are to be developed by and for practitioners. The knowledge and experience of service users and their organisations are likely to have a helpful role to play in supporting better integrated and coordinated practice in human services.

Administrative barriers to integrated practice

Long-term human service users can frequently be on the receiving end of at least four different major services: health, social care, housing and benefits. Like the rest of us, they are also likely to turn to and have contact with many more. Not only do workers in these four specific services have separate different training, but many may not have training at all. Each of these services has different histories, cultures and traditions, goals, organisational structures, chains of command and philosophical approaches. Some may be locally provided, others under central control. They fall under different government departments, as well as different local organisations and systems. All these issues have implications for the practice of their particular practitioners, as well as for integrated and interprofessional and interagency practice. Thus the National Health Service is still essentially a universalist service, free at the point of delivery. Local authority social care, on the other hand, in spite of its increasing desire to make a 'universal offer', continues to be a means- and needs-tested residual service. There have long been serious shortages of housing provision and its provision and management have increasingly been outsourced. Meanwhile benefits policy and practice have increasingly been framed in terms of containing 'abuse' and reducing the numbers in receipt of disability and incapacity benefits. These different approaches, principles and organisational arrangements have major implications for the various practitioners, the potential for cooperation and coordination between them and of course for the support service users are able to access.

From service users' experience, there are other significant consequences for practice and coordination created by the different locations and professional backgrounds of practitioners. One of these is the tendency of services to divide service users into administrative categories and to be structured and organised accordingly. An important recent example of this is the breaking up of social work into social work with families and children, overseen by the Department for Children, Schools and Families (now the Department for Education), and social work with adults, still housed in the Department of Health. But this does not take account, for example, of the fact that disabled people may also be parents and children include disabled children. Thus while people actually frequently cross over such bureaucratic divides – they may have physical impairments, as well as use mental health services, or be deaf and have learning difficulties – their allocation to different departments, services and practitioners creates barriers and divisions between practitioners and between practice and service users. Another problem occurs during times of transition, for example when an individual moves from the status of child and young person to adult, or from adult to 'older person'. At such points, the professionals working with people, and often the entitlements they have, may change. Services are notoriously inept at ensuring continuity and good support through these periods. Practitioners may change or have to refer to different services, and in both cases, new problems are often created.

Key learning points

Ensuring continuity and good support between different agencies and professionals.

- Different professionals need to be sensitive to and gain an understanding of the different ethos and cultures of other professions to maximise the effectiveness of their work with them for service users.
- All professionals benefit from recognising that while they come from a particular professional perspective, with a specific role and responsibility, service users see the world in terms of their overall holistic needs and situation and professionals need to take this as their starting point.
- Service users are increasingly being expected and want to experience professional practice as a process of 'co-production' in which they are equally involved. All professional and interprofessional activity will benefit from recognition of this.

Case study

A service user with learning difficulties was admitted to a hospice. Some staff began to express their concerns that they hadn't had training in how to work with someone with learning difficulties and that this hadn't cropped up before. They called for specialist training. But one social worker who was experienced in working with disabled people argued against this. She felt that nurses and other staff were seeing this person as in some way inherently different and needing a different response, rather than recognising the commonality of their needs, rights and experience. She highlighted the importance of supporting their access needs, ensuring that they were kept properly informed of what was happening and able like any other service user to give their informed consent. But at the same time, she said, 'I think at the heart of this desire for more training is a sense that this person is different to the rest of us – "other". Such "training" would reinforce people's sense of distance between them and her, not reduce it.'

The complex and overlapping nature of people's actual identities is one of the reasons why *Shaping Our Lives* and a number of other service-user controlled organisations have come to work with a wide range of service users, instead of working with just one group, like mental health service users, or being 'impairment-specific' as many traditional disability charities have been. This has made it possible for them to see the many things these different groups have in common, as well as differences which distinguish them.

There are undoubted tensions between the commonalities and differences that may exist between different individuals and groups. The trend in services like health and social care, however, seems to have been towards specialism and away from genericism, justified by the argument that this is most likely to recognise and serve the particular needs of different groups. Service users have mixed views about this (Beresford, 2007). However, lines of demarcation tend to be drawn according to professional and organisational issues rather than service-user preferences. It is crucial that service users are fully and actively involved in any reorganisation of services – both within and between agencies. Among other issues this could address key concerns relating to interprofessional working, including:

- how information will be shared and what arrangements will be established to ensure informed consent
- how different agencies and professionals propose to put the rights and interests of service users at the centre of their interprofessional activities
- how this will be monitored and reviewed, by whom and when.

Service users also highlight the tendency of services and professionals to see people as sets of isolated symptoms or 'needs', rather than recognising and relating to the whole person. This is sometimes encouraged by both the structuring and value base of occupational roles in human services. Trends to the division of labour and narrowing and commodification of caring roles can discourage people from being seen in the round. Thus recent tendencies, for example, in policing, nursing and social care have all contributed to the narrowing of professional roles to more managerialist, organising functions and the creation of ancillary roles taking a more 'hands-on' role. Yet from service users' experience, it is often the routine and mundane ongoing contact that they can have with workers which encourages the relationships which they tend to see as fundamental to positive practice.

What these organisational, professional and structural issues highlight from service users' perspectives is that if agencies and practitioners are to work better together, high-level change, different kinds of roles and changed face-to-face relationships are *all* likely to be needed, if service users are to be ensured appropriate, seamless and uninterrupted support.

The dominance of medicalised individual models

It is not only the ways in which agencies and professions are organised which can affect and limit their

191

ability to work well together. The values and philosophies underpinning them also have an important bearing. Health and social care have tended to be based predominantly on individualised understandings of people and their problems. Over the twentieth century these were increasingly overlaid with medicalised understandings. Such medicalised individual interpretations and explanations of people, with their origins in physical and psychiatric medicine, have spread to dominate public services much more generally, although this is often implicit rather than explicit in their working. Historically understanding of groups like disabled people, mental health service users, older people, people with chronic and life-limiting conditions and people with learning difficulties have tended to be framed in terms of them having a personal problem, in terms of their incapacity, deficiencies and pathology. They tend to be understood in terms of what they can't do rather than what they can do. This has had massive ramifications for human service practice. We can see it institutionalised in the increasing trend to respond to problems experienced and identified in children and young people through their inclusion in a growing range of psychiatric diagnostic categories like ADHD (attention-deficit hyperactivity disorder) and the evidenced over-prescription of major tranquilisers to older people in institutional provision.

Such service users' historical experience of public provision has tended to be characterised by two features. Firstly, the tendency to segregate and lump people in such groups together in separate, often institutional, provision. Thus they have often been cut off from more mainstream services, reinforcing prevailing assumptions and stereotypes about them among their workers. Secondly, dedicated services and professions and occupations which have been developed to work with them have tended to frame their understanding of them in individualistic terms as needing help and care because of their 'incapacity' and 'vulnerability'. Such individualistic interpretations have also encouraged the making of moral judgements, often implicitly in occupational and professional practice. This has particularly applied to groups where an element of culpability has been felt to explain their failure to conform, notably, among young and unemployed people and people living on welfare benefits.

Key learning points

Reframing different professionals' views on service users:

- to be sensitive to difference and diversity among service users while recognising their commonalities, shared rights and entitlements
- to learn from and build on service users' valuing of social rather than individualised models for understanding and working with them
- to see service users as active participants in interprofessional working, who have now developed their own organisations, movements, bodies of knowledge and user-led services and support
- to recognise service users as an additional partner in interprofessional working.

Case study

Palliative care is an area where multi-agency and interprofessional practice is well developed. It also has a strong tradition of working in an holistic way. However, a study of service users views of specialist palliative care social work practice highlighted the far-reaching problems created by inconsistencies between medicalised individual and social approaches to practice in this setting. For example, while service users saw social work support as particularly helpful when difficult emotion issues began to emerge for them, because the referral system was largely led by medical staff, referrals tended to be related to the perceived seriousness of *physical* symptoms (Beresford *et al.*, 2007).

Exercise 14.2

Consider how you would work with service users and other professionals and agencies involved to provide a holistic and person-centred response to the service user's needs.

Such individualised interpretations of people may offer only a partial picture, placing a disproportionate emphasis on the individual, rather than taking account of them in their broader context and circumstances, but it can also create underlying tensions between different professional perspectives. This is particularly highlighted in the case of social work, although it is also evident in the competing approaches of psychiatry and psychology. There are also instances of policy-makers deliberately seeking to modify the conceptual basis of a helpful profession. An important instance was the removal of probation officer training from social work education in the 1990s and its realignment with more individualised correctional approaches (Smith, 2005). The defining characteristic of social work is its inherently *social* approach – even though some case work traditions have been more indebted to psychiatric approaches. Thus social work essentially seeks to address the individual in their social setting, taking account of both and paying attention to their interrelations.

Service users value the social approach of social workers, but they quickly become aware that this is not the prevailing model in use and that human service workers coming from other perspectives tend not to attach the same emphasis or have the same understanding of broader social and situational issues. This leads to a related and no less important issue that service users repeatedly highlight, particularly in the context of multidisciplinary and multi-agency work. This is the operation of a hierarchy of power and credibility between different professionals. This is frequently talked about in relation to community mental health teams (CMHTs), but applies in many other contexts too. Here, service users are conscious of the professional dominance of psychiatry, the tendency for nursing staff to be subordinate and of social workers often to challenge such inequalities of status and power and to come into conflict with other professionals for this reason. Some teams work in much more egalitarian ways, but traditional medical dominance reflected in differentials in reward and recognition continue to operate to create more fundamental barriers to truly collaborative and equal working. Such inequalities still seem to be perpetuated in professional education and training, reinforcing inequalities for the future.

Many service users particularly value the social workers' role as advocate, with both their own and other agencies and with other professionals. They frequently align themselves with social workers'

Exercise 14.3

By what means and approaches can each professional group change their approaches to working with service users to ensure that they are more equal and inclusive?

perspectives, especially since in a field like mental health, for instance, they are not as directly involved in actual medical treatment aspects of their experience of services, which may for example include the administration of major tranquillisers and depot injections, both willingly and against their will.

How do inequalities of power and status between agencies and professions affect service users?

Service users quickly become sensitive to medical dominance in health and social care services and occupations and the way that this can result in them, their rights and wants, not being fully understood or recognised. Interagency and interprofessional working can be the site of such conflicts, but can also provide opportunities for resolving them, especially where the concerns of service users are actively incorporated in their processes.

How can such inequalities be highlighted and addressed?

Ways forward for collaborative practice

As we have seen, a number of overarching obstacles to positive interagency and interprofessional practice can be identified from the perspectives of service users. These include:

- administrative and organisational barriers
- the reduction of service users to abstracted needs and characteristics
- the dominance of the medical model and the subordination of social approaches
- inequalities of power and status between professions and occupations.

All of these can lead to tensions and conflicts between different agencies, services and workers, which in turn can have damaging and disruptive effects for service users.

Including service users

Service users, however, not only offer a critique of the barriers facing collaborative practice. They also offer ways forward from their own ideas and discussions for overcoming these difficulties and developing a unified and unifying approach to practice.

Key learning points

A different way of approaching collaborative working between agencies and professions is for both to be shaped much more by service users and their organisations. This approach offers a key route to harmonising them all with the rights and wants of service users and in turn with each other. The perspectives of service users:

- offer common core values and principles
- share goals and objectives
- make it possible to build on shared user experience and knowledge.

That is what the second part of this chapter now focuses on. Several key components for such change emerge. All are key elements in the theory and practice of service-user organisations and movements. They include:

- the philosophy of independent living
- developing social/barriers-based models to underpin practice
- rights, responsibilities and entitlements
- user involvement in education and training
- valuing user knowledge and experience in practitioners
- ensuring equal access to service users in its fullest sense
- developing effective and inclusive involvement in agencies and workforce.

These taken together provide a basis from service-users' perspectives for consistent and positive practice across the different human service roles and agencies with which this book is concerned. While issues of organisation, communication and coordination will also need to be addressed, this is more likely to be achieved if grounded in this way.

We can now look at each of these in turn. We begin with two key ideas and approaches that have been developed by service users and their movements. The first of these is the social model of disability. This was developed by the disabled people's movement but has subsequently been widened in both its meaning and application, to provide a theoretical base for practice with much wider relevance.

Key learning points

Research and consultations with social work and social care service users repeatedly highlight the importance they attach to a range of human qualities which they associate with good practice. These include warmth, empathy, compassion, openness and honesty, flexibility, listening, reliability, being non-judgemental and treating people as equals. While they talk of these as human *qualities*, what often seems to lie at their heart is the development of particular skills. They also see the quality of their relationship with the practitioner as key to good practice.

The philosophy of independent living

The philosophy of independent living was also originally inspired by the disabled people's movement. It follows from the social model of disability. It is based on a belief that disabled people should be enabled to live their lives on as equal terms as possible alongside non-disabled people. The philosophy of independent living turns traditional notions of independence on their head. It is not preoccupied with the individual, or narrow ideas of personal autonomy. It does not mean standing on your own two feet or managing on your own. Instead of seeing the service user as having a defect or deficiency requiring care, it highlights the need to ensure they have the support that they need to be autonomous and live their lives as fully as possible,

A Closer Look

Developing social/barriers-based models to underpin practice

The social model of disability represents a fundamental break from traditional individualised Western understandings of disability, which tend to be interpreted in personal 'tragedy' terms. The social model draws a distinction between the (perceived) impairment – intellectual, physical or sensory – which may affect the individual, and disability, the negative societal reaction to people seen as having such impairments. It does not see disability simply in deficit terms as a problem of the person. For the first time, the social model highlighted the oppression and discrimination experienced by disabled people (Oliver, 1996; Oliver and Zarb, 1989; Thomas, 2007). Since then much work has been done to explore the nature of impairment as well as of disability and to make better sense of the interrelations of the two.

The social model makes clear the barriers faced by disabled and other people, restricting their lives and undermining their opportunities and quality of life.

It has highlighted the way in which such traditional medicalised individual understandings have dominated public and policy understandings of disability as well as professional responses to it, and the inhibiting effects they have had on such agency and professional roles. A barrier or social model approach, including attitudinal, physical and communication barriers, is increasingly being seen as having relevance across a growing range of welfare policy users (Thomas, 2007), including people with experience of poverty, drug and alcohol problems, chronic and life-limiting conditions, where societal reactions are no less important than individually experienced problems or impairments. The social model of disability is increasingly informing public policy officially in the UK, although its actual impact is open to question (ODI, 2008). Certainly it provides a coherent and consistent model, which takes account of both personal and social factors, to inform human service practice and agencies. It is likely to encourage more effective and helpful collaboration, underpinned by a shared model of understanding.

on equal terms and interdependently with others (Morris, 1993). This support is not expected to come from family members required to be unpaid or 'informal carers'. It rejects the concept of care and replaces it with the idea of support. It sees independence as meaning autonomous decision making rather than the physical capacity to carry out all activities of daily living unaided (Campbell and Oliver, 1996; Morris, 2004). Instead of people being assessed on the basis of what they can't do to qualify for 'care', under this model, support is provided to enable them to live their lives as fully as possible. There are two interrelated and key aspects to the philosophy of independent living:

1. Ensuring people the support that they need under their control to be able to live their lives as fully as they can, on as equal terms as possible, with non-disabled people.
2. Equalising their access to mainstream policy and services like housing, health, education and employment.

This emphasises the relevance of independent living as a value base across public policy, as well as

specifically in relation to human services. In England, a governmental Independent Living Strategy with cross-departmental support signed up to these values (ODI, 2008), although again it needs to be said that public services are still a long way from being organised and provided on a basis consistent with this.

Rights, responsibilities and entitlements

Human services have traditionally framed their users in terms of their *needs*. Such needs have tended to be defined by others on behalf of service users. Distinctions have also been drawn between 'needs' and 'wants', with

Exercise 14.4

What role does interprofessional working have to play in ensuring the independence and empowerment of service users to the greatest extent possible?

What skills do professionals need to try to ensure this in their interprofessional working?

wants taken to mean what service users might prefer, but not necessarily what policy-makers and professionals regard as appropriate to provide for service users. Disabled people and other service users increasingly expressed their dissatisfaction with others defining their needs for them (Oliver and Barnes, 1998). While there has been a developing discussion from left of centre social policy writers arguing the value of 'need' as a formative concept, this is not a view that has generally been accepted by commentators coming from service-user movements (Doyal and Gough, 1991; Oliver, 1996).

Instead, the disabled people's and service-user movements have tended to frame their demands and objectives in terms of their rights not needs, requiring support and change, rather than care and welfare. They are concerned with the achievement of both their civil and human rights, collective as well as individual rights. To achieve these goals and values, service-user movements have developed new approaches to collective working. These place an emphasis on self-organisation – developing their own 'user-controlled' organisations – as well as on participation and people 'speaking for themselves'. But they also take account of people's feelings and needs for support in the process. To make this possible they have increasingly highlighted ideas of inclusion and empowerment (Campbell, 1996; Campbell and Oliver, 1996).

Goals of achieving and safeguarding people's civil and human rights can be seen to offer a more accountable and less normative basis for human service roles and services than the concept of need. They also highlight the need for particular care, consistency and accountability where such roles are concerned with restricting rights (as are, for example, the roles of social worker, psychiatrist and police), as well as with supporting them.

and service cultures than through involving service users in occupational education and training (Beresford, 1994). This has led to the widespread development of 'user-led training', 'user trainers' and 'training for user trainers'. This makes it possible for workers to learn from people with direct experience of services, to find out more about what they want from services and how these can be most helpful for them. It also makes it possible, sometimes for the first time, for workers to relate to service users in positive, equal and active roles, rather than in the often passive and dependent role of patients or clients.

Service-user organisations have pressed for such involvement to extend through all aspects of training; from providing direct input in professional and in-service training to being involved in developing course curricula, providing course materials and, indeed, selecting, evaluating and assessing courses and students. All these have become established in professional social work training and education. The new social work degree qualification introduced in 2003 required the involvement of service users in all stages and aspects of the qualification (Branfield *et al.*, 2007; Levin 2004). This has subsequently been extended to post-qualifying social work education and training (Branfield, 2009). Other occupations, from allied health professions to the police, have also introduced user involvement into their training programmes. The challenge is to ensure that such involvement develops coherently and systematically within and across professions and occupations. What it makes possible and provides a stimulus for is consistency and coherence – both of values and aims, within and between them, encouraging collaboration from the bottom-up, between both practitioners and agencies.

User involvement in education and training

A continuing message from service users and their organisations over the years is that there are few more effective ways of changing and improving practice

Valuing user knowledge and experience in practitioners

One of the characteristics of traditional practice and agencies has been that they have been constructed top-down, rather than bottom-up, drawing little on the understanding of their end users. There is often

Exercise 14.5

What might service users experience as positive in their contacts with the many agencies they may be involved with? What might they experience as negatives?

minimal overlap between service providers and service users and this can work to the detriment of both. It does not make for improved understanding of service users, or encourage the most appropriate practice and service provision. User involvement in training offers some corrective to this. However, service users and their organisations also argue the importance of encouraging the valuing of service-user experience and the recruitment of people with such experience to become workers in such services.

Clearly this would only apply where such experience did not clearly debar them from recruitment, as for example in the case of people with serious criminal convictions seeking to join the police, or child abusers being considered for work in child protection, They would also need to have the other necessary skills and qualities, in addition to direct experience. Service users make clear that they see shared direct experience as a valuable quality in practitioners. The addition of a common strand of experience is clearly likely to encourage shared understanding, empathy and compassion between different occupations. Unfortunately, significant barriers to the inclusion of such experience still seem to exist (Snow, 2002). However, encouraging the recruitment of suitable workers with experience as service users is likely to provide an improved basis for common understanding and shared principles and values between different services and agencies.

Ensuring equal access to service users

Many forms of exclusion and bias continue to operate in services. The introduction of the disability equality duty, anti-disability discrimination and new equality legislation all signify this. Some groups face particular barriers accessing services or experience inferior

treatment from them. We know, for example, that a number of black and minority ethnic communities tend to have inferior treatment in the mental health system and are more likely to be subject to its forensic, compulsory and restrictive provisions (Mental Health Foundation, 2009; Rutherford and Duggan, 2007). They are also less likely to access valued services, like specialist palliative care. Common standards of access and inclusion are key if there is to be effective interagency and interprofessional practice. Key to this is the need to develop effective policies and practices for access for all agencies and occupations. In this way it will be possible to ensure that they both operate inclusively individually and together in relation to each other. Access is much more than a matter of enabling wheelchair users to negotiate physical environments, important and essential though this is. What's needed are the development of policies and practices for access which make it possible in its fullest sense. Such a comprehensive approach to access demands provisions for:

- physical access
- cultural access
- communication access.

Developing effective and inclusive involvement in agencies and workforce

Pressure and provisions for user involvement in public provision have mushroomed, particularly in human services like health and social care, in recent years. We have already seen how this has developed in professional and occupational education and training. But it has also taken root in a wide range of other spheres, including planning, management, standard setting, research and evaluation and practice development. Service users and their organisations complain that such involvement can often be tokenistic and patchy. Its impact has also varied between different professions and services. It continues, for example, to be underdeveloped in medical professions, in contrast with social work, while being particularly high profile in policy areas like social care and regeneration.

However, an effective strategic approach to user involvement can be expected to encourage common standards and consistent approaches which can only help in interagency and interprofessional work. By connecting provision and practice closely and directly with the perspectives of service users, it makes possible greater coherence and consistency between them. This is rooted in the priorities of service users and the achievement of their rights and wants.

Conclusion

Effective user involvement – in all its senses – provides a basis for positive and improved interagency and interprofessional practice for the future. It is likely to include the key elements of:

- building on service users' ideas, models and values
- being rights-based
- drawing on user-led education and co-learning
- valuing service-user experience and knowledge
- ensuring access and inclusion.

Most importantly, **service users and their organisations will routinely be regarded as part of the team** that needs to work together. Improved collaboration and participation is not only about connecting with other professions and agencies. Crucially it means seeing engaging with service users as key for both process and outcomes – means and ends.

As a key starting point for involving service users equally in interprofessional working and making it possible for all professionals to engage with service users on equal terms, it needs to be recognised that this is not merely a technical or mechanical task. Such involvement and equal working is not something that is amenable to simplistic checklists or 'toolkits', although this has increasingly become the expectation as human services have become dominated by managerialist and consumerist thinking.

Involvement is not only about reasserting our common humanity as professionals and service users, but also about making it more possible. What it can then help achieve is shared understanding between professionals and service users. It helps do this by highlighting the importance of:

- more equal relationships
- more inclusive ways of working that prioritise diversity
- challenging the dominance of managerialist/bureaucratic approaches over professional practice
- professional practice framed in terms of people's lives, not the services they use
- more holistic, social models of understanding people and of professional practice
- more rights-based approaches to practice
- linking with and supporting service users' own user-controlled organisations.

All of these principles will not only help achieve better, more participatory professional practice, but also help all professionals committed to interprofessional working advance it more effectively.

Further reading

Beresford, P. and Croft, S. (1993) *Citizen Involvement: A Practical Guide for Change*, Basingstoke: Palgrave Macmillan.

Beresford, P., Adshead, L. and Croft, S. (2007) *Palliative Care, Social Work and Service Users: Making Life Possible*, London: Jessica Kingsley Publishers.

Beresford, P., Fleming, J., Glynn, M., Bewley, C., Croft, S., Branfield, F., Postle, K. (2011) *Supporting People: Towards a Person-Centred Approach*, Bristol: Policy Press.

Branfield, F., Beresford, P. with Andrews, E. J., Chambers, P., Staddon, P., Wise, G. and Williams-Findlay, B. (2006) *Making User Involvement Work: Supporting Service User Networking and Knowledge*, York: Joseph Rowntree Foundation, York Publishing Services.

Useful websites

www.shapingourlives.org.uk

Shaping Our Lives: the national service users and disabled people's organisation and network.

www.solnetwork.org.uk

Networking website SOLNET

References

Aspis, S. (1997) Self-advocacy for people with learning difficulties; does it have a future? *Disability and Society* 12 (4), 647–54.

Beresford, P. (1994) *Changing The Culture, Involving Service Users in Social Work Education*, London: Central Council of Education and Training in Social Work, Paper 32.2.

Beresford, P. (1999) Making participation possible: movements of disabled people and psychiatric system survivors, in T. Jordan, and A. Lent (eds) *Storming the Millennium: The New Politics of Change*, London: Lawrence and Wishart.

Beresford, P. (2005), 'Service user': regressive or liberatory terminology?, *Current Issues, Disability and Society* 20 (4), 469–77.

Beresford, P. (2007) *The Changing Roles and Tasks of Social Work from Service Users' Perspectives: A Literature-informed Discussion Paper*, London: General Social Care Council, www.gscc.org.uk/NR/...B915.../SoLSUliteraturereviewreportMarch07.pdf, accessed 22 December 2009.

Beresford, P., Adshead, L. and Croft, S. (2007) *Palliative Care, Social Work and Service Users: Making Life Possible*, London: Jessica Kingsley Publishers.

Beresford, P. and Croft, S. (1993) *Citizen Involvement: A Practical Guide for Change*, Basingstoke: Macmillan.

Beresford, P. and Harding, T. (eds) (1993) *A Challenge to Change: Practical Experiences of Building User-led Services*, London: National Institute for Social Work.

Branfield, F. (2009) *Developing User Involvement in Social Work Education*, Workforce Development Report 29, London: Social Care Institute for Excellence.

Branfield, F., Beresford, P. and Levin, E. (2007) *Common Aims: A Strategy to Support Service User Involvement in Social Work Education*, Position Paper 7, London: SCIE.

Campbell, P. (1996) The history of the user movement in the United Kingdom, in T. Heller, J. Reynolds, R. Gomm, R. Muston, and S. Pattison (eds) *Mental Health Matters: A Reader*, Basingstoke: Macmillan.

Campbell, J. and Oliver, M. (1996), *Disability Politics: Understanding Our Past, Changing Our Future*, Basingstoke: Macmillan.

Carter, T. and P. Beresford (2000) *Age and Change: Models of Involvement for Older People*, York: York Publishing in association with Joseph Rowntree Foundation.

Charlton, J. I. (1998) *Nothing about Us without Us: Disability, Oppression and Empowerment*, CA: University of California Press, Berkeley.

Coleridge, P. (1993) *Disability, Liberation and Development*, Oxford: Oxfam in association with Action on Disability and Development.

Doyal, L. and Gough, I. (1991) *A Theory of Human Need*, Basingstoke: Palgrave Macmillan.

Levin, E. (2004) *Involving Service Users and Carers in Social Work Education*, SCIE Guide 4, London: Social Care Institute for Excellence.

Mayer, J. E. and Timms, N. (1970) *The Client Speaks: Working Class Impressions of Casework*, London: Routledge.

Mental Health Foundation (2009) *Increase in Use of Compulsion Worrying Says Mental Health Foundation*, 15 October, http://www.mentalhealth.org.uk/media/news-releases/news-releases-2009/15-october-2009/, accessed 12 October 2010.

Morris, J. (1993) *Independent Lives?: Community Care and Disabled People*, Basingstoke: Macmillan.

Morris, J. (1996) *Encounters with Strangers: Feminism and Disability*, London: Women's Press.

Morris, J. (2004) Community care: a disempowering framework, *Disability and Society* 19 (5), 427–42.

ODI (2008) *The Independent Living Strategy: A Cross-government Strategy about Independent Living for Disabled People*, London: Office for Disability Issues.

Oliver, M. (1996) *Understanding Disability: From Theory to Practice*, Basingstoke: Macmillan.

Oliver, M. and Barnes, C. (1998) *Disabled People and Social Policy: From Exclusion to Inclusion*, Harlow: Addison Wesley Longman.

Oliver, M. and Zarb, G. (1989) The politics of disability: a new approach, *Disability, Handicap and Society* 4 (3), 221–40.

Priestley, M. (1999) *Disability Politics and Community Care*, London: Jessica Kingsley Publishers.

Rutherford, M. and Duggan, S. (2007) *Forensic Mental Health Services: Facts and Figures on Current Provision*, London: Sainsbury Centre for Mental Health.

Smith, D. (2005) Probation and social work, *British Journal of Social Work* 35 (5), 621–37.

Snow, R. (2002) *Stronger than Ever: Report of the First National Conference of Survivor Workers UK*, Stockport: Asylum.

Thomas, C. (2007) *Sociologies of Disability and Illness: Contested Ideas in Disability Studies and Medical Sociology*, Basingstoke: Palgrave Macmillan.

Chapter 15
Member of the team? Carers' experience of interprofessional working: key issues in current policy and practice

Carmel Byers and Creating Links[1]

Chapter summary

Interprofessional working and the involvement of service users and carers in the design, delivery and provision of services they use have both been in the forefront of government policy and legislation in the children and family and adult policy agenda and are now key requirements for agencies providing social services (Department of Health, 2010; Quinney, 2006). However, until the present (December 2011), very little has been written on carers' perspectives on interprofessional working and their part in this. The issue of professionals working together in the interests of the service user and carer is fundamental to, for example, social work practice in the National Occupational Standards (Topss, General Social Care Council, 2002) and (GSCC) Codes of Practice (2002), and has gained even more prominence as a result of the findings of the Laming Inquiry (Department of Health, 2003) which identified the failures of the professionals to work together and communicate effectively, emphasising the need for a more 'joined-up' approach to effective collaborative working between agencies and within multi-agency teams. Other professions similarly emphasise the importance of engaging in interprofessional working in their equivalent Codes. If, according to these policy directives, carers and the people they care for are to have a meaningful involvement in planning, service provision and delivery of the services they receive, it could be expected that they would be seen as equal partners in the interprofessional team. However, evidence from research studies points to a considerable gap between the policy directives relating to greater participation and involvement of users and carers and the reality of current practice (Hardy *et al.*, 2001; Roulstone and Hudson, 2007; Walker and Dewar, 2001).

This chapter draws on the experiences of informal carers in order to gain an understanding of how interprofessional working is perceived by those on the receiving end of social services,

---

[1] 'Creating Links' is a group for people who use services and carers and is involved in all aspects of social work education at the University of Hertfordshire.

and whether they consider themselves part of the care team. Carers were consulted on their perspectives of working with various professional groups and to what extent they considered themselves involved and included in decision-making processes. Included were those with caring responsibilities for people with learning disabilities, people with mental health needs, older people, parent carers and also foster carers. Carers associated with carers organisations in Hertfordshire were consulted individually and in groups, as were the members of 'Creating Links', people using services and carers group involved in all aspects of social work education at the University of Hertfordshire who were also directly involved in the facilitation of the consultations and in compilation of this chapter. The consultation also includes the perspectives of foster carers who differ from informal carers in that they are generally self-employed and part of the care service provision, receiving payment and training for the care work they do. However, their perspectives on interprofessional working bear many similarities to those of informal carers. The areas discussed in this chapter are developed further in the next chapter, written by the same authors.

In order to ensure confidentiality, no individuals are identified in the chapter. Indications for good practice drawn from the carers' perspectives are identified throughout. Carers were made aware of the purpose and the nature of the book, and the content of the chapter, to which they agreed.

Learning objectives

This chapter will cover:

- how and why current policy directives in health and social care emphasise that carers and the people they care for should have a meaningful involvement in planning, provision and delivery of the services they receive and why this may not be being met in many areas
- how the principles and practice of carer-focused interprofessional working can be based on different agencies appreciating the place of carers as a key part of the arrangements for assessing needs and developing plans
- why the views and experiences of carers are so important in health and social care, and have to actively be sought and valued
- how to take into account key issues for carers in being part of service delivery – information exchange and communication sharing; taking a holistic approach to the needs of carers and service users; the influence of different values and assumptions of professionals across agencies; and having a lead professional who takes account of these areas
- the indicators for satisfactory involvement of carers include feeling that information is shared, feeling included in decision making, feeling that there is someone who can be contacted when needed and feeling that the service is responsive to their needs.

Current information on carer involvement

Current evidence suggests that carer involvement and participation is limited, highlighting a considerable gap between the policy directives and the reality of current practice (Bliss, 2006; Hardy *et al.*, 2001; Roulstone and Hudson, 2007; Walker and Dewar, 2001).

Studies researching carers' involvement and interprofessional teamwork cover a range of service user and carer groups, including older people, people with conditions such as dementia and cancer and disabled children, located in settings such as a hospital and the home, with services provided by statutory and voluntary agencies, including interprofessional and interagency working. Studies explore a range of models of involvement in decision making relating to various aspects of care and medical needs, including assessment and care management processes and discharge planning.

Despite this wide variation in settings, service user and carer groups and perspectives, certain common themes emerge which would appear to be confirmed by the carers participating in the consultation in this chapter.

It is important to note that there is evidence of improved practice in interprofessional working, with greater professional awareness of supporting service users and carers, resulting in easier access to some services (Abbott et al., 2005; Roulstone and Hudson, 2007), and that the amount of consultation is increasing (Princess Royal Trust for Carers, 2002). However, a number of studies also identify that carers and the people they care for often feel excluded from decision making and planning, feeling 'taken for granted' and dissatisfied with the level of involvement (Abbott et al., 2005; Hardy et al., 2001; Hingley-Jones and Allain, 2008; Huby et al., 2007; Roulstone and Hudson, 2007; Walker and Dewar, 2001). A recent report from the Princess Royal Trust for Carers highlights how carers have to fight to gain some recognition as 'partners in care', and how too often, carers feel that they are left with all the caring responsibilities and little recognition or support (Princess Royal Trust, 2009).

Earlier projects undertaken by The Princess Royal Trust for Carers (2002) have highlighted carers' concerns about the nature and quality of consultation, with carers expressing ambivalence and criticism of involvement processes with statutory service providers. In the experience of some carers, consultation was perceived as negative because of poor and indifferent practices, including not taking account of the pressures and strains typical in carers' lives when setting times and dates of meetings, and the principle of prompt feedback being disregarded (Princess Royal Trust for Carers, 2002; Roulstone and Hudson, 2007).

A range of factors have been identified in considering the possible explanations for the gap between the ideals of service user and carer involvement and the realities of practice. Firstly, power sharing has been highlighted as a possible difficulty; power dynamics in public institutions and agencies may undermine alternative viewpoints that conflict with the professional and organisational position. Managerialist agendas and the differences in the perspectives, language, priorities and perceptions of service users, carers, professionals and managerial providers can lead to dissatisfaction and conflict resulting in a lack of agreement of what constitutes satisfactory outcomes. This can lead to service user and carer views not being considered sufficiently and a lack of commitment from some organisations to participation and involvement (Carr, 2004, 2007; Tew, 2005).

Another aspect of organisational power dynamics may be seen in the impact of managerialism in particular on statutory services, with the shifting of power from professionals to managers and frequent organisational restructuring, undermining the progressive and liberatory values inherent in service user and carer empowerment (Beresford and Croft, 2004).

Secondly, professional assumptions about service user and carer competence in decision making and

Key learning points

Indications for satisfactory involvement

Walker and Dewar (2001) identify four markers that carers have suggested as indications for satisfactory involvement:

- feeling that information is shared
- feeling included in decision making
- feeling that there is someone who can be contacted when needed
- feeling that the service is responsive to their needs.

The importance of a lead professional who takes responsibility as a central coordinator of professionals and agencies who is a named person who can be contacted by the carer when needed is highlighted in a number of studies and will be discussed in the next chapter.

Exercise 15.1

What elements of interprofessional practice are important to ensure that the four markers indicating satisfactory involvement identified by Walker and Dewar are achieved?

expectations can make it difficult for users to be heard or have an impact on decisions (Carr, 2004; Fernandez *et al.*, 2007). Studies have generally come to similar conclusions concerning what carers want from the professionals with whom they work in order to feel involved in planning and decision making and part of the interprofessional team (Preston Shoot, 2003).

Many of the findings in the literature concerning the difficulties and conflicts in achieving successful involvement and what constitutes good practice are also identified by the carers in this consultation and listed in the **'Key Learning Points'** section in this chapter.

Most studies are in agreement with Vickridge (1998) that good professional practice can be achieved by working cooperatively across agencies, but that it only becomes 'user-centred' when users and carers are fully involved both in defining what they need from the service and being involved in the planning and development of services to meet that need. The high importance to carers of effective consultation and communication in achieving this is paramount (Hingley-Jones and Allain, 2008). In order to achieve this, professionals need to have not just an obligatory involvement as part of their job, but a personal belief in the value of service user and carer involvement (Sitzia *et al.*, 2006).

Who are the carers?

According to Carers Trust:

A carer is someone of any age who provides unpaid support to family or friends who could not manage without this help. This could be caring for a relative, partner or friend who is ill, frail, disabled or has mental health or substance misuse problems.

(Carers Trust, http://www.carers.org/what-carer)

This definition relates to those known as 'informal' carers who are generally family members who are unpaid and with no formal training. There is some disagreement over this term, as they may have had little choice in the matter of becoming carers (Beesley, 2006). However, it is important to acknowledge that not all those who find themselves in the position of looking after a family member, friend or neighbour in the community may consider themselves a carer, but rather see their role as part of their family or community responsibilities.

Different professionals may well perceive carers in a variety of ways which may impact on interprofessional working (Carers UK, 2009a; Macpherson *et al.*, 2008). Twigg and Aitkin (1994) conceptualise carers in distinct ways which include being viewed as a resource valued only in terms of their ability to provide support for the person cared for, being viewed as a co-worker whose well-being is addressed solely to ensure that the caring role remains sustainable and being viewed as a client, entitled to support in their own right. These concepts of carers would still appear to be currently valid.

Although research is limited in England and Wales on the correlation between informal care and

A closer look

Numbers of carers and current trends

It is estimated that each year, two million people become carers. According to Carers UK (www.carersuk.org) over three in five people in the UK, 10 per cent of the total population, will become carers at some time in their lives (Carers UK, 2009b). According to the last census in 2001, there were approximately six million informal carers. Reliance on carers' willingness to provide care by social services and the NHS is estimated to be worth £87 billion a year (Census 2001). In addition, research by Carers UK in 2002 found that carers contribute around £1 billion per year support in the community through setting up and running self-help groups for carers, campaigning and running projects charities and other activities. These figures are likely to increase, and it is estimated that the number of carers needed by 2037 will rise by 60 per cent to 3.4 million.

(Carers UK, 2001; Princess Royal Trust, 2009)

ethnicity (Young *et al.*, 2005), a recent report by Carers UK states that there are over 500,000 Black, Asian and Minority Ethnic (BAME) carers in England and that 10 per cent of all carers providing round-the-clock care are from BAME communities (Carers UK, 2011). Evidence suggests that certain BAME groups have been shown to be three times more likely to provide care compared with white British counterparts. There are high incidences of caring, particularly among Bangladeshi, Pakistani and Indian groups, but lower access to support. Almost twice as many Pakistani women are carers when compared to the national average (Carers UK, 2011; Gunaratnam, 2007; Princess Royal Trust, 2009; Young *et al.*, 2005). BAME carers face additional difficulties due to language barriers, stereotyping around caring and difficulties accessing culturally appropriate services, which puts them at greater risk of ill health, poverty, loss of employment and social exclusion. There is evidence of particular social and economic disadvantage for non-white ethnic groups who are considerably more likely to be experiencing financial hardship (Carers UK, 2011; Yeandle *et al.*, 2007). All this poses challenges for interprofessional working in the light of the complexities of disability, ethnicity and diverse user needs, which may result in multiple oppressions.

What is meant by involvement and participation?

In order for the professionals and the service user and carer to feel part of the team, there need to be clear indications of what is understood by involvement and participation by both carers and professionals. Despite the emphasis in recent years on service users and carers being involved in and participating in the planning, delivery and provision of services they use, there does not appear to be a commonly agreed definition of what is meant by involvement and participation (Roulstone *et al.*, 2006). Huby and colleagues consider that this can be taken to mean 'service-user centredness' but this may not necessarily imply active participation (Huby *et al.*, 2007). According to

Roulstone *et al.* (2006), there is not yet a consensus on what carer participation means, and that this can be construed as ranging from consultation to direct involvement in shaping the outcome of the services carers use. The participation of carers and service users should lead to outcomes that they consider they require from the service (Vickridge, 1998).

The lack of an agreed definition of carer involvement and participation leads to a lack of clarity over the objectives of carer involvement. If there are no agreed objectives for carer involvement, then it is difficult to evaluate the success or otherwise of carer participation either by the service users and carers or by the professionals (Hingley-Jones and Allain, 2008).

The degree of carer involvement and participation may also be affected by professional motivation, willingness and commitment to the agenda of involvement and participation, and this may vary markedly between professionals and professional groups. Sitzia *et al.* (2006) indicate that 'obligatory' involvement as part of the professional's role was counterproductive when not coupled with a 'personal belief' in the value of service user and carer involvement. Professionals may adopt terms like 'involvement and participation', but understanding of these terms may be superficial (Walker and Dewar, 2001).

An important consideration arises as to how far carers want to be involved in decisions regarding the people they care for. A significant proportion of service users and carers may wish to be involved in some decisions regarding the people they care for, but not in others. Some may embrace this in all its aspects, and others for various reasons may not want to be involved at all levels of assessment and decision making, preferring the professional team to take the lead role on particular aspects of their care. In considering whether carers are part of the interprofessional team, it may therefore be important to note that participation and involvement can be defined at whatever level the service users and carers are comfortable with, and should be negotiated between the service users and carers and the interprofessional team (Huby *et al.*, 2007). This serves to illustrate the challenges and complexities for interprofessional working in effectively supporting carer participation (Roulstone and Hudson, 2007).

What is meant by the interprofessional team?

Two definitions that appear to relate well to the qualities of interprofessional teams are identified by Payne (2000), based on the work of Brill in 1976:

A team is a group of people each of whom possesses particular expertise; each of whom is responsible for making individual decisions, who together hold a common purpose; who meet together to communicate, collaborate and consolidate knowledge, from which plans are made, actions determined and future decisions influenced.

(Brill, 1976 cited in Payne, 2000, p. 6)

A team has five basic characteristics ... the sharing of a common interest; to have a common aim and set of values; to have common objectives and/or tasks; for members to have designated roles and/or tasks; the feeling of membership and loyalty to the group.

(Redman, 1996, cited in Payne, 2000, p. 7)

A closer look

Questions to be considered in interprofessional practice with carers

- How do the carers perceive themselves and their caring role?
- How do the professionals perceive the carer and their role?
- What are the objectives of carer involvement from the perspective of the carer and that of the professional?
- Are the objectives clear for both?
- How far does the carer wish to be involved in decisions?
- What level of involvement is the carer comfortable with?
- What are satisfactory outcomes from the perspective of the carer, and that of the professional? Is there a conflict?

Background: policy developments promoting user and carer involvement

A wide range of policy and practice initiatives have been focused on the participation and involvement of informal carers in decision making, service assessment, provision and review. The goal of promoting maximum choice and greater independence for service users and carers is central to recent health and community care policies; the aim of which is to create health and social services that are accountable to users, responsive to their needs and through which users have greater control over what happens to them (Department of Health, 1990; Hardy *et al.*, 2001; Walker and Dewar, 2001). As community care depends on the goodwill and good health of informal carers, it is in the interests of health and social service providers to value, support and involve service users and carers in the decision-making process, and this continues to be a fundamental objective of government policy (Henwood, 1998; Walker and Dewar, 2001). This need for recognition has been incorporated into the Carers (Recognition and Services) Act 1995, which acknowledges the need for carers to have their needs assessed in their own right, and for that assessment to influence decisions about future care. Similarly the Community Care (Direct Payments) Act 1996 aims to include carers by allowing them to purchase services they are assessed as needing to support them in the caring role.

More recently the National Carers Strategy (Department of Health, 1999), the Community Care Delayed Discharge Act 2003, Carers and Disabled Children Act (2000) and the Carers (Equal Opportunities) Act 2004 have all played their part in giving greater significance to carer involvement and participation in planning, assessment and review of support, and the promotion of joined-up policy with the aim of seamless working across professional and service boundaries (Department of Health, 1999a, b, 2000, 2001b, c). The key goal of the New Deal for Carers Strategy 2008 was the recognition of carers both as expert partners and as individuals in their own right with their own life aspirations (Department of Health, 2008a).

Although there are limitations, the professional facilitation of the participation of informal carers in service design, review and delivery are now key statutory expectations with substantive rights attached (Department of Health, 2010). The role of professional cooperation and willingness to see carers as equal partners is a key factor in achieving these objectives.

Similarly, recent legislation and policy in the area of child and family social work focusing on prevention and support has also emphasised the importance of involvement and participation, requiring the creation of a more integrated service for children and families. The Children Act 2004, which emerged from the Green Paper Every Child Matters (Department for Education and Skills, 2003), itself a government response to the findings of the Laming inquiry (Department of Health,

2003), stated the need for more integrated interprofessional working including multi-agency teams. New legislation and policy developments (Children Act 2004 and Health Act 1999) have powers that support integrated working with disabled children with the aim of reducing fragmentation and bureaucracy. More recently, policy has been summarised in Aiming High for Disabled Children; transforming services for disabled children and their families (Department for Education and Skills, Department for Children, Schools and Families and HM Treasury 2007). These policies have shaped interprofessional working with disabled children and their families moving to integrated practice led by a key worker.

Despite progress towards increased levels of participation, carers' organisations and recent research continue to highlight a gap between policy and practice. Studies show that meaningful involvement remains limited, with carers continuing to feel excluded from the decision-making process and disappointed with their level of involvement (Hardy *et al.*, 2001; Princes Royal Trust, 2004; Rethink, 2003; Walker and Dewar, 2001).

Possible explanations for this have cited managerialist agendas, of which performance management culture is a part. This may encourage local authority and other social service agencies to put emphasis on output rather than outcome (Hardy *et al.*, 2001; Roulstone and Hudson, 2007). For example, success in community care assessments for these organisations may be based more on the organisational process and systems in place than the extent to which the processes deliver choice, opportunity and independence for service users and carers. The emphasis on 'throughput' coupled with the lack of resources and uncertainties in funding may limit the quality of carer involvement, participation and power sharing (Roulstone and Hudson, 2007).

Key learning points

Requirement for the involvement and participation of carers

The requirement for the involvement and participation of carers is clearly stated in the practice guidance accompanying the Carers and Disabled Children Act 2000. This makes clear in its guiding principles the need for a shift in practice regarding:

- holistic integrated family-based assessment that sees carers and cared-for people as partners in the caring relationship
- greater recognition of carers, and listening to their needs in addressing outcomes that would follow from the assessment process. (Department of Health, 2001a, p. 2)

The wider guidance makes clear the need for:

- multi-agency information sharing
- maximum local authority coordination in joining up care and carer provision with wider legislation guidance and services. (Department of Health, 2001a)

Exercise 15.2

What might be the practice elements that professionals should take into account when working interprofessionally, in order to achieve the four key points identified in the practice guidance for the Carers and Disabled Children Act 2000?

Carers' perspectives of interprofessional working

Many of the issues identified so far are confirmed by carers involved in the consultation. Carers' experiences, expectations and concerns, some of which are not new and have been raised in other studies, will now be discussed in the second part of this chapter under the following themes:

- information and communication
- taking a holistic approach
- values and assumptions.

Other issues identified as significant by the carers arising from these themes are related to power, control and agency agendas, implications for working together in meetings and other forums, and strategies to include carers as part of the interprofessional team. These themes will be explored in the next chapter.

Indications for good professional practice as identified by the carers have been drawn from the above themes and listed in each section.

Information and communication

Sharing information between professionals and carers

The importance of providing information emerges repeatedly in studies of service user and carer satisfaction and good practice (Bliss, 2006; Carers UK, 2006; Vickridge, 1998). Practical information, as well as advice and support, is essential to carers. Service users and carers generally place issues of information and good communication high on the list of what they require from professionals (Bliss, 2006; Robinson and Banks, 2009). This has even greater significance when considering interprofessional working. Information sharing is clearly a key element and fundamental to ensuring good communication between professionals and service users and carers. Concerns about communication and information sharing have long been considered problematic, with studies across service-user groups identifying that carers often receive insufficient information, particularly in relation to their caring tasks, including medical issues, physical care and advice concerning services (Carers UK, 2006; Keely and Clarke, 2002; Rethink, 2003).

Similarly, carers for both adults and children participating in our consultation highlighted significant areas of concern regarding the sharing and dissemination of information, both to themselves and the people they care for. Two particular areas of concern were identified. Firstly, the quality and accuracy of the information that they and the people they care for receive from professionals, and secondly, the quality and accuracy of the information that professionals disseminate and share with each other.

Quality and accuracy of received information

Professional knowledge and understanding of government directives, policy and legislation, resources and services available, may be understood and interpreted differently by professionals from a variety of health and social service agencies. The experience of carers showed that departments and agencies frequently contradicted each other's perception, and sometimes shared inaccurate information. Carers received conflicting information regarding their rights, and reported variations in interpretations of policy, entitlement and eligibility criteria depending on the professional with whom they were involved at a particular time. This often resulted in conflicting and confusing advice.

Professional language and jargon was frequently used and interpreted differently by professionals in different contexts. Some professionals may be lacking in specific areas of specialist knowledge, and hold differing professional views and perceptions of a carer's situation and needs, and this may lead to inaccuracies and variations in the information that is disseminated. Carers expect honesty and transparency from all professionals with whom they are working, and while it is understood that professionals may not have all the information that carers require, it is expected that they will do the necessary research, and provide the required information within an acceptable period of time.

Frequently there was no clear information available about what carers were entitled to. This is further complicated by the 'postcode lottery', variations in the availability of services in certain areas, resulting in carers engaging in an exhausting process of continuous phone calls to try to obtain information. Carers and parent carers could ill afford the time taken trying to search for this information. Professionals themselves were reported as being unclear about the roles of other professionals and the services that could be provided by them.

Clearly, conflicting information is confusing for carers. Examples given included receiving diagnoses by different professionals which were considered confusing. Two parent carers reported receiving a variety of professional views of their child's difficulties, including Asperger's syndrome, high-functioning autism, developmental disorder and evidence of social and communication difficulties. While these diagnoses can be seen as behaviours relating to autistic spectrum disorder, the variation in terms and lack of explanations can be confusing and worrying for carers and may paralyse the decision-making process, delaying access to services and influencing the level of services offered.

Quality and accuracy of information that professionals disseminate and share with other professionals

The importance of effective communication between professionals is stressed in the policies and guidance outlined in the previous section. However, carers reported experiences that suggested a lack of communication between health and social work professionals, for example general practitioners not passing on information to social services. Carers reported that not infrequently inaccuracies and a lack of clarity in the information that professionals disseminate to one another can result in what one carer described as 'Chinese whispers', with information undergoing changes and distortions as it is passed on. Carers expressed concern that even though a professional may have no specific training in the needs of that particular service-user group, their view of the needs of a carer may automatically be accepted by other professionals.

Although some advances are currently being made in this field, a lack of communication including the giving of conflicting, inaccurate and contradicting information between and within departments was also highlighted by carers, both in adult and children and family services.

Information passed between professionals is largely done through correspondence and written reports and carers reported several occasions when this information had been inaccurate. One carer sent a report back to the professional who wrote it, as statements had been attributed to the carer that were in fact made by the person she was caring for and vice versa. After the carer pointed this out, the professional concerned acknowledged this and amended the report. This example illustrates the importance of having all reports sent to the carer and service user for checking for accuracy. It is important, however, for professionals to be aware of the literacy skills and language and communication needs of the carers, in order not to assume that all is understood.

Carers and parent carers wanted to be in possession of copies of all relevant documents, so that they had all the necessary information to hand in case of losses. While this is generally accepted practice, and largely does take place, there were still reports of files, reports, documents and letters getting lost, or not being received. It is important for the professional to be aware of literacy levels. One carer reported that she would always request a printout from hospital or GP appointments, in order to be able to take accurate information to another professional. This she found far more useful than verbal reports and discussions.

These experiences concurred with findings of earlier studies concerning the need to improve communication and information sharing between agencies and professionals (Bliss, 2006; Carers UK, 2006; Vickridge, 1998) and to ensure accurate recording that can be communicated to other professionals. High staff turnover makes this particularly relevant for some areas of the service, where it is not uncommon for service users to have a number of different social workers in one year.

Information may not always be passed on to other professionals when workers leave the agency. On a number of occasions carers expressed concern at the lack of preparation by professionals who had not accessed the relevant information, resulting in carers and those they care for having to repeat their story yet again. One of the results of poor coordination between professionals is carers having to 'relive' and retell their stories again to different professionals. Information was frequently requested several times over by different professionals and this was perceived as intrusive. One carer considered that the information requested was 'stuff you wouldn't tell your close friend'. This can be an exhausting process needing considerable courage and effort, and carers may feel that these efforts and the energy expended 'goes down the drain'.

One parent carer described how following the departure of her social worker, the newly allocated worker began to explore various options which had already been investigated by the previous worker. The fact that this information had not been passed on was frustrating for the carer who felt that she was having to 'start over again'. A carer reported that the person she was caring for who uses mental health services had been removed from a GPs list without other professionals being informed, with the result that his treatment had been delayed. This delay was compounded by the lack of communication between the medical professionals and social workers with whom he was involved, and made worse by the high turnover of staff. In the words of one parent carer,

A closer look

The importance of communication and information sharing

Similar to the findings of other studies (Cleaver *et al.*, 2004; McGill *et al.*, 2006). Carers were concerned that professionals do not always refer them to an appropriate service, and that they were frequently not updated with the current progress on their situation, including when they might expect to receive a service. Carers stressed the importance of being updated regularly. The use of electronic methods such as texting or email were suggested as possible methods.

Carers suggested that some of the difficulties outlined in this section on information and communication could be overcome by the creation of a central base where service users and carers could find the information they need.

The carers' experiences confirm the current evidence that the lack of information disempowers carers and service users, excludes them and increases feelings of isolation.

Exercise 15.3

Given the importance of clear communication:

- What might be the difficulties and barriers that professionals should be aware of which impede the process of good communication with service users, carers and other professionals?
- What may cause these difficulties to arise?
- How might they be addressed?

'professionals will come and go, but me and my daughter are in it for life'.

Confidentiality

The question of effective information sharing clearly raises issues of the complexities of confidentiality. It is also important for professionals to understand issues of confidentiality, what should be shared and the impact of the Data Protection Act. A complex relationship exists between professionals, service users and carers that can give rise to potential conflicts of interest between them regarding confidentiality. Professionals need to make carefully weighed decisions regarding information sharing (Roulstone and Hudson, 2007).

Concerns about confidentiality included a carer who reported incidents where confidential reports had been faxed to her workplace, a carer who had received confidential phone calls regarding the person she was looking after at her workplace after requesting communications should be received only at home, and a foster carer who received confidential review and school reports on a young person who was no longer in her care.

Exercise 15.4

Confidentiality

- What might be the complexities inherent in ensuring confidentiality when working interprofessionally?
- How might these be addressed to facilitate appropriate information sharing?

Key learning points

Implications for good practice:

■ All reports and assessments should be shared, and communications confirmed in writing, with consideration given to language, literacy and alternative forms of communication, ensuring information is understood.

■ Discuss options available rather than just leaving written information, or a leaflet about a service.

■ Following an appointment, provide a report or printout for carers to take home and keep (health professionals in particular), which can if required on a future occasion be shown to another professional, making it easier for carers to pass on information.

■ Effective report writing skills with training on what to write and how to compile useful and accurate reports.

■ Professionals should have a clear understanding about the role of other professionals and be able to give information about the services that can be provided by them.

■ Agencies and their computer systems should be able to communicate with each other to improve coordination and accuracy of information.

■ Engage in adequate preparation, reading files, passing on relevant information and listening, so carers and service users don't have to re-tell their stories and 'start over again' a number of times at considerable emotional cost.

■ Maintain good communication, with follow-up visits and feedback on progress (of services).

■ Information sharing between professionals should take place, with due consideration given to issues of confidentiality and data protection.

■ If a professional does not have the information required, they should be prepared to find out and feed back to the carer and service user.

Taking a holistic approach

Taking a holistic approach to a carer's situation and the people they care for was considered an important element of interprofessional working. Carers identified that professionals tend to focus on the elements of a situation relevant to their particular professional perspective, resulting in poor coordination between services. In the case of disabled children's services, parent carers highlighted that often significant reports were written by professionals assigned to their child, who did not have the in-depth knowledge of their situation that a support worker was likely to have due to their closer relationship. Similarly, parent carers expressed concerns regarding service managers attending panels and similar forums when they did not have direct knowledge of their child, yet took important decisions regarding resources and care plans.

As one carer observed: 'You can have 10 reports by 10 different people but the appropriate service is still not available.' Shared ownership of the decision-making process is more likely to meet the holistic needs of individuals (Poxton, 2004).

As identified in the previous section, the lack of holistic understanding of the carers' situation could involve the carer and the person they are caring for in the frequent repetition of their histories, which is often painful and emotionally draining.

In order to avoid this, carers were reluctant to contact duty workers who were not familiar with their situations, considering this 'a waste of time'. Where cases were held 'on duty', carers were concerned that there was a danger of themselves and the people they were caring for being seen as a 'file number'.

Taking both a holistic and a personalised approach involves recognising the strengths that carers and parent carers possess. However, the current managerialist agendas and anxiety about not meeting eligibility criteria and resource limitations can frequently lead to both carers and professionals maximising or medicalising needs in order to get a service, or to prevent a reduction in a service already being provided. Having to portray their situation as a 'worst-case scenario' in order to do this was demoralising for carers and their families, who may have put in great efforts to their situation and be feeling positive and encouraged about the progress of the person they are caring for. While recognising that diagnoses are a very necessary element in indicating service needs and future planning, the need for professionals to attach 'labels' to service users and for carers and parent carers to seek 'labels' from professionals without which a service may not be provided can further contribute to feelings of disempowerment.

Carers gave examples where hours of allocated support were reduced when situations were going

Key learning points

Implications for good practice:

- A personalisation approach should be prevalent with the aim of encouraging professionals to take a holistic view of the carer and all elements of their situation.
- To gain a more holistic understanding of the carer and the person they are caring for, files and computer records should be read.
- One professional should act as the lead worker and should have a good knowledge of the individual and disseminate accurate information to other professionals involved.
- Parents and carers are the expert on their own child. Professionals should support this by contributing with the breadth of their knowledge.
- Adopt a strengths-based approach, work with and focus on supporting personal resources, build confidence and focus on ways of helping the carer and service user to feel encouraged and positive.

well due to their efforts, even though this provision had been identified as necessary in assessments.

This would appear to contradict good practice in working towards a personalised strengths-based approach, and supporting and recognising the considerable personal resources that families dedicate to their caring role. Instead of supporting and celebrating success, carers are demoralised by the highlighting of deficiencies and deficit in order to be given or continue to be given a service.

As one carer commented: 'if they think you can cope, you are a low priority.'

Values and assumptions

Interprofessional working can frequently be hampered by professionals who operate from different professional and personal value perspectives. The carers consulted reflected that this is still an issue impeding good practice. Professionals can make varying assumptions, for example, on the grounds of diagnosis, age and disability as identified by Peter Beresford (Chapter 14) and Suzy Croft (Chapter 12) in this book. Carers were keen to point out that their situations were diverse and that they do not necessarily have similar needs just because they are caring for someone who shares a similar diagnosis, condition, gender, age group, ethnic background or culture. Although there is greater professional awareness of the importance of recognising cultural and religious diversity, there is evidence of cultural stereotyping and expectations for example that family and friends would 'look after their own' (Carers UK, 2011; Gunaratnam, 2007).

Expectations, assumptions and judgements made by professionals concerning carers' marriages, the nature and quality of their personal relationships and other lifestyle issues were frequently made with little evidence to support these assumptions. Similarly, some professionals may be quick to make 'judgements' which labelled carers and stigmatised them as 'trouble-makers', particularly if they made any complaints concerning the service. Carers were concerned that this reputation would circulate around the professional teams, affecting the service they may receive.

The level of service user and carer involvement may be influenced by the values held by professional groups. Some professional and personal value bases may give less importance to involvement and participation, and therefore be less motivated for various reasons to engage in promoting this (Sitzia et al., 2006). A personal commitment and a belief in service user and carer involvement and participation by professionals are necessary in order for this to be successful. If professional value bases give less prominence to this, then it is less likely to be implemented.

Key learning points

Implications for good practice:

- Don't make assumptions, judgements, or comments on diagnoses, marriages and personal relationships based on little evidence to support them.
- Work towards overcoming professional differences in perception.
- See the carer as a person, not a condition or file number.
- Make a genuine connection with service users and carers.
- Value carer's involvement and participation.

Conclusion

The implications for practice identified by the carers in this consultation reflect issues that have been identified as important for good practice in carer participation and involvement elsewhere (Princess Royal Trust for carers, 2006). The carers consulted and the issues raised in this chapter have confirmed the findings of previous research studies, that despite policy directives, **carer participation in and involvement with the interprofessional teams is still limited**, and there are still concerns over a number of issues, including the **lack of effective communication and information-sharing**. Resource issues, managerialist agendas and organisational and structural issues amongst wider agendas have had a part in this. Although it should be noted that significant progress has been made in recent years, with service users and carers taking a more collaborative role, and **professionals increasingly acknowledging service users and carers as the experts in their own lives**, a number of issues still remain a concern for carers. These will be explored in the following chapter.

Acknowledgements

With grateful thanks for the help, advice and support of members of the Creating Links–People Using Services and Carers group, Carers in Hertfordshire and Parents in Action, as well as individual carers who gave up their time to contribute their knowledge and perspectives to this and the following chapter. The contributions of all those involved were much appreciated and valued.

Further reading

Roulstone, A. and Hudson, V. (2007) Carer participation in England, Wales and N Ireland: a challenge for interprofessional working, *Journal of Interprofessional Care* 21 (3) 303–17.

Kirton, D., Beecham, J. and Ogilvie, K. (2007) Still the poor relations? Perspectives on valuing and listening to foster carers, *Adoption and Fostering* 31 (3), 6–17.

Abbott, D., Watson, D. and Townsley, R. (2005) The proof of the pudding; what difference does multi-agency working make to families with disabled children with complex health care needs? *Child and Family Social Work* 10, 229–38.

Hingley-Jones, H. and Allain, L. (2008) Integrating services for disabled children and their families in two English Local Authorities, *Journal of Interprofessional Care* 22 (5), 534–44.

Beesley, L. (2006) *Informal Care in England*, London: The Kings Fund.

Bruce, D. and Paterson, A. (2000) Barriers to community support for the dementia carer: a qualitative study, *International Journal of Geriatric Psychiatry* 15, 451–7.

Carr, S., (2010) *SCIE Report 36: Enabling Risk, Ensuring Safety: Self-directed Support and Personal Budgets*, London: SCIE.

Cleaver, H., Walker, S., Scott, J., Cleaver, D., Rose, W., Ward, H. and Pithouse, A., (2008) *The Integrated Children's System Enhancing Social Work and Inter-Agency Practice*, London: Jessica Kingsley Publishers.

Cooper, H. and Spencer-Dawe, E. (2006) Involving service users in interprofessional education; narrowing the gap between theory and practice, *Journal of Interprofessional Care* 20 (6), 603–17.

Department for Education and Skills (2004) *The Common Assessment Framework*, www.education.gov.uk.

Department of Health, Department of the Environment, Transport and the Regions (1999) *Better Care, Higher Standards, A Charter for Long Term Care*, London: DoH DETR.

Department of Health (2001) *Health Service Circular Better Care, Higher Standards: Guidance for 2001/02*, London: DoH.

Department for Education and Skills and HM Treasury (2007) *Aiming High for Disabled Children* http://www.education.gov.uk/childrenandyoungpeople/sen/ahdc.

Kirton, D., Beecham, J. and Ogilvie, K., (2007) Still the poor relations? Perspectives on valuing and listening to foster carers, *Adoption and Fostering* 31 (3), 6–17.

Twigg, J. and Atkin, K. (1994) *Carers perceived: Policy and Practice in Informal Care*, Buckingham: Open University Press.

Victor, L., (2009) *A Systematic Review of Interventions for Carers in the UK: Outcomes and Explanatory Evidence, November 2009*, Princess Royal Trust for Carers, Woodford Green, Essex.

Useful websites

Resources with a range of information and publications for carers, service users and professionals

www.carers.org.

The Princess Royal Trust for Carers

www.crossroads.org.uk

Crossroads – Caring for Carers

www.carersuk.org

Carers UK

www.scie.org.uk

Social Care Institute for Excellence

www.rethink.org

Rethink; Severe Mental Illness Charity

References

Abbott, D., Watson, D. and Townsley, R. (2005) The proof of the pudding; what difference does multi-agency working make to families with disabled children with complex health care needs? *Child and Family Social Work* 10, 29–38.

Beresford, P. and Croft, C. (2004) Service users and practitioners reunited: the key component for social work reform, *British Journal of Social Work* 34, 53–68.

Bliss, J. (2006) What do informal carers need from district nursing services? *British Journal of Community Nursing* 11 (6), 251–6.

Carers UK (2001) *It Could BeYou; A Report on the Chances of Becoming a Carer,* London: Carers UK, www.carersuk.org.

Carers UK (2006) *In the Know; The Importance of Information for Carers,* London: Carers UK, www.carersuk.org.

Carers UK (2009a) *The Equality Bill and Carers,* London: Carers UK, www.carersuk.org.

Carers UK (2009b) *Facts about Carers, Policy briefing,* June 2009, London: Carers UK.

Carers UK (2011) *Half a Million Voices; Improving Support for BAME Carers,* London: Carers UK, www.carersuk.org.

The Carers (Recognition and Services Act 1995, www.legislation.gov.uk.

The Carers and Disabled Children Act 2000, www.legislation.gov.uk.

The Carers (Equal Opportunities) Act 2004, www.legislation.gov.uk.

Carr, S. (2004), *SCIE Position Paper 3; Has Service User Participation made a Difference to Social Care Services?*, London: SCIE/Policy Press.

Carr, S. (2007) Participation, power, conflict and change: theorising dynamics of service user participation in the social care system of England and Wales, *Critical Social Policy* 27, 266–76.

Census (2001) Office for National Statistics, www.statistics.gov.uk.

The Children Act 2004, www.legislation.gov.uk.

Cleaver, H., Walker, S., with Meadows, P. (2004) *Assessing Children's Needs and Circumstances, the Impact of the Assessment Framework,* London: Jessica Kingsley Publishers.

The Community Care (Direct Payments) Act 1996, www.legislation.gov.uk.

The Community Care Delayed Discharge Act 2003, www.legislation.gov.uk.

Department for Education and Skills (2003) *Every Child Matters,* www.education.gov.uk.

Department of Health (1990) NHS and Community Care Act, www.legislation.gov.uk.

Department of Health (1999a) *Caring about Carers; A National Strategy for Carers,* London: DoH.

Department of Health (1999b) *Better Care, Higher Standards,* London: DoH.

Department of Health (2000) *Carers and Disabled Children Act: 2000,* www.legislation.gov.uk.

Department of Health (2001a) *Carers and Disabled Children Act 2000. Carers and People with Parental Responsibility for Disabled Children Practice Guidance,* www.dh.gov.uk.

Department of Health (2001b) *Valuing People; A New Strategy for Learning Disability for the 21st Century,* London: HMSO.

Department of Health (2001c) *Carers and People with Parental Responsibility for Disabled Children; Practice Guidance Accompanying the* Carers and Disabled Children Act 2000, London: DoH.

Department of Health (2003) *The Victoria Climbié Inquiry; Report of an Inquiry by Lord Laming,* London: DoH.

Department of Health (2008a) *A New Deal for Carers, Health and Social Care Taskforce Report,* London: DoH.

Department of Health (2008b) *Carers at the Heart of 21st Century Families and Communities: A Caring System on Your Side, A Life of Your Own,* HM Government: DOH.

Department of Health (2010), *Recognised, Valued and Supported: Next Steps for the Carers Strategy, DoH Guidance 2010, electronic version only at* www.dh.gov.uk.

Department of Health, Department for Children Schools and Families (2008) *Aiming High for Disabled Children: Transforming Services for Disabled Children and their Families,* London: DfES and HM Treasury

Fernandez, J. L., Kendall, J., Davey, V., and Knapp, M. (2007) Direct payments in England; factors linked to variations in local provision, *Journal of Social Policy* 36 (1), 97–121.

General Social Care Council (2002) *Code of Practice for Social Care Workers and Code of Practice for Employers of Social Care Workers,* updated 2010, www.gscc.org.uk.

Gunaratnam, Y. (2007) Breaking the silence; black and minority ethnic carers and service provision, in J. Bornat, J. Johnson, C. Pereira, D. Pilgrim and F. Williams (eds),

Community Care: A Reader, Milton Keynes: Open University Press.

Hardy, B., Young, R. and Wistow, G. (2001) Dimensions of choice in the assessment and care management process; the views of older people, carers and care managers, *Health and Social Care in the Community* 7 (9), 483–91.

The Health Act 1999, www.legislation.gov.uk.

Henwood, M., (1998) *The Community Care Development Programme; Building Partnerships for Success; An Evaluation Report for the Department of Health,* London: DoH.

Hingley-Jones, H. and Allain, L. (2008) Integrating services for disabled children and their families in two English Local Authorities, *Journal of Interprofessional Care* 22 (5), 534–44.

Huby, G., Holt Brook, J., Thompson, A. and Tierney A. (2007) Capturing the concealed; interprofessional practice and older patients' participation in decision-making about discharge after acute hospitalization, *Journal of Interprofessional Care* 21 (1), 55–67.

Keeley, B. and Clarke, M. (2002). *Carers Speak Out Project: Report on Findings and Recommendations.* Woodford Green, Essex: Princess Royal Trust for Carer.

Macpherson, R., Collins, G. N., Slade, M. and Lerescu, T. (2008) The relationships between user, carer and staff perceptions of need in an assertive outreach team, *Journal of Mental Health* 17 (5), 452–61.

McGill, P., Papachristoforou, E., and Cooper, V. (2006) Support for family carers of children and young people with developmental disabilities and challenging behaviour, *Child Care Health and Development* 32 (2), 159–65.

Payne, M. (2000) *Teamwork in Multi-professional Care,* Basingstoke: Palgrave.

Poxton, R. (2004) What makes effective partnerships between health and social care?, in I., Glasby and E. Peck (eds.) *Care Trusts; Partnership Working in Action,* Abingdon: Radcliffe Medical Press.

Preston-Shoot, M. (2003) Only connect: Client, carer and professional perspectives on community care assessment processes, *Research, Policy and Planning* 21 (3), 23–35.

Princess Royal Trust for Carers (2002) *Carers Speak Out Project,* Princess Royal Trust for Carers, Woodford Green, Essex.

Princess Royal Trust for Carers (2006) *Consultation with Carers: Good Practice Guide,* Princess Royal Trust for Carers, Woodford Green, Essex. http://www.carers.org/our-publications.

Princess Royal Trust for Carers/Crossroads for Carers. (2009) *Putting People First Without Putting Carers Second,* Woodford Green, Essex: Princess Royal Trust.

Quinney, A. (2006) *Collaborative Social Work Practice,* Exeter: Learning Matters.

Rethink (2003) *Who Cares? The Experiences of Mental Health Carers Accessing Services and Information,* London: Rethink.

Robinson, J. and Banks, P. (2005 updated 2009) *The Business of Caring; The Kings Fund Inquiry into Care Services for Older People in London,* London: The Kings Fund.

Roulstone, A. Hudson, V., Kearney, J., Martin, A. and Warren, J. (2006) *Working Together: Carer Participation in England, Wales and Northern Ireland,* Stakeholder Participation Position Paper 05, www.scie.org.uk.

Roulstone, A. and Hudson, V. (2007) Carer participation in England Wales and N Ireland: a challenge for interprofessional working, *Journal of Interprofessional Care* 21 (3), 303–17.

Sitzia, J., Cotterell, P. and Richardson, A. (2006) Interprofessional collaboration with service users in the development of cancer services: The Cancer Partnership Project, *Journal of Interprofessional Care* 20 (1), 60–74.

Tew, J. (2005) Power relations, social order and mental distress, in J. Tew (ed.) *Social Perspectives in Mental Heath,* London: Jessica Kingsley Publishers.

Topss UK Partnership (2002) *National Occupational Standards for Social Work,* www.skillsforcare.org.uk.

Vickridge, R. (1998) Collaborative working for good practice in palliative care, *Journal of Interprofessional Care* 12, 63–7.

Walker, E. and Dewar, B. J. (2001) How do we facilitate carers' involvement in decision making? *Journal of Advanced Nursing* 34 (3), 329–37.

Yeandle, S., Bennet, C., Buckner, L., Fry, G. and Price, C. (2007) *Diversity in Caring: Towards Quality for Carers,* University of Leeds, London: Carers UK.

Young, H., Grundy, E. and Kalogirou, S. (2005) Who cares? Geographic variation in unpaid caregiving in England and Wales: Evidence from the 2001 Census, *Population Trends* 120, 23–34.

Chapter 16

The barriers presented by power, control and agency agendas on carer participation in interprofessional working: promoting inclusionary practice[1]

Carmel Byers and Creating Links[1]

Chapter summary

In the previous chapter, our consultation with carers identified practice issues that, despite policy directives and best practice initiatives, posed difficulties for carers in their attempts to work in partnership with professionals and be valued as members of the interprofessional team. This chapter continues to explore the experiences of informal carers associated with carers organisations in Hertfordshire, foster carers and the Creating Links people using services and carers group (see Chapter 15) in order to gain their view of the effectiveness of interprofessional working and how far they consider themselves to be part of the care team.

Building on the issues of communication, holistic approaches and values discussed in the last chapter, structural barriers that impede carers' participation will be explored here, the three most significant of which, as identified by the carers in the consultation, are issues of power, control and the impact of agency agendas.

Learning objectives

This chapter will cover:

- how carers of both adults and children can feel caught up in the difficulties between professional hierarchies and disputes between agencies, and how this might be rectified
- how professional opinions given by a person in a position of greater professional power may carry more weight in decision making than others who may have more in-depth knowledge gained over a significant period of time, by less powerful professionals or carers, and the effects of this on the carers

▶

---

[1]'Creating Links' is a service users and carers group involved in all aspects of social work education at the University of Hertfordshire.

■ carers' expressed wishes to have a single point of contact in order to avoid duplication and improve coordination between agencies and professionals by way of the identification of a named and trusted health or social care professional

■ the importance of carers and service users being able to bring a person to support them, such as a family member or a friend, to professional and interprofessional meetings

■ how the use of professional jargon, acronyms or other inappropriate use of terminology in the presence of the service user/carer can be disempowering and even frightening for them if not explained sufficiently or set in context

■ how aiding carers to fully participate in plans requires proactive consideration of practical arrangements as to how their caring needs can be met to enable them to participate fully in interprofessional planning, assessments and reviews.

The quality and nature of interprofessional and inter-agency working relationships can affect and influence whether a service user or carer will receive a service from a particular agency, with carers feeling caught up in the professional differences, hierarchies and disputes between agencies. The importance of professionals respecting the position of other professionals has been highlighted as an important element for success (Walker and Dewar, 2001).

In our consultation with service users in developing the content of this and the previous chapter, an example was given by a carer who reported difficulties between the adult care team who were supporting the husband she was caring for, and the housing department who had been requested to make some adaptations to their home. The lack of communication and interagency friction over resourcing caused considerable delays to the adaptations being made exacerbating the already difficult caring situation with her husband. Professional rivalries and a lack of cooperation in some instances are evident between certain professionals and agencies, with the carer expressing this as 'it is like they (the different agencies) are saying to each other – who are you to tell me (what to do)'?

Professionals who are effective brokers, and have good working relationships and networks with particular agencies, may be more successful at obtaining a service or resource for their service users than those with weaker networks. Carers were concerned that this contributed to the arbitrary nature of the allocation of resources and services. Carers suggested that it is often down to the effort made by individual workers whether a service was received or not. As one carer expressed, 'it is a matter of luck if you get a good social worker and if they work hard for you'.

Professional hierarchies are reported as influencing decision making, with some professionals in more powerful positions retaining undue influence as far as carers were concerned.

This has been identified in a number of studies, particularly in areas of medicine and psychiatry [as identified by Peter Beresford (Chapter 14) and Suzy Croft (Chapter 12) in this book]. Examples were cited in which professional opinions given after a brief contact with a service user or carer by a person in a position of professional power may carry more weight in decision making than the more in-depth knowledge gained over a significant period of time, by less powerful professionals.

The need for a lead professional

The need to avoid duplication and improve coordination between agencies by identifying a named person as a single point of contact who is a trusted health or social care professional both in adult and children services is frequently identified in studies as a necessary requirement for successful interprofessional working and the promotion of carer involvement in decision making and access to services (Bliss, 2006; Hingley-Jones and Allain, 2008; Vickridge, 1998; Walker and Dewar, 2001). Evidence points to general levels of dissatisfaction with services received by parent and family carers (McGill *et al.*, 2006), suggesting that one person acting as a lead professional could contribute positively to favourable outcomes. Research by Abbott *et al.* (2005) with families of disabled children identified that families may have contact with at least 10 different professionals and over the course of a year and attend at least 20 appointments at hospitals and clinics. The number of professionals who may be involved in supporting a disabled child in the community can often lead to a lack of continuity and coordination and may leave families uncertain about who to contact regarding specific problems. The Common Assessment Framework (Department for Education and Skills, 2004) recognised these concerns in the requirement for a designated 'lead professional' to undertake a coordination role. However, despite the provision of a key worker, a large proportion of families in Abbott's study still felt that they had no one to turn to for emotional support (Abbott *et al.*, 2005).

This would appear to be confirmed by carers and parent carers in the consultation who identified concerns over the difficulty of getting professionals to work together in an honest and transparent manner, highlighting the importance of having one professional taking lead responsibility, facilitating coordination between the various professionals and their agencies, with a decision made in the interprofessional team as to who this will be and who will deputise for them if the lead is unable to attend a meeting.

Professionals are sometimes reluctant to assume a lead role, which can result in no single person taking responsibility. Carers reported that designated lead professionals did not always take the 'lead', which in some cases could lead to 'buck-passing' between agencies, resulting in delays in decision making and the provision of services, as professionals await decisions from other colleagues or agencies.

Exercise 16.1

What issues does this case study raise regarding inter professional working including power and agency agendas?

This case study illustrates a number of issues highlighted by carers in this chapter, including:

- the impact of professional hierarchies
- carers feeling their views are disregarded by professionals
- assumptions and misunderstandings about the carers intentions
- a lack of interagency coordination
- lack of in-depth knowledge of the service user and carer's situation by the decision-makers.

Case study

A foster carer's experience – Peter
All names have been changed to ensure confidentiality.

Peter is 12 years old. His mother requested that he be accommodated due to her severe difficulties. Because this was a voluntary arrangement, and no Care Order was in place, Peter did not have a social worker. A professional assistant was allocated to provide support.

Before his placement with foster carers Barbara and Ray, Peter had 11 different placements in four years. He attended a school for children with emotional and behavioural difficulties.

Peter was accommodated with Barbara and Ray with a view to a long-term placement. In the first few months of his placement, Peter presented no major difficulties, and showed signs of improved behaviour at school and in the foster home. However, after six or seven months, there was a rapid deterioration in his behaviour both in the foster home and in school. The foster carers discovered that this had been the pattern with his previous placement breakdowns.

Peter found it difficult to accept any kind of discipline. Small everyday situations had the potential to develop into major incidents, where Peter would put himself in dangerous situations, such as climbing out of windows. He found it difficult to adjust to family life, for example refusing to join in with activities and outings. He would also make unfounded accusations against authority figures including teachers and carers and had difficulty in making friends, isolating him from his peers.

Although Peter would express remorse after the incidents, he took no responsibility for his actions. He was excluded from school after a serious incident involving school property.

Barbara and Ray were concerned at the level of supervision required for Peter in order to keep him safe. Their family life was seriously affected by Peter's behaviour to the extent that they felt that foster care was not effective in meeting his needs. However, they were reluctant to terminate the placement without a suitable solution being found for him.

Barbara and Ray requested a crisis meeting. A number of meetings followed, including four closed Panel meetings to decide on a future placement for Peter and allocate funding.

A range of professionals were involved, including:

The Local Authority Children Schools and Families service:

- Team manager
- Professional assistant support worker
- Peter's social worker (allocated after concerns were raised at a crisis meeting)
- Barbara and Ray's supervising social worker from the Family Support team, Child and Adult Mental Health Services (CAMHS)
- Social worker (who had considerable knowledge of Peter's history, but had seen him only intermittently due to Peter's frequent moves)
- Psychiatrist (report requested by the Panel. After a short consultation a diagnosis of attention-deficit hyperactive disorder was given, and medication prescribed).

Education:

- Advisory teacher

Other:

- Respite Unit, Befriender who visited weekly, involvement of Peter's school and a special educational unit which Peter attended following his exclusion from school.

Barbara and Ray's perception of the process of resolving Peter's issues

Barbara and Ray felt they were not listened to regarding their view of Peter's situation, even though they were experienced foster carers and despite their experience of his living with them for several months. They felt strongly that Peter had difficulty living in a family environment, and his complex needs would be best addressed by a resource with a therapeutic provision. They did not want to terminate the placement until a solution was found that would meet Peter's needs, as they were anxious not to subject Peter to further placement breakdowns. However, their position was misunderstood by the professionals who assumed that as they had not terminated the placement outright, they would continue with the placement with some extra support.

The social worker from CAMHS, who had known Peter for a number of years and had an in-depth knowledge of his situation, supported Barbara and Ray's view that Peter could not cope in a family environment. However, the recommendations in her report submitted to the Panel meeting were not acted upon. The Panel requested a psychiatric opinion, and a diagnosis of attention-deficit hyperactive disorder (ADHD) was accepted after a short assessment. Medication was prescribed that made little difference and in fact caused Peter sleep disturbances.

Barbara and Ray were very concerned that Peter's needs were not recognised or understood, that the various provisions suggested by the Panel were not appropriate to meet his complex therapeutic needs and that Peter would remain in the cycle of placement breakdown.

The situation began to move towards an effective resolution with the allocation of a social worker who listened to Barbara and Ray as professional foster carers, acted as 'lead professional' and took on a coordinating role together with advocating and providing effective representation of Peter's needs to the Panel, and coordinating the gradual, effective and well-planned transfer of Peter to his new placement in a therapeutic setting, making what could have been another damaging placement breakdown into a successful move, positively viewed by Peter and the foster carers.

The process took two years from Peter's initial placement with Barbara and Ray until he was finally placed in a unit that could provide for his needs.

A closer look

Addressing the needs of carers with disabled children – lead professional roles

McGill and colleagues (2006), in their study of support for family carers of children with developmental difficulties, suggest that parents of disabled children with challenging behaviour are often not receiving support that they consider helpful. The study also found concerns similar to those expressed by Barbara and Ray, regarding the frequent use of medication despite a lack of evidence of its effectiveness for particular children. The issue of resources was a significant one for the agency, given that Peter's final placement was out of the county, and was most likely to be a key consideration for the Panel in planning Peter's future. McGill and colleagues raise concerns over equality of access where rationing is apparent, particularly in relation to residential provision, arguing that it is possible that families who do not receive adequate support may be less likely to achieve the outcomes they are seeking than those who 'make a nuisance' of themselves, or who are more articulate with financial and psychological resources (McGill et al., 2006). The successful outcome facilitated by the social worker acting as lead professional in Peter's situation demonstrates that effective interagency and interprofessional coordination can facilitate the desired outcomes.

Research by Kirton and colleagues (2007) on the extent to which foster carers are considered 'colleagues' by other professionals and agencies, corroborates a number of issues arising out of the experiences of Barbara, Ray and Peter. The study found a varied response as to whether foster carers felt valued and listened to by professionals and that it depended largely on the relationship with the social worker, and a wide variation in the nature of the policies and practices of agencies which had a significant influence over the foster carers' perceptions. The study found evidence of low status, lack of consultation and participation in decision making and even forms of 'clientisation'. As identified earlier in these chapters, the importance of effective communication between foster carers and their agencies was again highlighted here.

Key learning points

Implications for good practice:

- a lead professional should be selected who can undertake a coordinating role, is proactive and able to offer emotional support
- be aware of professional tensions and conflicts between agencies that may impede service delivery
- develop effective 'brokering' skills
- be aware of professional power hierarchies in decision-making.

Working together in meetings and forums

As can be seen from the case study, in order for carers to feel included in decision making, they need to have an effective voice in interprofessional meetings and forums. Meetings are the most used forum for collaborative working, generally involve a number of professionals and can be the only opportunity carers may have to meet together and discuss current and future care needs. However, in their study of carers involvement in decision making, Walker and Dewar (2001) found that carers were disappointed by their experiences of meetings; that decisions had been made without carers being present; that they could not raise issues they wanted to discuss and that professionals gave the impression of wanting the meeting dealt with as quickly as possible. In addition, there were no mechanisms in place to check if carers were satisfied with the outcomes. The interruption of meetings by pagers and by people leaving to answer phone calls were accepted by some professionals as part of working life, but this can suggest to carers that professionals are distracted by other matters (Walker and Dewar, 2001). Across the service-user groups there were observations that on occasions, professionals had had preliminary discussions before meeting the carer and the service user. Decisions may therefore have been made before the family had been involved. Research by Hingley-Jones and Allain (2008), studying integrated services for disabled children and their families, similarly identified that parent carers had to fight to get a place at the discussion table, with quick judgements being made on very little information which would not have occurred had parents been present. Parents wanted to be included in all discussions about their children and service developments (Hingley-Jones and Allain, 2008). Similar findings apply to other service-user groups, that unless carers feel listened to and involved in the decision-making process, they are unlikely to access appropriate support (Bliss, 2006). The carers in our consultation expressed similar views.

Attendance at meetings can pose considerable difficulties for carers and the people they care for. Transport issues, caring responsibilities and the lack of available replacement care can prevent attendance. The number of professionals involved in meetings, deciding who should attend and the difficulties in arranging acceptable dates and times can contribute to the delaying of vital decisions that need to be made. Meetings are frequently arranged and sometimes rearranged to suit the convenience of the professionals rather than the carer and service user, which contributed to carers' feelings of exclusion from the team.

The consultation identified a lack of understanding of professional roles, compounded by the use of professional language and jargon, and the use of initials and acronyms for agencies that not only the carers and service users may not understand, but also the professionals themselves.

Professional meetings can be stressful events for carers and service users. Carers considered that when attending meetings they should be able to bring a person to support them, such as a family member or a friend. Information given or recorded at these meetings may not be remembered by the carer or service-user participants. Carers often reported that they only thought of what they wanted to say once they had left the meeting room (Walker and Dewar, 2001). This can result in carers not having a clear recollection of what was discussed and recorded, reinforcing the importance of distributing copies of notes of meetings to ensure that the content and decisions are clear to all.

Carers and parent carers agreed that well-run meetings were very useful. Meetings that were well chaired, set timescales and generally 'got things moving' generally had satisfactory outcomes. There were also reports where meetings made less progress because the facilitator had changed, the new one did not know the case and where the Panel or Chair was not familiar with the situation; as identified earlier when discussing holistic approaches, decisions were often made by senior managers who had little knowledge of a carers or service users' situation. Where professionals did not work well together, the resulting delays in decision making could be considerable and very frustrating for carers.

Meetings with professionals sometimes did not offer carers an opportunity to talk privately about their concerns. Carers may not want to discuss their difficulties and worries in front of the person they are caring for, and there are occasions in meetings where professionals do not demonstrate sufficient awareness and sensitivity regarding the feelings of the service user. Similarly, parent carers reported that frequently there is no opportunity to have a conversation with professionals without their child being present. Some topics are inappropriate to discuss in front of the child, such as financial issues, the stresses of caring or relationships with a partner. An opportunity for carers to express their feelings away from the person they are caring for would address this, however although it is possible to request a separate meeting, in the experience of the carers this was generally not readily available. The use of terminology used inappropriately in the presence of the service user, whether adult or child, can be undermining and even frightening for that person if it is not explained sufficiently or understood in a particular context.

Exercise 16.2

How can professionals ensure that carers:

- have a voice in meetings
- are involved in decision making
- are satisfied with the outcome?

The use of information technology, including web cameras and conference calls, was suggested as a means of enabling meetings to take place more easily. For carers and service users with access to this technology, webcams could be used to keep in touch with professionals, making more time for visits to those

Key learning points

Implications for practice:

- Pre-meeting preparation: carers make a list of questions and identify what, from their perspective, would be a satisfactory outcome.
- Carers and parent carers being present when decisions are made, with transparency in the decision-making process. Carers or service users to be able to bring a friend or family member for support.
- An opportunity for carers to have some meeting time without the person they are caring for being present.
- Arranging meeting times suitable for carers and service users, with consideration given to transport and replacement care needs.
- Set timescales for meetings; how long they will take and when the next one will take place.
- Chair or facilitator to have some knowledge of the carers' situation where possible.
- Follow-up check to ensure that the service user and carer felt satisfied with the outcomes of the meeting.
- Creative use of technology where attendance is difficult for service users and carers, such as the use of webcams and conference calls.

that do not have this technology. There were some concerns, however, as to whether this would work well in the social care setting where direct communication and contact is of importance.

A closer look

Carers as a resource or a full part of the interprofessional team?

Carers confirmed the findings of recent research (Abbott *et al.*, 2005; Hardy *et al.*, 2001; Hingley-Jones and Allain, 2008; Huby *et al.*, 2007; Roulstone and Hudson, 2007; Walker and Dewar, 2001) that they felt were treated as a resource rather than a person in their own right who was part of the care team. Most wanted more involvement in care planning, a more effective voice in decision making, and not to be regarded as just someone who was 'invited' to meetings. A recent report from the Princess Royal Trust for Carers highlights how carers have to fight to gain some recognition as 'partners in care', and how too often, carers feel that they are left with all the caring responsibilities and little recognition or support (Princess Royal Trust 2009), a situation familiar to the carers in the consultation. Professionals may sometimes communicate a lack of trust in carers, who may have to fight for the right to resources including direct payments and individual budgets. Evidence suggests that carers are poorly represented among recipients of direct payments, which when accessed can give greater flexibility, and that professionals may not offer direct payments to users and carers because of attitude barriers influenced by perceptions of risk and vulnerability (Carr, 2010; Fernández *et al.*, 2007).

Carers as part of the interprofessional team?

Although there are clear indications in policy to regard service users and carers as 'experts by experience', and carers and parent carers generally consider themselves in this way, their general view is that they are not recognised as such, their expertise often being disregarded. They are often not awarded the same respect as other professionals involved in the team, who may be divided on whether carers should be regarded as 'colleagues' (Kirton *et al.*, 2007). Even though there is an expectation that carers will be able to provide professionals with extensive knowledge about the person they are caring for, their views and perspectives often carry little weight in the decision-making process.

Examples of exclusion from the team included an incident where a carer had been bypassed by an agency home carer employed to provide support for her disabled husband. The home carer had communicated directly with the social worker over a minor incident that occurred in the home, rather than initially trying to resolve the matter with the carer herself who as a result felt excluded, marginalised and disempowered.

Feelings of exclusion extended to foster carers and children's services. Foster carers in particular felt excluded from the lives of young people in their care once they reached the age of 18 years, regardless of their developmental age. Exclusion from the professional care team and important aspects in the life of the young person could result in a lack of continuity leading to feelings of disempowerment both for the foster carers and the young person. One foster carer reported her frustration at not being informed of appointments made by professionals for the young person she was looking after. This resulted in the young person forgetting to attend the appointments and meetings, with detrimental effects. Foster carers also expressed concern that although they were still providing considerable support to the young people in their care, they were not invited to Leaving Care meetings, and so unable to support them effectively with the transition to independent life. Other frustrations included a carer not being allowed to accompany a young person with high-dependency learning disabilities into her appointment at a doctors' surgery. While it is necessary to respect the adult status of young service users, carers felt that 'blanket' policies limiting their involvement when the young people they were caring for reached the age of 18, often regardless of developmental age, excluded them from the professional team.

Parent carers of disabled children participating in our consultation generally did not experience themselves as part of the interprofessional team. Not infrequently the parent carers felt that they were regarded by professionals as a 'disabled family'. Where children were away at school or residential facility, a parent carer may be viewed by professionals as only a part-time parent. One parent carer whose child was at a residential school described being made to feel like a 'weekend woman', rather than her child's mother, with the resulting experience of exclusion from the team caring for her child. The number of professionals visiting a family can feel invasive. The family home no longer feels like home, but becomes a 'workplace', where others come to work. Parent carers also expressed concern over the role of fathers who for various reasons were frequently not seen by professionals and whose views were therefore often not taken into account.

While there was a clear desire for a genuine connection with professional workers, there were also concerns about the lack of clarity concerning boundaries, with certain professionals having relationships with a family described as 'too cosy', for example, over-familiarity, over-long visits and phone calls, which did not feel comfortable and could encourage collusive relationships.

> ### Key learning points
>
> - Carers should be seen as part of the care team and their expertise respected.
> - Carers should be offered more involvement in care planning and decision making.
> - Carers should have more control of their situations, and trust from practitioners particularly in relation to individual budgets and direct payments.
> - There should be flexibility and consideration of developmental age to be taken into consideration when children reach 18, so that carers and parent carers are not excluded from a supportive role.
> - There should be recognition and involvement of parent carers of children at residential schools and units.
> - Professional training and supervision should embed a culture of personalisation.
> - Professional boundaries should be recognised and respected.

Conclusion

While it is recognised that the views of professionals were not included in this consultation, and that the purpose was to report the views of carers only, this consultation suggests that despite evidence of considerable progress in the area of interprofessional and collaborative working, **there is still some way to go before carers feel part of the team**. Many of the issues highlighted by carers in this consultation in relation to interprofessional working and implications for good practice are not new and have been raised a number of times by service users and carers in other studies forming part of practice guidance (Rethink, 2003; Victor, 2009).

As identified in this and the previous chapter, various explanations have been offered for the current situation including **the impact of managerial agendas, professional value systems, lack of time and limited resources**. Some of the issues raised may be addressed by the implementation of the New Deal for Carers, Health and Social Care Taskforce report (Department of Health, 2008), whose proposals include a strategy for providing improved information to carers, increased availability of care breaks, the provision of better services and support for carers, including the introduction of a specialist carer's service in every area which would aim to provide **early identification of carers and promote advocacy, empowerment, involvement and ongoing emotional support**.

Involving carers in health and social work education, including interprofessional learning, can contribute a greater awareness of the needs of carers and promote good practice (Cooper and Spencer-Dawe, 2006). In our experience at the University of Hertfordshire, people who use services and carer involvement in education are generally highly evaluated by students, who have commented that the sharing of carers' experiences has given them a greater understanding of the realities of their everyday lives.

In conclusion, as indicated by Carr (2004) and Roulstone and Hudson (2007), in order for service users and carers' voices to be heard effectively in the interprofessional team, **their involvement and contributions will need to become part of regular practice, and result in observable change**. As the case study illustrates, successful outcomes are more likely to be achieved when professionals work in partnership with each other and ensure the participation of service users and carers. For carers to be able to consider themselves as part of the interprofessional team, their **involvement needs to be actively encouraged and valued** and result in the outcomes that they are seeking.

Reference

Abbott, D., Watson, D. and Townsley, R. (2005) The proof of the pudding; What difference does multi-agency working make to families with disabled children with complex health care needs? *Child and Family Social Work* 10, 229–38.

Bliss, J. (2006) What do informal carers need from district nursing services? *British Journal of Community Nursing* 11 (6), 251–6.

Carr, S. (2004) *SCIE Position Paper 3; Has Service User Participation Made a Difference to Social Care Services?* London: SCIE/Policy Press.

Carr, S. (2010) *SCIE Report 36: Enabling Risk, Ensuring Safety: Self-directed Support and Personal Budgets,* London: SCIE.

Cooper, H. and Spencer-Dawe, E. (2006) Involving service users in interprofessional education; narrowing the gap between theory and practice, *Journal of Interprofessional Care* 20 (6), 603–17.

Department for Education and Skills (2004) *Common Assessment Framework,* London: DfES.

Department of Health (2008) *New Deal For Carers: Revision of the Prime Minister's 1999 Strategy for Carers,* Health and Social Care Taskforce Report, London: Department of Health.

Fernández, J. L., Kendall, J., Davey, V. and Knapp, M. (2007) Direct payments in England; factors linked to variations in local provision, *Journal of Social Policy* 36 (1), 97–121.

Hardy, B., Young, R. and Wistow, G. (2001) Dimensions of choice in the assessment and care management process; the views of older people, carers and care managers, *Health and Social Care in the Community* (9), 483–91.

Hingley-Jones, H. and Allain, L. (2008) Integrating services for disabled children and their families in two English Local Authorities, *Journal of Interprofessional Care* 22 (5), 534–44.

Huby, G., Holt Brook, J., Thompson, A. and Tierney, A. (2007) Capturing the concealed; interprofessional practice and older patients' participation in decision-making about discharge after acute hospitalisation, *Journal of Interprofessional Care* 21 (1), 55–67.

Kirton, D., Beecham, J. and Ogilvie, K. (2007) Still the poor relation? Perspectives on valuing and listening to foster carers, *Adoption and Fostering* 31 (3), 6–17.

McGill, P., Papachristoforou, E. and Cooper, V. (2006) Support for family carers of children and young people with developmental disabilities and challenging behaviour, *Child Care Health and Development* 32 (2), 159–65.

Princess Royal Trust for Carers/Crossroads for Carers (2009) *Putting People First without Putting Carers Second,* Woodford Green, Essex: Princess Royal Trust for Carers.

Rethink (2003) *Who Cares? The Experiences of Mental Health Carers Accessing Services and Information.* London: Rethink.

Roulstone, A. and Hudson, V. (2007) Carer participation in England Wales and N Ireland: a challenge for interprofessional working, *Journal of Interprofessional Care* 21 (3), 303–17.

Sitzia, J., Cotterell, P. and Richardson, A. (2006) Interprofessional collaboration with service users in the development of cancer services: The Cancer Partnership Project, *Journal of Interprofessional Care* 20 (1), 60–74.

Vickridge, R. (1998) Collaborative working for good practice in palliative care, *Journal of Interprofessional Care* 12, 63–7.

Victor, L. (2009) *A Systematic Review of Interventions for Carers in the UK: Outcomes and Explanatory Evidence, November 2009,* Woodford Green, Essex: Princess Royal Trust for Carers. http://www.carers.org/our-publications

Walker, E. and Dewar, B. J. (2001) How do we facilitate carers' involvement in decision making? *Journal of Advanced Nursing* 34 (3), 329–37.

Chapter 17
Teachers and education

Mary Rees

Chapter summary

This chapter focuses on interprofessional practice through the eyes and experience of the teacher. It takes three key themes for schools and teachers:

- their professional role and training
- the organisation and accountability of the education system
- their relationships with families and parents

and considers them in the light of:

- legislative imperatives
- opportunities, barriers and dilemmas
- what can/should good practice look like?

The chapter draws on a number of research projects on interprofessional practice conducted in local authorities including the impact of interprofessional practice on outcomes for children with additional needs; professionals' perceptions of the nature and extent of sexual exploitation in the county and the development of interprofessional practice for practitioners. It uses case studies and fictionalised accounts from this unpublished research to illuminate the landscape and to offer scope for the reader to analyse and respond to some of the points. Through working with practitioners in my research much has been learned about the process and outcomes of interprofessional practice. A key point emerging from studies has been that effective interprofessional practice can really make a difference in outcomes for children, although sometimes practitioners struggle in developing new skills and strategies. As a teacher, I am conscious of the tensions in the education system of working in this new way but also of the willingness of teachers to develop their own professional skills in order to do their best for their pupils and families.

Learning objectives

This chapter will cover:

- how teachers not only have a role in the formal education of the child, but also consider the child within the family, and other professional groups

▶

- the Teacher Development Agency's (TDA) Professional Standards for Teachers (2007), which emphasises the need for the teacher having a commitment to collaboration and cooperative working

- why and how teachers have a duty to the children they teach and to the wider social purposes for which teaching is done

- how many of the problems that children have in school, for example behaviour difficulties, are caused by a complex set of factors such as parenting issues, mental health or family difficulties, requiring coordinated intervention from a number of agencies

- the implications for schools having become more autonomous in their management of budgets and staffing, and how the wider coordination of services by local authorities has declined, and how current initiatives meaning schools becoming academies gives them more and more autonomy, presenting challenges in ensuring schools take a broader role in the coordinated care and education of children and young people

- how the conceptual framework of 'knotworking' is explored as a way of helping agencies and professionals consider a more sustainable model of interprofessional practice than many current ones.

Introduction

Education as a discipline is a wide area, encompassing for example early years provision, primary and secondary schools and further and higher education. Space does not permit specific reference to all age phases, and the generic descriptor 'schools and teachers' is used unless referring to a particular phase.

Education is a constantly changing field as political parties adopt differing policy trajectories that in turn lead to different operational frameworks and new organisational trends. The reader is advised to refer to government websites for the latest policy statements as some of the following specific documents referenced may well be superseded by the time of going to press. However, I have tried to steer a course through the ups and downs of policy changes in order to tell a story that is less susceptible to political whims and more focused on the needs of the child and the role of teachers in realising that aim.

Children's practitioners value the contribution that a range of colleagues make to children and young people's lives, and they form effective relationships across the children's workforce. Their integrated practice is based on a willingness to bring their own expertise to

bear on the pursuit of shared goals, and a respect for the expertise of others.

(GSCC, GTCE, NMC[1], 2007, joint statement)

This joint statement agreed by the then professional ruling bodies for social work, education and health – GSCC, the GTCE and the NMC – reinforces some of the the policies and practice advocated in the Every Child Matters Green Paper and subsequently set out in the Children Act 2004. In particular, in this quotation, the need for the three professions and their professionals to work together. This in turn was in part responding to the Laming Report following the death of Victoria Climbié. The Report investigating this tragic and high profile case concluded that the different services were operating within discrete frameworks and organisations (Laming, 2003). This led to a failure to share information on children and families and consequently to have a complete picture of the child and the family. What was needed was for services to work together, sharing information and building up a more holistic picture of the child and the family. For example, rather than schools having a role only in education of the child, leaving social services for example to consider the child within the family, professional groups would work together, sharing information, addressing needs as they arose. Existing professional boundaries and responsibilities

---

[1] GSCC, GTCE, NMC refer to the General Social Care Council, the General Teaching Council for England, and the Nursing and Midwifery Council.

A closer look

Teachers have a key contribution to make to the five Every Child Matters outcomes:

- **Being healthy** so that they are physically, mentally, emotionally and sexually healthy, have healthy lifestyles and choose not to take illegal drugs.
- **Staying safe** from maltreatment, neglect, violence, sexual exploitation, accidental injury and death, bullying and discrimination, crime and anti-social behaviour in and out of school, have security and stability and are cared for.
- **Enjoying and achieving** so that they are ready for school, attend and enjoy school, achieve stretching national educational standards at primary and secondary school, achieve personal and social development and enjoy recreation.

- **Making a positive contribution** so that they engage in decision making, support their community and environment, engage in law-abiding and positive behaviour in and out of school, develop positive relationships, choose not to bully and discriminate, develop self-confidence, successfully deal with significant life changes and challenges and develop enterprising behaviour.
- **Achieving economic well-being** so that they engage in further education, employment or training on leaving school, are ready for employment, live in decent homes and sustainable communities, have access to transport and material goods, live in households free from low income.

See http://www.education.gov.uk/

might blur so that, for example, schools would play their part in having responsibility for all of the five outcomes from Every Child Matters (ECM) (DFES, 2003).

The professional bodies' joint statement set out above belies the complexity of interprofessional practice and also, in common with many such policy statements, focuses on the 'what must be done' rather than the 'how should it be done'. In particular, when further examined the 'shared goals' may look very different from the perspective of any one of the professionals working together.

What does this mean for schools and teachers? In a major research project exploring teachers' lives and effectiveness across 100 schools and 300 teachers, Day and colleagues observed the following:

> The vision is one of universal services to which every child has access, and which involve educational professionals working closely with health and social service professionals to provide an integrated, multidisciplinary service . . . The Every Child Matters outcomes . . . are major implications for the way that teachers see their work. These outcomes are substantially different from the narrower results driven agenda with which many teachers are currently working.
>
> (Day *et al.*, 2007, p. 12)

While the early years sector has traditionally worked with other services, being more involved with

Key learning points

Professional role and training:

- The role of the teacher has extended in response to policy changes.
- Teachers are often at the centre of interprofessional practice.
- Teachers develop the skills needed to extend their role in a number of ways, both formal and informal.

the child and the family and thus having contact with perhaps health visitors and social services, the challenges not only for teachers but also for the schools in which they work have been great.

National Professional Standards

The teacher's professional role and the expertise referred to in the joint statement are embodied in the document *Professional Standards for Teachers*, published by the TDA in 2007. The standards are arranged in three interrelated sections covering professional attributes, professional knowledge and understanding and professional skills. The framework itself also sets out the progression of a teacher through a career path from Qualified Teacher Status (QTS) to Advanced Skills Teachers. There are separate standards for head

Key learning points

Standards relevant to collaborative practice as teachers move through their career are:

- have a commitment to collaboration and cooperative working (at Qualified Teacher status)
- have a commitment to collaboration and cooperative working where appropriate (Core standards)
- have sufficient depth of knowledge and experience to be able to give advice on the development and well-being of children and young people (post-threshold).

Well-being is the term used to signify the learner's rights in relation to the five ECM outcomes set out above.

Exercise 17.1

Identify where interprofessional practice is addressed in your own professional standards, both at initial training stage and in your later professional development standards. What kinds of evidence could you provide to show that you can meet those standards in your own practice?

teachers and deputy head teachers. At each stage, teachers are required to provide evidence that they have met the standards.

It can be noted that there is little explicit mention of interprofessional practice, and even less in the standards for Qualified Teacher Status. And yet becoming a teacher 'means more than acquiring technical knowledge and expertise. It means becoming a teacher morally, through one's commitment to the children one teaches and to the wider social purposes for which teaching is done' (Hargreaves and Jacka, 2010, p. 4).

The teacher's professional role: a new role in assessment and intervention

Much of the move towards interprofessional practice is centred around the concept of early intervention, the rationale that if a child's additional needs are assessed and addressed at an early stage, they will not escalate and cause greater problems as time goes on. 'It is always better to prevent failure than to tackle a crisis later' (DCSF, 2007, p. 5).

However, these needs and the means to meet them might fall outside the usual remit of a school's expertise. Many of the problems that children have in school, for example behaviour difficulties, are in fact the result of complex and diverse factors that may have as their root parenting issues, mental health or family difficulties, requiring intervention from a number of agencies. As a drive towards early intervention for vulnerable children and young people, rather than a direct referral to Social Services, a process is put in place which acknowledges and facilitates an approach which can involve different services and can, it is hoped, prevent the escalation of problems. A multi-agency assessment, the Common Assessment Framework (CAF) is undertaken, leading to the formation of a Team Around the Child (TAC) consisting of a range of professionals, matching the needs of the child.

Details of this, including implementation guidance and training materials, can be found at www.dfes.gov/ISA/sharing_Assessment/caf.cfm. Two important roles within that team are the CAF instigator, who first identifies the need for intervention, and the lead professional, the person who coordinates, monitors and evaluates the impact of the intervention. Both of these roles are commonly taken by teachers in school, either the Special Educational Needs Coordinator (SENCo) or Inclusion Coordinator (InCo), in secondary schools or often the head teacher in primary schools. The case

Case study

A child with learning and behavioural difficulties was assessed by the educational psychologist who called in the behaviour support team. They came in quickly and worked with him regularly. The school also referred the child to the counselling service. He was seen within three months for two blocks of counselling. Both the child and his parents are now more engaged with school. Although he still has learning difficulties, the child is now far more settled in a classroom situation and has started to make progress. Over a two-year period of intervention with this child, all of the support services remained responsive.

A closer look

The view from the edge

'If we have a dilemma – and we do because we are on the edge'

(Interview response)

I can't sleep. I just keep going over and over what's happening to Ellie. As I was leaving school yesterday afternoon there they were, the boys, well young men really, in their early twenties some of them, hanging around calling to the girls from their cars, loud music, smoking, drinking. Why don't the police move them on? Why can't the school stop them? Mostly the girls just walk by and ignore them. Not Ellie though. I saw her come out, not 14 yet but looking 20, make up, skirt rolled right up. Straight into the car. She tried to get her friends to come too but they walked off. The car drove off, tyres screeching, music blaring. Where

to? Somewhere out of the way – a park? Someone's house? Last time she was brought home it was from a hotel. Her stepdad hit her then. Nothing happened she said. No sex, no drugs. 'I went because I wanted to', she said, 'and you can't stop me'.

That's the problem of course, not realising that you're being exploited. Loving all the attention, feeling wanted. Mum's tried to stop her – takes her mobile away so she can't communicate with the men but they just buy her a new one. I could do without all this going round in my head at two o'clock in the morning! But the truth is I know that, as a professional, I have a responsibility to support Ellie and her family, to help them resolve this situation. I want Ellie to see that she has choices, to help her find ways of raising her self-esteem that don't depend on the approval and attention of these men.

Exercise 17.2

List the professionals, agencies and services that schools commonly work with.

Consider the role you would expect these to play where a child may have behaviour/emotional difficulties identified by the school the child attends; first, for a child of 6 years; second, for a young person of 14 years of age.

study on the opposite page from a head teacher shows how effective timely and responsive intervention can be in meeting the needs of children.

Opportunities and dilemmas

For teachers and schools, if the initial problem appears to lie outside the school's usual remit of teaching, learning and attainment, knowing how to respond can be more difficult and teachers can feel uncertain about how to act. The case example above is a fictionalised account from a practitioner who clearly feels at the boundary of her professional knowledge and expertise. How would you respond to such a scenario?

Implicit in effective interprofessional practice is a need not only for each professional to feel secure in

their own professional knowledge but also to be aware of the roles and expertise of others and to extend their own knowledge into different fields. For example, as a teacher I should be secure in my expertise in the pedagogy of teaching and learning, in content knowledge and also in what Shulman termed pedagogic content knowledge (Shulman and Hatch, 2005). This is the core of my professional knowledge. However, I may feel less secure in practice relating to children's wellbeing in a more holistic way. Of course teachers have always been concerned for their children in a wider sense. Nell Noddings has written about care as an integral part of the teacher's role – taking the concept of *caring about* further into *caring for* (Noddings, 1984). Ronald King wrote about a primary teacher's relationship with pupils as being more than that of pedagogical authority – he called it 'a professional affection' (King, 1978). But faced with the kinds of dilemmas framed above how can they know what to do? How can teachers and schools extend their professional knowledge to confidently make judgements concerning issues which seem to lie outside the boundaries within which they normally work? One way is for Children's Services to define and publish thresholds or tiers of need. Within these frameworks are criteria which enable a range of practitioners to assess whether the situation should be met by universal services, by more than one service (hence the need for a CAF) or should be directly referred to social services. Although these can be enormously helpful starting points, the evaluation of the National Children's Trust Pathfinders found that there was also a need to ensure that their use did not undermine the philosophy of a multi-agency approach (Siraj-Blatchford and Siraj-Blatchford, 2009, p. 35). The task of fitting unique and often complex situations into a generic framework can become an end in itself and mitigate against the holistic view the framework is endeavouring to provide.

What can good practice look like? Professional learning in an interprofessional context

Most adults think they know what a teacher does; whether that understanding is accurate or not, they have fixed ideas about the boundaries they work within. Often there are misconceptions. Similarly in our understanding of the roles of health professionals or social workers, there is sometimes uncertainty regarding their professional knowledge and expertise. For example, a social worker friend of mine was horrified that as a teacher I had not had more child development in my training. Eraut categorises professional knowledge into 'C' codified knowledge; stored in publications and in the case of teaching, embedded in the standards and curricula, and 'P', personal knowledge, 'in terms of what people bring to practical situations that enables them to think and perform. Such personal knowledge is not only acquired through the use of public knowledge, but also constructed from personal experience and reflection'(Eraut, 1999, p. 77). In this way, theory is built up, either in one organisation or co-constructed in a multi-agency setting. In order for this to happen, professionals must articulate their practice, not only for other professionals in their own services but across services. Opportunities can be provided for them to do this in training as well as in practice. Organisational features of interprofessional practice such as Multi-agency teams (MATs) and multi-agency networks can themselves be good examples of staff

Exercise 17.3

Professional learning can occur in many different contexts, for example informal conversations, meetings with groups of colleagues, participation in multi-agency groups, from books and articles in professional and peer-reviewed journals and courses and training events.

What is your personal knowledge and what is your codified knowledge of interprofessional practice and what kinds of experiences led to that learning?

development. Other examples of professional development in an interprofessional context can also be very effective in building up an understanding of other agencies and services. An extensive research study into interagency training around safeguarding found that the outcomes of training across the sample were significant and positive: 'the knowledge of the substantive topic; attitudes to service users; and self-efficacy in relation to knowledge of safeguarding policies and procedures as well as in working with service users, all increased' (Carpenter *et al.*, 2010, p. ii).

The use of in-service interprofessional training to develop interprofessional practice can then serve to not only inform but also to provides opportunities to develop Eraut's 'Personal knowledge' where professionals share experiences and gain insights into each other's perspectives.

Legislation

The role and purpose of schools has for some years been driven by a standards agenda whereby pupils, staff and governors have all been evaluated in terms

Key learning points

The organisation and accountability of the education system

- The ways in which schools work within the education system influence their capacity to respond to an interprofessional agenda.
- Children's centres provide a useful model for interprofessional practice.
- Effective interprofessional relationships are not always those that are developed over time.

of standards (attainment levels) set by government. Pupil performance has been judged by the results of statutory tests and published in league tables so that schools can be evaluated against other schools. The results of this have been a highly focused curriculum based on attainment, and also a lack of collaboration between schools as they compete with each other. However, the Every Child Matters policy shifts the focus and schools now have to demonstrate how they are contributing to all five outcomes. Ofsted inspectors now, for example, in their inspection of the target of 'staying safe' evaluate not only the behaviour and attendance of pupils but also how provision contributes to the learners' capacity to stay safe and healthy, staying safe including children being 'safe from crime and anti-social behaviour' (Ofsted, 2005 in Roche and Tucker, 2007, p. 222) 'Perhaps what we are witnessing here is a fundamental shift in responsibility for the care and education of the young, where schools are judged against learner behaviours both in the specific institution and wider community' (Roche and Tucker, 2007, p. 222).

This shift necessitates not only the development of new roles and identities in the education sector but also reorganisation. Schools (particularly in the secondary sector) in some ways have become more and more autonomous, for example in their management of budgets and staffing, while the role of local authorities has declined and schools have been shaped and controlled by government through their Inspection regimes. For example, National Curriculum provision and inspection frameworks have resulted in a more centralised control and schools have become more competitive. Current initiatives in the form of schools taking on Academy status has given them more and more autonomy. There are also basic elements of the organisation of schools that militate against them taking a broader role in the care and education of children and young people. For example, the hours and pattern of provision including school holidays have always been limiting to collaboration with other services, and the geographical distance between schools and other services does not always facilitate good communication.

Opportunities for development

Two major organisational changes have sought to support the new integration of services and implement policy. The co-location of services within these organisations aimed to provide 'one-stop shops' for families and ease of communication for their professionals, thus ensuring more effective localised provision. Two examples of this policy are Children's Centres for children and families within the early years age group, and extended school consortia that offer a range of provision across schools. The placing of agencies together has a number of aims, a prime one being ease of communication as poor communication between professionals was one of the failings initially identified in the Laming Report. These initiatives, designed to maximise effective communication, have thus far had mixed reviews. Initial studies have highlighted that, as intended, both sets of organisations have customised their structures and ways of working, The Think Family policy encourages services to work together to provide a more holistic service for families in, for example, Family Intervention projects. The decline in services offered to schools by local authorities and the rise of academies may drive schools to collaborate more on joint commissioning of services and, in commissioning them, have a greater interest in working with them to ensure impact and value for money.

However, co-locating services does not in itself facilitate communication. Much depends on the leadership and management skills of the managers, and it is also important not to lose the professional identities of the practitioners themselves. These identities are revealed through knowledge, values and, most visibly, a professional language. Professional vocabulary can be a real barrier to effective communication across services unless time is taken to share and explain jargon. However, equally important in interprofessional communication is the need for each service to maintain its own identity, through for example narratives and stories that illustrate the often unarticulated meaning that practitioners attribute to their professional beings.

Practitioners working in interprofessional contexts such as this report the benefits of working in this way, although there are potentially some practical

Case study

A police officer attached to an integrated service centre had the following experience.

'We had a case where the Police were called out to a domestic violence incident between a mother and grandmother. In cases where children are in any way involved, it comes through to me and I can look up on Integrated Children's' Services databases to see if other agencies are involved. In this case there were worries that the nine-year-old child was not attending school. After further investigation, it transpired that Mum had mental health problems and the child was staying at home to look after her. Anyway, in the end we got Young Carers involved who are supporting the child, Mum is also receiving support from Adult Care Services. So that's great, if I wasn't here that wouldn't happen. It's good that I'm based here because I'm building up my knowledge from the other professionals and also I'm a point of contact for my police colleagues who can tap into other expertise through the centre. I love it here, I can really make a difference.

I've got a year's secondment to this team but I don't know what will happen after that. It's my performance review next week and I don't know what my sergeant is going to say – she doesn't know anything about what I do here. I don't know if this scheme will continue as it is now. It will be evaluated but the different services will evaluate it against different criteria. Children's services will want to know if there are fewer referrals to social services but the police will look at things like response rates and crime figures.'

challenges in working away from one's own mainstream discipline. The case study of a police officer (above) exemplifies some of these benefits and challenges.

Exercise 17.4

From the school perspective, what agencies would you liaise with over the issues in the case study above, and to what purpose? From the child's perspective, what would their experience be throughout this in terms of interprofessional practice?

Children's centres

The aim of development of children's centres was that they could provide a focal point for rationalising a wide range of existing community based initiatives, building vital links between education, employment, health and social services, including Jobcentre Plus to help join up and return to work with the child care provided (2002 Interdepartmental Review in Curtis and Burton, 2009).

As such they formed an important plank in the then Labour Government's aim to aid disadvantaged families and reduce child poverty and built on earlier initiatives such as the Sure Start programme and Early Excellence Centres. Aimed initially at families with young children, many have developed into models of excellent integrated practice. They provide a core offer of activities

and support for families including timely access to targeted and specialist services. Hence their managers have learned to lead teams of different professionals from different agencies. 'The role entails being multi-faceted at every level. . . . and is a massive shift away from the traditional framework of delivering services to one that emphasises being flexible, locally responsive and locally accountable' (Curtis and Burton, 2009, p. 287).

Extended schools

Extended schools have a similar rationale and genesis to children's centres. Drawing on the experience of community schools in Scotland, they aimed to provide a greater level of resource for children and families. There are different models of extended school – each developing its provision according to the needs of its community. However, as Cummings and colleagues (2007) surmised from their research, even those providing a full range of extended services are a long way from the community schools in Scotland. The very idea of the school being at the centre of the community it serves still remains the case for many primary schools, but the policy changes on 'choice' for families in their secondary school means that most children now travel to their secondary school. The advent of specialist schools and colleges exacerbates that distancing of the family from the school. Evaluations of extended schools have been positive, in particular the access to social care and health expertise that the organisation and the (to some extent pooled) budgets can provide. The benefits of social care professionals identified from an evaluation of extended schools cited characteristics which echo the aims of multi-agency practice.

> The three main benefits of social care professionals working with extended schools highlighted were: earlier identification of needs and quicker access to services; a better understanding and knowledge of roles and responsibilities between social care and education colleagues; and a more coherent, holistic package of support.
>
> (Wilkin *et al.*, 2008, p. 30)

A closer look

Opportunities to build interprofessional relationships

Many schools build up relationships with other professionals over time. One head teacher in our research said, 'there's a few professionals – I put their numbers on speed dial'.

'My advice (to head teachers new in post) is to make contact with three key people' (head teacher).

Personal relationships with other professionals are often key to effective interprofessional practice. An early study into common operational features of effective integrated working found that 'Integrated working in the areas nominated as good practice was fundamentally based on personal relationships that, although currently effective, may not be sustainable over time' (DCSF, 2007, p. 1).

The research concluded that although localised and co-located services could be the first step to a fully integrated practice, there were risks. These conclusions were that these risks were as follows:

- As one respondent stated, 'It is totally dependent on individuals and changes in personnel could cause it to falter'.
- Islands of good practice created could become a different sort of silo.
- 'The benefits of localised integrated working are likely to be limited by the personal sphere of influence of the team and the children that are served by that team' (DCSF, 2007, p. 4).

A different way of being

Interprofessional relationships are usually built on trust, on trusting another practitioner's professional judgement, their communication skills and professional interpersonal skills. Although professional trust is commonly built up over time, sustained professional relationships are not always viable as staff move on, organisational frameworks change and geographical areas can differ. In such cases working relationships can be established which are less dependent on individuals and more focused on the child. Engestrom constructed a conceptual framework of 'knotworking' that is helpful in considering a more sustainable model of interprofessional practice.

> knotworking signifies an activity that captures a pulsating movement, in which different aspects or threads are connected that would not have been connected otherwise. During knotworking, the actors assemble often in an improvised, collaborative activity, without clear institutional boundaries.
>
> (Engestrom in Daniels *et al.*, 2010, p. 188)

This model has two advantages. First, it enables us to perceive of teams around the child not as static teams, but of changing individuals and services, according to needs. Secondly this framing of interprofessional activity as a dynamic process, constantly changing as it adapts to new contexts, resonates well with the need to follow the child and families changing needs and to follow the child's trajectory (DCSF, 2007). The school or Children's Centre can be a natural space for this to happen, but the individual participants in interprofessional practice itself will shift and evolve as the needs dictate.

Relationships with parents

Legislation

Schools' relationships with parents and families have changed substantially since the days when a white line was marked in the playground beyond which it was made clear that parents must not

Key learning points

- Communication between schools and parents varies according to age phase.
- New roles developed in schools can be used to strengthen relationships with parents.

Exercise 17.5

List all the communication (verbal and written) between a familiar school and home over the course of the term. Note which way (home–school or school–home) and the purpose of the communication. Which of the five ECM outcomes is the principal focus?

step. Similarly, the naming of that relationship has encompassed labels such as 'partners', 'collaborators', 'supporters', revealing the diversity of those relationships, how they are perceived by both parties, and how they evolve as the pupil progresses through the different phases of schooling. Parents have historically been seen as fundraisers for schools, in the form of participants in Parent–Teacher Associations (often a misnomer as parents have been much more involved than teachers). Although in primary schools there is now much more contact between parents and school, in secondary schools parents are more formally 'invited' to attend consultation evenings and communication tends to be more fragmented. The power of those relationships has shifted somewhat in recent years. Policy promoting 'choice' in schools has meant that parents can select the school for their child on the basis of published National Curriculum attainment results. Parents continue to monitor those results, questioning and holding the school to account through parent governors, elected by parents and also at the open annual governor meeting.

In its responsibility to enable children to meet the ECM outcomes and its part in early intervention strategies the school has developed a wider role. This shift in role and focus requires schools to liase with parents about a far more open agenda. It may require them to discuss sensitive family issues, raising the possibility of support needed from a variety of services. Crucially, it may require the school to initiate a common assessment and subsequently convene and monitor the team of professionals providing support, with a teacher often taking on the lead professional role. The associated administrative and professional responsibility can seem daunting to schools developing different sets of skills to address a new context.

Opportunities

There are new activities and new roles in schools which can support these developments. Current interventions in literacy and numeracy rely heavily on parental support and offer opportunities to work with parents; many schools now run workshops to enable parents to become more aware of and involved in their children's education. Parent support workers attached to schools can bridge the space between the authority of the teacher and the needs of families. However, the focus of most of the communication between home and school is the child's learning and immediate organisational and personal factors which influence that. A survey of interactions between parents and teachers in primary schools found that the most common reasons for contact (whether by letter, phone or person) were homework, behaviour, absence and illness (Holden and Cullingford, 2003). In the ten schools surveyed, parents and teachers spent an average of 27–35 minutes per week in personal contact. The deputy head and the Year six teacher had the most contact. So it appears that there is contact, often at a sustained level, between home and school. A senior leader in a primary school has the potential to have a relationship with parents over eight crucial years of a child's life. These relationships often extend beyond a focus of the child's attainment and build a mutual trust.

A developing role: schools and teachers as partners in children's services

Interprofessional practice is relatively new to all services and organisations and schools and teachers face the same challenges as others in making it work. Jyrkama offers a framework for the analysis of agency which can be useful in analysing the progress of change (Jyrkama, 2007). He names six modalities which can be used to frame the role of teachers as part of multi-agency provision in children's services.

- Osata: knowing how to do something. A familiarity with the frameworks and administrative requirements of national and local systems is important. How and when that knowledge is gained and updated is and will continue to be dependent upon the sector and the local authority.
- Kyeta: being able to do something. The skills necessary for this kind of work both with other professionals and with parents are not always embedded in training, both initial and in-service. Reflection on the roles and identity of teachers is an important part of that process.
- Voida: having a possibility to do something. The organisational features enabling interagency practice are in place, both at a structural and organisational level.
- Taytya: having to do something. The legislation that is in place is constantly changing. Being obliged to working closely with other professionals may be a legislative requirement, but more compelling for teachers is perhaps their professional responsibility if, as is suggested, this results in better outcomes for their children.
- Haluta: wanting to do something. Teachers want to do the best for their pupils. They have often been frustrated at their inability to impact on aspects outside their 'traditional' school and learning roles and working together with other agencies can enable them to address issues in a much more holistic way.
- Tuntea: feeling, experiencing, appreciating something. How can teachers know that together with other professionals, they have made a difference to children's lives? And how can that difference be recognised? A different way of working requires a different way of evaluating success. It is that evaluation that will enable teachers to continue to develop their practice and motivate them to continue to collaborate closely with other services and practitioners.

Conclusion

This chapter is written against a landscape **of constantly evolving policy and practice which impacts on the role that schools and teachers have in interprofessional practice.** Such a dynamic context presents particular challenges as well as opportunities for development. Teachers have always been solution-focused, investigating what is the best way to teach a particular curriculum, why a pupil finds it difficult to learn something, what is the best way of teaching a particular child to read etc. In its review of research on interagency practice in 2007, NFER concluded that interagency practice can build capacity in resolving problems. There were also 'benefits in terms of increased understanding and trust between agencies which can lead to willingness to take risks and enhanced potential for innovation and improved outcomes' (Atkinson *et al.*, 2007). **In taking on a wider role schools and teachers bring considerable skill and understanding to a common endeavour of improving outcomes for children and young people.** The script for a new way of working has been given through policy directives and will now become embedded in teachers' professional lives.

Further reading

Education 3–13 is an international research journal covering primary, elementary and early years education, published by Routledge.

Useful websites

www.nfer.ac.uk

The National Foundation for Educational Research is the UK's largest research organisation for education and children's services, research reports are often available free from the website.

www.education.gov.uk

The DfE (current title, historically named DfEE, DCSF) publicises current government policy.

www.tda.gov.uk

The Teacher Development Agency (TDA) publishes documents relating to current teacher roles.

References

Anning, A., Cottrell, D., Frost, N., Green, J. and Robinson, M. (2006) *Developing Multi-professional Teamwork for Integrated Children's Services*, Maidenhead: Open University Press.

Atkinson, M., Jones, M. and Lamont, E. (2007) *Multi-agency Working and its Implications for Practice: A Review of the Literature*, Slough: NFER.

Cabinet Office (2002) Inter-departmental childcare review – delivering for children and families, in Curtis, L. and Burton, D. (2009) Naïve change agent or canny political collaborator? The change in leadership role from nursery school to Children's Centre. *Education 3-13*, Vol 37, No. 3. 287–99.

Carpenter, J., Hackett, S., Patsios, D. and Szilassy, E. (2010) *The Outcomes of Inter-agency Training to Safeguard Children*, London: Department for Children, Schools and Families.

Cummings, C., Dyson, A., Muijs, D., Papps, I., Pearson, D., Raffo, C., Tiplady, L. and Todd, L. (eds) (2007) *Evaluation of the Full Service Extended Schools Initiative, Research Report 852*, Manchester: University of Manchester.

Curtis, L. and Burton, D. (2009) Naïve change agent or canny political collaborator? The change in leadership role from nursery school to Children's Centre, *Education 3-13*, 37(3), 287–99.

Daniels, H., Edwards, A., Engestrom, Y., Gallaher, T. and Ludvigsen, R. (2010) *Activity Theory in Practice: Promoting Learning Across Boundaries and Agencies*, Abingdon: Routledge.

Day, C., Sammons, P., Stobart, G., Kington, A. and Gu, Q. (2007) *Teachers Matter: Connecting Work, Lives and Effectiveness*, Maidenhead: Open University Press.

DCSF (2007) *Effective Integrated Working: Findings of Concept of Operations Study*, London: DCSF.

DFES (2003) *Every Child Matters*, Cm. 5860, London: The Stationery Office.

Eraut, M. (1999) Non-formal Learning in the workplace, in A. Anning, D. Cottrell, N. Frost, J. Green, and M. Robinson, M. (eds) (2006) *Developing Multi-professional Teamwork for Integrated Children's Services*, Maidenhead: Open University Press.

GSCC, GTCE, NMC (2007) *Values Supporting Interprofessional Work with Children and Young People*, accessed through the UCET website, www.ucet.ac.uk/226

Hargreaves, A. and Jacka, N. (1995) Induction or seduction? Postmodern patterns in preparing to teach, *Peabody Journal of Education* 70(3), Spring 1995, 41–63.

Holden, A. and Cullingford, C. (2003) An analysis of parent/teacher relations in primary schools, *Education 3–13*, 31(3), 41–8.

Jyrkämä, J. (2007) Agency, and activity situations: elements towards studying the everyday of aging, in H. Daniels, A. Edwards, Y. Engestrom, T. Gallagher, and S. R. Ludvigsen, (eds) (2010) *Activity Theory in Practice, Promoting Learning through Boundaries and Agencies*, London: Routledge.

King, R. (1978) *All Things Bright and Beautiful: A Sociological Study of Infants' Classrooms*, Chichester: Wiley.

Laming, Lord (2003) The Victoria Climbié Inquiry, available at http://www.victoria-climbie-inquiry.org.uk/finreport/finreport.htm

Leadbetter, J. (2007) *Effective Integrated Working: Findings of Concept of Operations Study*, London: DFES.

Noddings, N. (1984) *Caring, a Feminine Approach to Ethics and Moral Education*, Berkely, CA: University of California Press.

Office for Standards in Education (2005) Every Child Matters-framework for the inspection of children's services, as cited in J. Roche, and S. A. Tucker, (2007) Every Child Matters: 'tinkering' or 'reforming' – an analysis of the development of the Children Act (2004) from an educational perspective. *Education 3–13*, Vol 35, No. 3, 213–23.

Phillips, D. K. and Carr, K. (2010) *Becoming a Teacher through Action Research*, Abingdon: Taylor and Francis.

Roche, J. and Tucker, S. A. (2007) Every Child Matters: 'tinkering' or 'reforming' – an analysis of the development of the Children Act (2004) from an educational perspective, *Education 3-13*, 35, 3, 213–23.

Shulman, L. S. and Hatch, T. (2005) *Into the Classroom: Developing the Scholarship of Teaching and Learning*, San Francisco, California: Jossey Bass.

Siraj-Blatchford, I. and Siraj-Blatchford, J. (2009) *Improving Development Outcomes for Children through Effective Practice in Integrating Early Years Services*, London: Centre for Excellence and Outcomes in Children and Young People's Services.

TDA (2007) *Professional Standards for Qualified Teacher Status and Regulations for Initial Teacher Training*, London: Training and Development Agency.

Wilkin, A., Muirfield, J., Lamont, E., Kinder, K. and Dyson, P. (2008) *The Value of Social Care Professionals Working in Extended Schools*, Slough: NFER.

Chapter 18
Medicine and teamworking

Liz Anderson and Angela Lennox

Chapter summary

This chapter will explore teamworking within the evolution of medical practice from its early beginnings to the present day. It will highlight the drivers and enablers of change and speculate on the future, including the impact of recent government reforms of the NHS and the evolution of professional regulation. We start by reflecting on the history of medicine and the key moments which have shaped today's medical practice in order to analyse the current and speculate on the future of role of doctors within team-based working and collaborative practice.

Learning objectives

This chapter will cover:

- the practice of medicine which has a long and influential history that has shaped the delivery of modern health care
- the pivotal role of being a diagnostician which has traditionally enabled doctors to practice autonomously and assume leadership roles
- how relationships between medics and other professionals are changing
- the need for doctors to be firmly committed to improving patient care through effective teamworking
- how modern day medical training embraces teamworking and collaborative practice
- new challenges for the twenty-first century doctor will include an increased accountability to the public and patients.

Introduction

In a recent address to a new intake of training doctors, Professor Sir Peter Rubin of the General Medical Council (GMC) entitled his reflections '*Not what we used to be*'. He outlined the enormous changes that have taken place within a profession that has had to move with the times to respond to advances in science, global health challenges and the demands of the general public (Ruebens, 2009). The role of the GMC from its early beginnings in 1858 featured heavily in the talk which recognised how the profession has been challenged in its ability to self-regulate (Irvine, 1997a, 2001; Southgate and Dauphinee, 1998) and has had to deal with the barrage of national discontent, with exposed malpractice by doctors, resulting in national inquiries into avoidable deaths (Smith, 1998). The outcomes of such inquiries identified teamworking environments which were at best dysfunctional and at worst autocratic, in which individuals were unable to question authority. Although findings point to 'general failings' in the NHS, the role of the doctor as dictatorial leader was one factor that led to the establishment of annual appraisal and revalidation; additionally, health care organisations were required to underpin all activities with robust clinical governance. These actions were reinforced by government policies which emphasised the importance of team-working to achieve high-quality, safe patient care (Department of Health, 2000a, 2001b).

Historical perspectives

At the turn of the nineteenth century medical training was not a university prerogative and the doctor learned through being an apprentice, mainly in hospitals. Medical schools arose through their affinity to hospitals at the turn of the twentieth century. The 1944 Goodenough Report changed the way doctors were trained, leading to a university degree as a requirement to ensure the acquisition of knowledge appropriate for the new era of science and research evidence (Goodenough Report,

1944). These academic underpinnings led to medical training comprising pre-clinical years of academic science-based study, followed by practical learning in the hospital and more recently in the community.

Until this point, admission to UK medical schools for women had been almost impossible with the first female Doctor, Elizabeth Garrett Anderson, achieving her admission through a difficult route of nurse training and access from the Society of Apothecaries in 1870.

Fundamental to these historical roots has been the evolution of self-regulation and professional autonomy as the key principles on which medical practice has evolved. It is widely believed that Hippocrates authored The Hippocratic Oath in the late fifth century BC, marking the earliest expression of medical ethics (Ludwig, 1967). The need for self-regulation was more fully articulated by medical practitioners in the early 1900s who believed that the complexity of the knowledge base and skills required, especially as technology advanced, would make regulation by non-professionals difficult; while autonomy provided doctors with the freedom to exercise their judgement in the best interest of the patient, without societal interference. Both principles are based on the premise that doctors will act competently and will put the interests of their patients in front of their own, as outlined by the World Medical Assembly (WMA) in the Declaration of Madrid 2009 World Medical Assembly (1987–2009).

Recent challenges to the leadership of medical professionals

As the general public reflected on how up to 35 babies needlessly died under the age of 1 year while undergoing heart surgery in Bristol Royal Infirmary, questions were asked about the autonomy and authority of the medical profession. The Bristol Royal Infirmary investigation identified a working environment which harked back to the era of God-like control of care by the medical profession. In his analysis of the situation Sir Ian Kennedy, inquiry leader, described concerns about the dominant powerful position of the surgeon 'pervading the culture of the theatre team'.

The public inquiry into the child heart operation scandal at Bristol concluded that within the health care team

> many failed to communicate with each other, and to work together effectively for the interests of their patients. There was a lack of leadership, and of teamwork . . . It is an account of a Hospital where there was a 'club culture; an imbalance of power, with too much control in the hands of a few individuals'
>
> *(DoH 2001a), paras 3–10.*

In 2000, just as the fall-out of the Bristol inquiry was being assimilated, Dr Harold Shipman was convicted of the murder of 15 of his patients. Shipman, a GP based in West Yorkshire took life and death decisions into his own hands. The investigation subsequently concluded that he had killed at least 215 of his patients between 1975 and 1998 and possibly up to 459 patients. Most of his victims were elderly women in good health. These findings left the general public bemused, shocked and asking questions of a profession in which they often had blind trust.

The privilege of autonomy for the medical profession goes hand in hand with the continuing responsibility for effective self-regulation. However, these and other high-profile abuses of professional autonomy resulted in the medical profession being accused of complicity and complacency, while the GMC was accused of putting doctors' interests in front of those of their patients, and regulatory procedures were judged as being seriously flawed (Smith, 1998).

Responding to public and professional criticism and acknowledging the conflicts arising from self-regulation, the GMC published the 'Duties of a Doctor' which set out the principles and values on which good practice is founded. The guidance is addressed to doctors, but it was also intended to inform the public on what to expect from doctors. Fundamental to this guidance is the recognition that doctors work in teams, setting out clarity on team-working responsibilities and personal accountability. Sir Donald Irvine, former President of the GMC, acknowledged that the position of doctors within the modern era is changing (Irvine, 1997a). Science has led to the emergence of new specialisms and patients want closer, open and honest relationships with their doctors: 'Doctors are no longer alone in the clinical management of patients. Multi-professional teamwork, the philosophy behind modern shared care, has to be reconciled with the personal nature of the doctor-patient relationship' (Irvine, 1997b, p. 1541).

The White Paper 'Trust, Assurance and Safety – The Regulation of Health Professionals in the 21st Century' proposed changes in the composition and functioning of the regulatory councils of health professionals (Department of Health, 2007c). The key proposals were that the GMC was required to (i) assure its independence of governance and

A closer look

GMC felt to be 'unfair and biased'

A survey of 264 patients who had complained to the profession's self-regulatory body found that 82% were not satisfied the process was impartial. Only six of the cases that had been concluded resulted in concrete action against a doctor; 85% of complainants were left with a more negative impression of the council.

The Guardian, 13 October (1999)

Exercise 18.1

Make a list of behaviours that you think would cause a doctor to be referred to the GMC:

- Are these unique to medicine?
- Is professional conduct an interprofessional issue?
- Why does each profession issue its own professional code of conduct?

A closer look

The shocking truth about a trusted GP

A *Daily Telegraph* article told of how patients trusted their GP (Dr Shipman) completely unaware that for 25 years he was killing his patients. The article describes the staggering scale of his activities, which resulted in hundreds of deaths. The author outlines the contrast between patients' perceptions of him as a competent professional, motivated by kindness and compassion to the stark realities of his behaviour.

Based on: *Daily Telegraph* June 2001

accountability; (ii) introduce an effective system of revalidation to demonstrate doctors' fitness to practise' which was to consist of two components: *relicensure* and specialist *recertification* and (iii) address concerns at local and national levels on tackling poor performance. The GMC further responded to public and professional disquiet by proposing the merger of Postgraduate Medical Education and Training Board (PMETB) with the GMC. Following an inquiry by Sir John Tooke this was established in 2010, with the result that the GMC now assumes responsibility for regulating all stages of medical education in the UK and across a doctor's career (Department of Health, 2008; MMC Inquiry, 2008).

The GMC medical training and teamworking

The GMC continually reviews how doctors are prepared for practice, and in 1993 called for a reduction in the factual content of the medical curriculum. Ten years later their report, *Tomorrow's doctors*, further reduced the requirement for basic science education while introducing elements of professionalism including preparation for teamworking and collaborative practice. The focus on the doctor–patient relationship also increased with the aim of achieving a partnership model of patient engagement. The most recent directives reiterate the need for medical students to learn about teamworking and emphasise the requirement for interprofessional learning (General Medical Council, 2009). These directives are less clear, however, on how the knowledge, skills and attitudes relating to teamworking and collaborative practice should be achieved and assessed. Huge variability therefore exists concerning how medical students are prepared for teamworking and collaborative practice and indeed whether it is assessed at all (Stone, 2010). Although the number of medical students completing undergraduate interprofessional education is growing in the UK (Anderson *et al.*, 2009; Barr and Ross, 2006), for many it is regarded as no more than a distraction from the purer science-based learning which underpins their ability to problem-solve symptoms and ultimately diagnose patients.

A closer look

Do students think differently as a result of interprofessional teaching?

I cannot help but think about the number of ward rounds conducted solely by medical staff. The course [IPE] has taught me the importance of integrating inputs from various other groups.

Interprofessional learning was a memorable and valuable teaching experience for me it's especially important for medical students to undergo the process since young students may feel that doctors are the most important members of the team. I firmly believe it is important to challenge these myths and stereotypes early in our education so that students learn positive teamworking strategies.

Extracts from IPE portfolios of final year University of Leicester medical student 2010.

Leading protagonists have sought solutions to improve clinical care through community multidisciplinary centres; for example, Drs Patrick and Marilyn Pietroni whose work at the Marylebone Centre Trust, London gave psychodynamic insights to cultivate a holistic understanding of interprofessional education and practice (Pietroni and Pietroni, 1996). In Leicester, the pioneering work of Dr Angela Lennox (joint author of this chapter) led to the design of a multidisciplinary health and social care centre to address the health needs of a disadvantaged inner city areas, opening Prince Phillip House in 1996. This was one of the first modern multidisciplinary health care centres in the UK which embraced teamworking practice with interprofessional learning (Cole, 2002). This initiative led to a doctor–nurse partnership to design a successful practice-based model of interprofessional education (Anderson and Lennox 2009; Lennox and Anderson 2007; Lennox and Petersen 1998) which enabled the local medical school to embed interprofessional education (IPE) within its curriculum. For those medical students who are trained to think broadly alongside other students and develop a true sense of being interprofessional we can postulate a willingness to ensure collaborative practice (Anderson *et al.*, 2009; Wakerhausen, 2009).

The inclusion of competence for interprofessional practice comes under the GMC directive to prepare tomorrow's doctors for 'professional practice'. Respect for patients and caring for colleagues are increasingly being taught under the themes of 'professionalism' which stems directly from the concerns we have highlighted relating to poor clinical performance and prompted by public concern (McNair, 2005; Pringle, 2000). These new curriculum changes remain challenging to deliver because so much of a medical student's clinical experience takes place within the acute setting, where the doctor is frequently stereotyped as 'powerful' and 'the leader' and where a patient-centred holistic team approach is easily lost (Howe *et al.*, 2002).

The medical profession and leadership

The GMC acknowledges that although doctors work within teams, many require knowledge and understanding of how to facilitate effective teamworking and how to lead and manage teams. Recent directives expect doctors to demonstrate an in-depth understanding of team working processes including 'making sure staff are clear about their individual and team objectives'; 'monitoring and reviewing a team's performance' and 'making sure that your team and the organisation learn from mistakes' (GMC 2006, p. 7). During 2009–2010 the GMC ran a series of consultations with 492 medical students on professionalism entitled '21st century doctor: your future, your choices'. The findings indicated that medical students want a clearer understanding of management and leadership competencies. They also highlighted the need for professionalism to become integrated into their core training, as well as the role and function of the GMC as their regulator. The NHS institute for Innovation and Improvement with the Academy of Medical Royal Colleges published its *medical leadership competency framework* for doctors in May 2008 (NHS Institute for innovation and improvement and AoME, 2008). The framework considers training required for doctors to become actively engaged with service design and innovation for change. One specific domain relates to how doctors work with others which includes other disciplines, organisations, patients, service users and the public. Teamworking is pivotal to this learning, portrayed as ensuring doctors develop networks, build and maintain relationships and creating environments within which others can contribute. The GMC has subsequently invited medical schools to increase the teaching of skills in leadership and management.

We could argue that the high status and leadership role of doctors within the UK is perpetuated from the moment of selection for entry to medical school. Medical students are set apart from other health care undergraduates by their prolonged training designed to produce competent, confident and self-assured doctors. Medical students are conditioned from the outset to achieve the highest standards of practice and to recognise that mistakes affect the morbidity and mortality of patients. The GMC stresses the unique status of medical students: 'Medical students have certain privileges and responsibilities different from those of other students. Because of this, different standards of professional behaviour are expected of them', (GMC, 2007, p. 4). The pressure to achieve perfection is constant and completion of training brings an image of authority which is hard to lose when other undergraduate health and social students perceive medical entrants as leaders (Hean *et al.*, 2006; Rudland and Mires, 2005).

This dominance of the medical profession in leading teams is being challenged. A range of research papers have attempted to analyse the changing role of the doctor in society and professional practice. In 2008 the King's Fund published *Understanding doctors – harnessing professionalism* (Levenson *et al.*, 2008) which describes the analysis of ten workshops consisting of 800 people, half of which were doctors. The aim was to capture the views of doctors and to consider these implications for them and the

Exercise 18.2

- How do you view leaders (these can be from any facet of life, e.g. a local MP, a Head Teacher)?
- Make a list of positive and negative attributes.
- Do any of these views relate to how you perceive doctors?

next generation. Outcomes included the need to articulate what is meant by 'modern medical professionalism' as well as to provide clarity on the role of the doctor. They generally welcomed the changing doctor–patient relationship to a more balanced, less authoritative role, alongside the increasing access to health care knowledge of their patients. There was also recognition by the medical profession that they are the most trusted of professionals and a desire to form better working relationships with health care partners and patients alike.

Learning from the past and moving to the future

Our starting point has led us to consider that doctors through historical roots, undergraduate selection, training and practice are placed into a position of team leadership which it is difficult for them to vacate. Medical practice requires doctors to be autonomous practitioners, who are efficient problem-solvers, decision-makers and responsible for the consequences of their actions. For many doctors, working in a team is still about other health care professionals being 'invited to contribute' to the medical team, which in the hospital setting typically consists of a consultant and the attached medical team (Reeves and Lewin, 2004). A hierarchical structure has been evident in operating theatres where according to research surgeons are often less willing to embrace a team-based approach to practise and see team briefings as a waste of their time, while other members of the team value them as opportunities to ensure safe practice (Lingard et al., 2006).

There remain concerns that the acute nature and fast pace of work within hospital environments provide fewer opportunities for collaboration and negotiated care. This is particularly true for emergency admission units, where doctors are required to make an initial diagnosis before other members of the team can be authorised to initiate their own professional input. There is no doubt that doctors do liaise with nurses, and when required, with other team members,

but how fully teamworking is embraced remains a concern. In their research on working in the acute ward, Reeves and Lewin describe doctors' team working as:

1. Initiated interactions with mainly the ward nurses to give instructions.
2. Focused and purposeful and time-limited.
3. The least likely professional group to interact with other professionals when working at the nurses' station.
4. Seeing their input at multidisciplinary team meetings as central and mostly being in control of these sessions. In essence practical constraints left many doctors limited to short 'unstructured and often opportunistic interactions' (Reeves and Lewin, 2004, p. 221).

This situation is perpetuated by the fact that patients are allocated to a named medical consultant throughout their hospital care and all other health care professionals interact with the patient under this organisational arrangement.

What of other areas of medical specialisms such as paediatrics, psychiatry and geriatrics? On the whole, areas where patients require the input of multidisciplinary teams have witnessed the emergence of good practice in interprofessional working. Many of these are driven by government policy, often initiated in response to past NHS whole system failures, for example 'Every Child Matters' and 'Safeguarding Adults' (Department for Education and Skills, 2003; Department of Health, 2010a). Similarly in mental health, the 'Care Plan Approach' (Department of Health, 1999) was set up to ensure joint working across a range of statutory agencies. In these specialist areas although doctors usually assume clinical leadership of the health and social care team, other members of the multidisciplinary team take on overall healthcare leadership and coordinating roles such as 'key worker' (Abbott et al., 2005). Indeed a key outcome of 'Every Child Matters' working practices is that the team should jointly identify suitable key workers (Department for Education and Skills, 2005).

Within primary care, GPs are legally required to assume leadership roles because they typically employ the clinical and administrative staff to run their GP practices. Patients are registered with an individual GP, not the practice, and it is the GP who is ultimately responsible for the care of the patient on their registered list. As with hospital care, all other primary care health care professionals interact with the patient under this structure. This role is reinforced by the fact that GPs are expected to provide leadership and advice to their staff across every aspect of decision making. GPs are also required to be skilled in running businesses. It is therefore difficult for GP independent contractors in the UK to take a non-leadership role in clinical and business decision making.

In some cases, the entrepreneurial leadership of GPs has resulted in efficient organisation of their practices through the team recruitment, facilities management (including the provision of IT infrastructure) and the implementation of clinical governance processes.

A closer look

Medical leadership in practice

Are medical-led teams a good thing? Consider this anonymised case.

Amber has five children; she is now 27 years old. She has had two partners with one surviving child from her first relationship; her second child dying aged four months from cot death. She is unemployed and lives in a cramped council flat. She trusts her GP and regularly sees the surgery for mostly social worries and concerns, e.g. housing problems, money worries. She fails to attend for her routine health checks (asthma and cervical cytology) and for her children's primary immunisations. Her GP and health visitor are the only professionals permitted into her home. This trust in her GP has, however, enabled the practice to opportunistically immunise her children and complete the health screens. The health visitor constantly liaises with the social worker involved because the family are recognised as a 'cause for concern' case load.

Effective teamworking

There is strong evidence that effective teamworking in primary care can improve the health and well-being of those with long-term conditions, witness the rise in the role of the practice nurse (Litaker et al., 2003). One example relates to the Quality and Outcomes Framework (QOF) Programme. Introduced in 2004, the QOF required GPs to develop the infrastructure to support the delivery of best practice for patients with long-term conditions. The outcome is impressive with almost 100 per cent participation of GP practices (NHS, 2010) and evidence has demonstrated that the QOF has already reduced inequalities in health (Kiran et al., 2010; NHS, 2010).

In contrast, the role of GPs in Practice-based Commissioning (PBC) proved much less successful. PBC commenced in 2005 as a central part of the government's health policy. Its aim was to give local clinicians much greater power and influence, working in partnership with PCTs, to shape how NHS resources were invested (Department of Health, 2009). The policy never reached its goal; in reality a lack of a shared vision between GPs and PCT managers, confusion over leadership roles and responsibilities and concerns over conflicts of interest of GPs resulted in a paucity of achievements with little improvement in patients' health (Curry et al., 2008).

What roles should doctors play in health care teams in the future? The drivers for change

Medical knowledge, skills and technology are expanding at an unprecedented rate. Furthermore it is estimated that by 2031 the number of over 75s in the UK will increase from 4.8m to 8.7m and with this an increased burden of disease (Office of National Statistics, 2011). This, together with the revolution in information technology, has huge implications for the medical profession and teamworking. To meet this increasing demand for NHS services while controlling increasing costs the British Government published a White Paper in July 2010 'Equity and excellence: Liberating the NHS' which set out its vision for the future of the NHS which focuses on cost-efficient productivity, and eliminating waste while continually improving the quality of care (Department of Health, 2010c). The government's vision aims to give patients and carers more choice and control over how care is delivered. Quality, innovation, productivity and prevention (QIPP) was developed to support this new direction. All QIPP activity is based on a combination of evidence from systematic reviews by the Cochrane Collaboration and practical examples of successful service transformation (Department of Health, 2010b). An outcome of QIPP is the identification of

the workforce required to efficiently deliver quality care across a range of care pathways.

The role of the doctor's participation in health care teams is therefore increasingly under review and driven by evidence-based outcomes. The future composition of teams will have less to do with historical practice and more to do with protocols which are proven to improve efficient health care delivery. In time, doctors will decreasingly be required to practise autonomously, but instead provide their expert knowledge and skills within a discrete, defined part of the care pathway. The growth of the advanced non-medical specialist role will also continue to challenge the dominance of the doctor leading the team. It is now commonplace to find advanced non-medical

A closer look

Changes in teamworking and the place of doctors

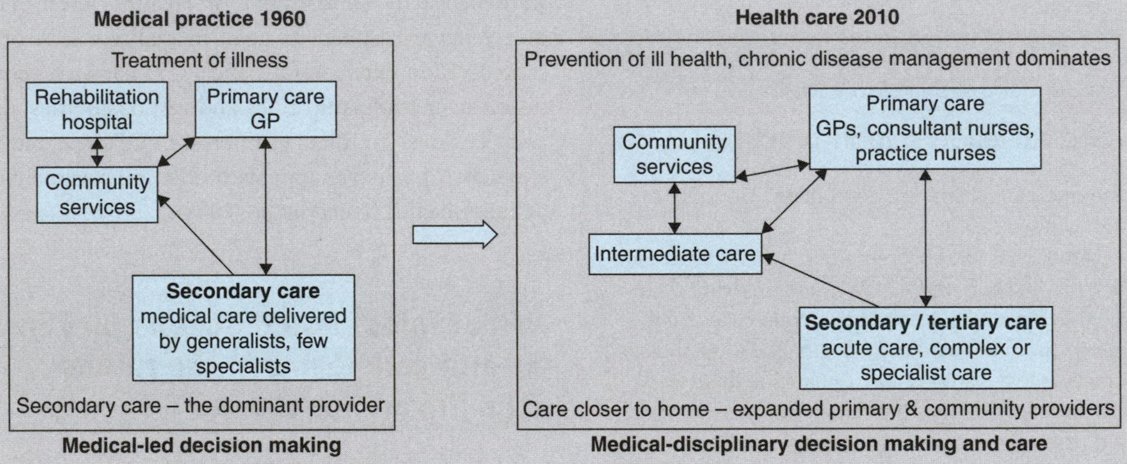

Figure 18.1 The changing healthcare landscape for the NHS

It is not just evidence-based care that is changing the face of medical practice; easy access to web-based knowledge for both the public and professionals is reducing the mystique and automatic respect afforded to doctors. The doctor–patient relationship has already changed over the decades from the 'passive, ignorant patient' of the Sir Lancelot Spratt era to that of the modern day doctor–patient relationship of mutual respect and understanding, with at times the doctor subsuming the non-expert role as for example, where a patient presents with detailed knowledge of a specific condition.

Increasing public knowledge of and engagement in health care, combined with an increasing intolerance of doctors who fail their patients, will further challenge the autonomous status enjoyed by the medical profession until now.

Against this background there are four recent and significant changes in the role of the doctor within health care teams:

- First – the NHS is undergoing a sustained shift in the access to health care from being hospital-based to within the community, closer to the patient's home. This has provided the GP generalist with an opportunity to take on highly specialist roles across a range of specialties, with service delivery in the community setting. In parallel the advanced medical practitioner is taking on many of the roles traditionally carried out by generalist GPs.
- Second – the publication in July 2010 of the White Paper 'Equity and excellence: liberating the NHS' (Department of Health, 2010c) sets out radical plans which will result in GPs being given much more responsibility for spending 80 per cent of the annual budget of the NHS. Hospitals are to be 'set free' from central control and an independent board will allow the NHS to be less influenced by politicians.
- Third – the White Paper describes radical plans for tackling public health challenges. Local government and communities will take a central role in improving health and well-being. Tackling inequalities in health and partnership working will be an essential component of service delivery.
- Fourth – the coalition government aims to drive up quality and extend patient choice by further opening up the NHS market to private and non-for-profit sectors (social enterprises and charities), so introducing competition where traditionally the NHS has had a monopoly over health care delivery.

As a result of these changes we can postulate that rising healthcare demands, new responsibilities, financial pressures, increasing regulatory requirements and the introduction of evidence-based care pathways will demand new ways of working within more efficiently structured, but flexible multidisciplinary health care teams.

practitioners working in specialist areas of medical practice across most hospital departments and community settings. For example, surgical assistants carrying out their own operating lists; nurse consultants in general practice trained to diagnose, prescribe and discharge patients; other specialist areas include palliative care, tissue viability, incontinence, cardiac failure, respiratory care and diabetes.

Conclusion

Reflecting on core knowledge, skills and responsibilities, it is not hard to see how for generations doctors have been leaders in health care and have been set apart, to some extent, from the rest of the clinical team. Furthermore the doctor's professional practice often results in significant health benefits to those who are helped or cured – power and authority indeed reinforced by patients who continue to extol doctors. Such a pivotal place in society attracts respect, including from colleagues from other professions who rely on their diagnostic and specialist skills. It follows that some doctors go on to believe they are the natural leaders of teams and many other

professionals have, to some extent, allowed this stance to persist.

With the pace of change over the last decade, and from the vantage point of looking back to the earliest medical practice and looking forward into the twenty-first century, we can conclude that doctors are more likely to practice within team-based structures, taking on leading roles only when it is right to do so. These changes are illustrated in Figure 18.1, which compares medical practice in 1960 with today.

Our evidence demonstrates that change is inevitable, based on historical patterns which more recently have been driven by public opinion, related policy directives and advances in our knowledge and understanding, as well as technology.

Doctors will remain in a pivotal leadership position as diagnosticians, but where patients require multidisciplinary follow-on care **doctors will be expected to encourage and engage with effective partnership working**. How change will unfold in the next decade is difficult to predict, especially as health and social care demands in the UK and in all affluent societies are at a crossroads; trying to achieve balance between what we would like to do and what we can afford.

In this chapter we have reflected on a historical journey which has placed doctors in leading roles within health care delivery and described the changing relationships they are assuming within the multidisciplinary teams that now support patients.

At the turn of the twenty-first century a leading member of the GMC, Sir Cyril Chantler, reflected on the constant concern for medicine today to consider the balance between how science and technology can overwhelm wisdom and the need for medicine to hold a place which balances science with humanity; often referred to as the art of practising medicine (Chantler, 2001). We can be certain that a profession brought to account for its authoritative attitude reflected long and hard on its humanity and seems content to embrace effective patient-centred team working from the stance of the responsibility which comes with being a doctor.

Further reading

Irvine, (2003). *The Doctors' Tale: Professionalism and Public Trust*. Radcliffe Publishing for further analysis of what it means to work professionally as a doctor.

Thistlethwaite, J. and Spencer, J. (2008) *Professionalism in Medicine*. Oxford: Radcliffe Publishing.

Hammick, M., Freeth, D., Copperman, J. and Goodsman, D. (2009) *Being Interprofessional*. Cambridge: Polity Press.

Useful websites

www.gmc-uk.org General Medical Council

www.kingsfund.org.uk King's Fund

www.medschools.ac.uk Medical Schools Council

www.bma.org.uk British Medical Association

www.dh.gov.uk Department of Health

www.asme.org.uk Association for the Study of Medical Education

www.who.org World Health Organization

www.caipe.org.uk CAIPE (UK Centre for the Advancement of Interprofessional Education)

References

Abbott, D., Townsely, R. and Watson, D. (2005) Multi-agency working in services for disabled children: what impact does it have on professionals? *Health and Social Care in the Community* 13 (2), 155–63.

Anderson, E. S. and Lennox, A. (2009) The Leicester Model of Interprofessional Education: developing, delivering and learning from student voices for 10 years, *Journal of Interprofessional Care* 23 (6), 557–73.

Anderson, E. S., Thorpe, L. N., Heney, D. and Petersen, S. (2009) Medical students benefit from learning about patient safety in an interprofessional team, *Medical Education,* 43, 542–52.

Barr, H. and Ross, F. (2006) Mainstreaming interprofessional education in the United Kingdom; a position paper, *Journal of Interprofessional Care* 20 (2), 96–104.

Chantler, C. (2001) Foreword, in M. Marinker *Medicine and Humanity,* London: Kings Fund.

Cole, A. (2002) A multi-disciplinary training programme on a deprived estate in Leicester, *Learning in Health and Social Care* 3 (94), 179–89.

Curry, N., Goodwin, N., Naylor, C. and Robertson, R. (2008) *Practice-based Commissioning. Reinvigorate, Replace or Abandon?* London: King's Fund, www.kingsfund.org.uk/publications/the_kings_fund_publications/pbc.html

Department of Health (1999) *A National Service Framework for Mental Health,* London: HMSO.

Department of Health (2000a) *The NHS Plan – A Plan for Investment, A Plan for Reform,* London: HMSO.

Department of Health (2001a) *The Kennedy Report. The Report of the Public Inquiry into Children's Heart Surgery at the Bristol Royal Infirmary 1984–1995: Learning from Bristol* (Cm 5207(II)), London: The Stationery Office.

Department of Health (2001b) *Working Together, Learning Together: A Framework for Lifelong Learning for the NHS,* London: The Stationery Office.

Department of Health (2007c) *Trust Assurance and Safety – The Regulation of the Health Professions in the 21st Century.* CM 7103, London: The Stationery Office, accessed 16 November 2010. http://www.dh.gov.uk/prod_consum_dh/groups/dh_digitalassets/@dh/@en/documents/digitalasset/dh_065947.pdf

Department of Health (2008) *Implementing the Tooke Report: Department of Health Update*, London: Department of Health. http://www.dh.gov.uk/en/Publicationsandstatistics/Publications/PublicationsPolicyAndGuidance/DH_090286

Department of Health (2009) *Clinical commissioning: Our Vision for Practice-based Commissioning,* London: Department of Health. http://www.dh.gov.uk/en/PublicationsandstatisticsPublications/PublicationsPolicyAndGuidance/DH_095692, accessed 12 January 2011.

Department of Health (2010a) *Clinical Governance and Adult Safeguarding: An Integrated Process,* London: Department of Health, http://www.dh.gov.uk/en/Publicationsand

statistics/Publications/PublicationsPolicyAndGuidance/ DH_112361, accessed 12 January 11.

Department of Health (2010b), *The NHS Quality, Innovation, Productivity and Prevention Challenge: An Introduction For Clinicians*, London: Department of Health.

Department of Health (2010c) *Equity and Excellence: Liberating the NHS,* London: The Stationery Office.

Department for Education and Skills (2003) Every Child Matters, London: The Stationery Office.

Department for Education and Skills (2005) *Common Core of Skills and Knowledge for the Children's Workforce*, Nottingham: DfES.

General Medical Council (2006) *Management for Doctors,* London: GMC.

General Medical Council (2007) *Medical Students: Professional Behaviour and Fitness to Practise, Guidance from the General Medical Council and the Medical Schools Council*, London: GMC.

General Medical Council (2009) *Tomorrow's Doctors. Outcomes and Standards for Undergraduate Medical Education*, London: GMC.

Goodenough Report (1944) *The Report of the Interdepartmental Committee of Medical Schools*, London: The Ministry of Health and Department of Health for Scotland.

Hean, S., Macleod-Clarke, J., Adams, K. and Humphries, D. (2006) Will opposites attract? Similarities and differences in students' perceptions of the stereotype profiles of other health and social care professional groups. *Journal of Interprofessional Care* 20 (2), 162–81.

Howe, A., Billingham, K. and Walter, C. (2002) In our own image – a multidisciplinary qualitative analysis of medical education, *Journal of Interprofessional Care* 16 (4), 380–9.

Irvine, D. (1997a) The performance of doctors: professionalism and self regulation in a changing world, *British Medical Journal* 314, 1540.

Irvine, D. (1997b) The performance of doctors II: maintaining good practice, protecting patients from poor performance, *British Medical Journal* 314, 1613–15.

Irvine, D. (2001) The changing relationship between the public and the medical profession, *JRSM* 94, 162–9.

Kiran, T., Hutchings, A., Dhalla, I. A., Furlong, C. and Jacobson, B. (2010) The association between quality of primary care, deprivation and cardiovascular outcomes: a cross-sectional study using data from the UK Quality and Outcomes Framework. *Journal of Epidemiology and Community Health* 64, 927–34, http://jech.bmj.com/ content/64/10/927.abstract aff 5.

Lennox, A. and Anderson, E. S. (2007) *The Leicester Model of Interprofessional Education. A Practical Guide to Implementation in Health and Social Care Education*, The

Higher Education Academy for Medicine, Dentistry and Veterinary Medicine. Special Report 9.

Lennox, A. and Petersen, P. (1998) Development and evaluation of a community-based, multi-agency course for medical students: descriptive study, *British Medical Journal* 316, 596–9.

Levenson, R., Dewar, S. and Shepherd, S. (2008) *Understanding Doctors – Harnessing Professionalism,* London: Kings Fund and Royal College of Physicians.

Lingard, L., Whyte, S., Espin, S., Baker, G. R., Orser, B. and Doran, D. (2006) Toward safer interprofessional communication: constructing a model of 'utility' from preoperative team briefings, *Journal of Interprofessional Care* 20, 1–13.

Litaker, D., Moin, L. C., Planavsky, L., Kippes, C., Methta, N. and Frolkis, J. (2003) Physician-nurse practitioner in chromic disease management: the impact on costs, clinical effectiveness, and patients' perception of care. *Journal of Interprofessional Care* 17 (3), 223–7.

Ludwig, Edelstein (1967) The Hippocratic Oath: text, translation and interpretation, *Supplements to the Bulletin of the History of Medicine*, No. 1, Baltimore: The Johns Hopkins Press. Reprinted in *Ancient Medicine: Selected Papers of Ludwig Edelstein,* Baltimore: The Johns Hopkins Press, 1967.

McNair, R. (2005) The case for educating medical students in professionalism as the core content of interprofessional education, *Medical Education* 39, 456–64.

MMC Inquiry (2008) *Aspiring to Excellence: Findings and Final Recommendations of the Independent Inquiry into Modernising Medical Careers*, led by Professor Sir John Tooke, Aldridge Press, Chiswick, London: Aldridge Press

National Health Service (2010). The Quality and Outcomes Framework 2009/10: Accessed Dec 21st 2011: http:// www.ic.nhs.uk/statistics-and-data-collections/audits-and-performance/the-quality-and-outcomes-framework/the-quality-and-outcomes-framework-2009-10

NHS Institute for Innovation and Improvement and AoME (2008) *Medical Leadership Competency Framework. Enhancing Engagement in Medical Leadership,* Warwick: Academy of Medical Colleges and NHS Institute for Innovation and Improvement.

Office of National Statistics (2011) http://www.statistics.gov. uk/pdfdir/age0910.pdf, accessed 3 March 2011.

Pietroni, J. and Pietroni, P. (1996) *Innovations in Community Care and Primary Care,* Edinburgh: Churchill Livingstone.

Pringle, M. (2000) The Shipman inquiry: implications for the public's trust in doctors, *British Journal of General Practice* 50, 355–6.

Reeves, S. and Lewin, S. (2004). Interprofessional collaboration in the hospital: strategies and meanings, *Journal of Health Services Research and Policy* 9 (4), 218–25.

Rudland, J. R. and Mires, G. (2005) Characteristics of doctor and nurses as perceived by students entering medical school: implication for shared teaching, *Medical Education* 39, 448–55.

Ruebens, P. (2009) '*Not what we used to be*'. Leicester Medical School, 22 September 2009.

Smith, R. (1998) Regulation of doctors and the Bristol inquiry, *British Medical Journal* 317, 1539–40.

Southgate, L. and Dauphinee, D. (1998) Continuing medical education: maintaining standards in British and Canadian medicine: the developing role of the regulatory body, *British Medical Journal* 316, 697–700.

Stone, J. (2010) Moving interprofessional learning forward through formal assessment, *Medical Education* 44, 396–403.

The Guardian (1999) Doctors' body 'biased against public'. Wednesday 13th October. Extract: Accessed 21st December 2011: http://www.guardian.co.uk/uk/1999/oct/13/sarahboseley1

The Daily Telegraph (June 2001) The Killing Fields of Harold Shipman. Extract from: accessed 21st December 2011: http://www.telegraph.co.uk/culture/4724155/The-Killing-Fields-of-Harold-Shipman.html.

Wakerhausen, S. (2009) Collaboration, professional identity and reflection across boundaries, *Journal of Interprofessional Care* 23 (5), 455–73.

World Medical Assembly (1987–2009) *Declaration of Madrid on Professional Autonomy and Self-Regulation*, http://www.wma.net/en/30publications/10policies/20archives/a21/index.html, accessed 12 January 2011.

Chapter 19
Occupational therapists

Chris McKenna and Cath Wright

Chapter summary

The aim of this chapter is to establish the purpose and meaning of interprofessional working from the point of view of the occupational therapist, as a student or whether they work in practice, research or academia. We will look at the origins of interprofessional learning within occupational therapy philosophy and history, as well as considering the current and future direction of services indicated by the College of Occupational Therapists. The links to the personal skills and qualities required for an individual to actively participate in interprofessional working are discussed critically and ideas for personal development are presented.

Learning objectives

This chapter will cover:

- the occupational therapy philosophy and interprofessional learning
- interprofessional issues in training
- collaborative working in a variety of contexts
- understanding the personal competencies, attitudes and values required for successful interprofessional working.

What is occupational therapy?

For an occupational therapist, defining who you are demonstrates the occupational therapy perspective on life. It is through our self-defining statement that we indicate how we fill our time, the skills we have and how we would like others to see us. When an occupational therapist indicates what their profession is, there follows the pregnant pause while the listener considers the statement. This is usually accompanied by the question 'what is that?' There then ensues a long and convoluted series of statements and examples which describe the activities of an occupational therapist.

One of the great difficulties in defining this profession is that occupational therapy exists not within any one particular context but as a process which can be applied within a range of differing and very diverse circumstances.

According to the College of Occupational Therapists, 'Occupational therapists help people engage as independently as possible in the activities (occupations) which enhance their health and wellbeing'.[1] While this provides a concise definition of the role of the occupational therapist it offers little to the observer who is attempting to understand what an occupational therapist actually does.

Definitions of occupational therapy

[occupational therapy is] enabling people to engage in a range of occupations and building peoples' capacity and ability to perform occupations.

(Curtin *et al.*, 2009)

[occupational therapy] aims to enable and empower people to be competent and confident in their daily lives, and thereby to enhance wellbeing and minimise the effects of dysfunction or environmental barriers.

(Duncan, 2006)

Occupational therapy evolved from the discussions of a range of professionals; individuals with their own skills which combined to form a cohesive group maintaining a similar philosophy: William Rush Dunton Jr (doctor), Susan Tracy (nurse), George Barton (architect) and Susan Johnson (arts and crafts teacher). Each brought their own thinking and skills to form a new organisation called the National Society for the Promotion of Occupational Therapy. The shared values and beliefs coalesced into a professional perspective paradigm.

A number of professional observers have noted that, as a relatively new profession, occupational therapy has undergone some changes from the early beginnings (Kielhofner, 2009). Its perspectives have evolved and changed, with adaptations leading through its pre-paradigmatic state to generating its own professional paradigm.

Philosophy

This process causes upheaval in the profession as it realigns itself. To some degree there was an attempt to follow the political and financial power of medicine as the occupational therapy profession generated its own underpinning philosophy. This has been partially rejected in the later part of the twentieth century and beyond with the return to its original roots of holism and organismic consideration.

This diversity of practice calls for a breadth of skills which is unique in health and social care practice. It transcends agencies and specialties because expertise is not embedded in medical specialisation or a sector of care but in the capacity to analyse activity and remove the obstacles preventing occupational performance regardless of the context (although some might suggest we bear in mind that context). A 'rights' perspective would view this approach as consistent with the expectations of disability legislation and the idea that people are entitled to be afforded the opportunity to live a 'normal' life.

Occupational therapy has several core values and beliefs which combine to form a philosophical base for the profession and which impact on interprofessional working.

[1]http://www.cot.org.uk/Homepage/About_Occupational_Therapy/, accessed 3 July 2009.

Occupation

Occupational therapy is based on the concept that activity is a central aspect of human experience and well-being. As such, occupational therapists believe that purposeful, balanced activity can be used as a healing force in treatment: 'Man through the use of his hands as they are energised by mind and will, can influence the state of his own health' (Reilly, 1962).

Occupation is not always an individual activity and this may demand the cooperation of individuals to ensure the interventions are successful without compromising the meaningful and purposeful nature of the occupation.

Holism

The occupational therapy profession believes that health is a dynamic multidimensional phenomenon, which comprises physical, psychological, emotional, social, cultural and spiritual aspects of the individual. As such occupational therapy maintains that the individual must be considered as a whole to maximise their potential and their response to treatment and intervention: 'The whole person must be considered in order to have a person who is as healthy as possible in all areas . . . of their life' (Mayers, 1990).

It would be negligent for the occupational therapist to intervene without engagement with other statutory and voluntary parties and advocates appropriate to the client's needs. This collaboration is integral to achieving a truly holistic approach.

Client-centred

The client-centred nature of occupational therapy requires that the client is the focus of the intervention. Implicit in this is the notion of interdisciplinary collaboration, in order to avoid what Parker (2006) refers to as 'professional rivalry and conflict over roles' as this could 'disadvantage the client' and to maximise the complementary skills available.

The occupational therapy profession believes that each individual is unique and that only when treated as an individual will they be motivated fully in treatment and maximise their potential. By taking a client-centred/client needs-led view of intervention, the occupational therapy profession advocates an individualised problem-solving approach as opposed to prescriptive intervention. 'New knowledge . . . will affirm the significance of the uniqueness, individuality and wholeness of each person' (Yerxa, 1994).

Empowerment

The occupational therapy profession believes that individuals should be given, where possible, control and choice within treatment and discharge planning. A relationship based on open discussion and negotiation is sought to promote mutual respect and cooperation. 'The future will bring increased emphasis on personal power, autonomy self-direction and self-responsibility' (Yerxa, 1994).

Working within a psychosocial model of practice can facilitate this approach; conversely, the medical model prohibits, to some extent, the amount of control given to the client. Occupational therapists can find themselves working within different models of practice; however, they should not lose sight of the desire to enable clients wherever possible.

Enablement

The belief that positive self-esteem and acknowledgement of abilities, strengths and potential enables an individual to make choices and seek control is a fundamental aspect of occupational therapy. Intervention is directed towards promoting these characteristics and, therefore, the support of colleagues is essential to reinforce positive behaviours. 'Occupational therapists should emphasise . . . participation and delight in one's own actions' (Yerxa, 1994).

Equality

The occupational therapy profession believes that all individuals should be treated with respect and as having equal value. Attitudinal, environmental and discriminatory barriers are challenged to promote well-being for all. While this is clearly not unique to occupational therapy it is nevertheless important in underpinning any intervention. It further establishes the ground rules for the interprofessional team and acknowledges the expertise of the client into their own unique context.

> Occupational therapists who are allies and advocates for persons with disabilities will help change society's attitudes from 'those people are inferior to these people are fundamentally human, just like the rest of us.
>
> (Yerxa, 1994)

Interprofessional issues in training

From the commencement of training the occupational therapy student receives a programme of modules that prepares them for practice. While the training offers fitness to practice at graduate competence level, more importantly it offers the novice practitioner the opportunity to consider the whole potential for practice.

Training in the formative years often provides 'black and white' professional guidelines which can construct strong professional barriers/boundaries. Training programmes then endeavour to demonstrate how the modular and specific professional content facilitates the students to critically appraise the many and varying practice possibilities and how to best work with colleagues to get the best outcome for their patients (College of Occupational Therapists, 2008).

Students in training will have a number of opportunities to explore these relationships in a theoretical and a practical way in health and social care programmes. This will increase their expectations of seeing this in practice and prepares them for engaging in interprofessional working.

From a project commissioned by the Department of Health into IPE (for Social Work), it emerged that the role of the practice educator/teacher was pivotal in facilitating interprofessional practice learning, a

A closer look

Occupational therapist training

Interprofessional learning helps me to be able to work interprofessionally in practice by providing knowledge of other professional roles, and understanding of their involvement in relation to the client's needs by providing an opportunity to experience other members of a multidisciplinary team working within their roles.

I feel that having an understanding of other professional roles helps to break down barriers between professionals, enhance communication between professional teams, provide effective care for clients and broaden knowledge of other available services.

Sophie Gibson, student

Exercise 19.2

Consider how your knowledge of other professions will help you to fulfil your role more effectively. How could this be measured?

role for which they were seemingly unprepared (Low and Barr, 2008, p. 5). This highlights the necessity of reinforcing to practice educators the importance of their role in facilitating the students understanding of the transfer of theory into practice.

The challenge for the individual is to develop confidence in one's own profession to allow boundaries to be dropped. This can only be achieved through an understanding of one's own discipline and those of colleagues.

Above all, individual occupational therapists need to have the confidence to speak out and the humility to listen.

While recognising that interprofessional working is advantageous, unfortunately in acute care where staff turnover is high, teams tend to be transient and staffing levels may mean that they do not 'belong' to one ward or clinical team. This can prove to be too challenging, and less collaborative multidisciplinary working (i.e. working in parallel, but not in partnership) becomes the accepted norm.

A closer look

The Reality of teamworking

In reality there are pockets of interprofessional working in acute hospital care, predominantly where there is a specialty in which the health care professionals recognise the complexity of the task and, therefore, the advantage of combining their expertise to address the problem.

This is most evident where a mature team exists that has worked together for some time, understands and trusts each other's roles, is used to learning together and the professionals are consistently accessible to each other. Innovation arises from such work and the patient experiences truly seamless health care. In our experience this has been most apparent in stroke rehabilitation, end of life care, amputee rehabilitation and ICU rehabilitation.

Sara Blackbourn,
Team Leader and Occupational Therapist

Collaborative working in context

Interprofessional working for occupational therapists should not be a new concept. Working together for the greater interest of the individual recipient is a long-standing feature of the profession (Joice and Coia, 1989). In order to fully engage in interprofessional working, the individual occupational therapist needs to have a sound understanding of why this is important as well as personal insight into their own working practices and available skills.

For some people in every profession, the concept of working together is just so simplistically common sense that for them the main frustration is when others appear to work against this, either directly or indirectly. In this section we explore why some individuals and teams struggle with interprofessional working as well as offering the reasons for engaging so that both types of reader can gain some insight.

The bottom line, if one is needed, is that for occupational therapists our professional body, The College of Occupational Therapists (COT), and our regulatory body, The Health Professions Council (HPC), require us to work in partnership:

5.3 You should respect the responsibilities, practices and roles of other people with whom you work.

5.3.2 You should recognise the need for multiprofessional and multi-agency collaboration to ensure that well co-ordinated services are delivered in the most effective way.

5.3.3 You have a duty to refer the care of a service user to another appropriate colleague if it becomes clear that the task is beyond your scope of practice. You should consult with other service providers when additional knowledge, expertise and/or support are required (HPC, 2008, standard 6).

5.3.4 If you and another practitioner are involved in the treatment of the same service user, you should work co-operatively, liaising with each other and agreeing areas of responsibility. This should be communicated to the service user and all relevant parties.

(College of Occupational Therapists, 2010)

7 You must communicate properly and effectively with service users and other practitioners. You must take all reasonable steps to make sure that you can communicate properly and effectively with service users. You must communicate appropriately, co-operate, and share your knowledge and expertise with other practitioners, for the benefit of service users.

(Health Professions Council, 2008)

The recent key drivers in health, social care and the third sector have sought to make services smarter, leaner, more efficient and overall improve the quality of the service to be received (Care Standards Act 2000; Health Act 2009, Health and Social Care Act 2008). The importance of listening to service users and carers in developing and monitoring services has officially been recognised as a high-value contribution, for example in the NHS Reform and Health Care Professions Act (Department of Health, 2002), and *Recovering ordinary lives: The strategy for occupational therapy in mental health services 2007–2017* (College of Occupational Therapists, 2006). The feedback from service users shows an overwhelming desire for professionals to communicate with each other as well as listening to and valuing the input from the individual and their significant others (Social Care Institute for Excellence, 2009).

Serious Case Reviews (SCR) have highlighted how, and where there are flaws in teamworking, incidents occur, in some cases with fatal consequences (Bristol Royal Infirmary Enquiry, 2001). Individual professionals also face a greater threat of litigation and professional conduct enquiries which can have an impact on a career or livelihood.

Interprofessional working and service users

Individual occupational therapists have encountered negative reactions to their interventions when they have failed to listen to the views of the individual and/or their carers and have been perceived to have delivered services with a heavy hand. For example,

Case study

An occupational therapist meets with a family with regard to a specialised seating system. Stephen, a three-year-old boy, has experienced an electric shock which has caused brain damage resulting in intellectual and physical impairment. Mum currently keeps Stephen resting on a bean bag all day. The occupational therapist suggests that in order to avoid deformity he be supplied with a chair which provides a good position and appropriate support.

As a consequence of Stephen's age it would be efficient to provide a chair which can be adapted to accommodate his future growth. These chairs are inevitably covered in lots of screws and handles to accommodate the necessary adjustments. Mum does not like this and, therefore, it is essential that some consensus is formed in order to avoid the chair being put in a cupboard, unused, because the chair made the Stephen's situation more easily noticeable.

Exercise 19.3

What personal skills or attributes do you require in order to be able to treat the client and their carers as a member of the team? How might these be developed?

providing rehabilitation equipment that was not what the individual wanted ('she made our house look like a hospital and made us have things we didn't need – we had managed without them before and had our own way that we were confident with and safe'), carrying out interventions with disregard to the information given by carers ('he never makes tea at home but she had him there making it').

Occupational therapists have long complained about the continuous need to explain what exactly an occupational therapist does to other professionals as well as to the public. As the profession is now moving into the third sector, voluntary agencies and other roles in emerging enterprises (Sealey, 1999) occupational therapists should brace themselves for continued verbal explanations. They should also recognise and value the positive way that they can communicate their role and values through effective interprofessional working. Being visible and modelling good practice as well as sharing and contributing can be a powerful way to showcase our profession.

We each have a significant role to play, as equals. Elitism between professionals is not healthy or productive and can lead to conflict (Kelly and Van Vlaenderen, 1996). For the recipients of services, the vulnerable and difficult to reach any conflict in teams can have a serious impact on the care and services they receive.

If working together in an interdependent way is so obviously beneficial, why do we need to be told to do it? Consideration of what stops individuals from communicating with others, from holding back information and in some cases actively sabotaging this best practice should help practitioners from falling into these negative practices. To enable individuals who see themselves as independent practitioners to come together, a foundation of trust and mutual respect must be created. Effort must be put into this process and it cannot be assumed that position,

A closer look

Service-user perspectives

During the early years of her life, Jessica has been under the professional care of many different services. Hardly a week has passed without at least one appointment or home visit and it can be problematic to fit these around other family commitments. Many areas of Jessica's development have been enhanced as a direct result of these interventions and provision of specialist equipment. I have found it most beneficial when the various services have been able to interact and this communication has led to a sense of cohesion in the treatments/therapies advised. I can then see them as a team, working together to help Jessica.

Julie, Mum

A closer look

Trusting each other

In modern accident and emergency departments, protocols are followed to assess individuals for equipment, such as walking aids, which have traditionally been the remit of the physiotherapist to provide. The physiotherapist has to trust that only those people who are deemed competent to follow the protocol are providing the equipment. If the physiotherapist feels that they have to reassess every individual then this is a duplication of effort and a demonstration of mistrust, with other staff members feeling their work is not valued.

This has been evidenced in practice as occupational therapists and physiotherapists working together become familiar with each other's role and are able to anticipate the other's interventions and enable the client accordingly. This understanding is born of trust, respect and a willingness to open professional boundaries.

Exercise 19.4

There are many situations that can cause these same feelings of mistrust – from the single assessment through to all sorts of treatment. Consider if you have inadvertently caused mistrust and how you might avoid it in future.

status, age or length of time in work can automatically ensure that you have the trust and respect of your colleagues. To gain trust professionals must demonstrate the key elements of competency and character (Covey, 2004). To demonstrate competency individuals need to show consistent, appropriate technical skills, critical thinking skills and interpersonal skills. Covey suggests that demonstration of integrity, maturity and 'abundance mentality' will collectively lead to a trustworthy character.

Mutual respect is earned through demonstrating an ability to listen to others, as well as showing that even if you hold a different point of view you will take the time to try to understand someone else's opinion (Covey, 2004). A policy of seeking first to understand another person before voicing your own opinion can go a long way to building respect (Covey, 2004). Working towards consensus, the win–win outcome may take time but is more productive in the end as sabotage is less likely to occur (Covey, 2004; van den Hove, 2004). There is a common misunderstanding that to compromise may resolve a dispute. Compromise could lead to one or more party feeling disenfranchised, which in turn may lead to their non-participation or, worse than this, they may actively try to sabotage outcomes.

Trusting each other to implement the best evidence-based practice and to do what we say we

will do is also a basis for interprofessional learning. To do this we should be prepared to explain why we feel interventions are valid, be seen to be contributing towards the evidence base and be happy to make explanations in a positive rather than in a defensive way. Each professional knows their own professional reasoning – helping others to understand it too can ease tension and mistrust – in recognising each other's professional strengths and working with them we can reduce the pressure on all professionals and be more efficient in our output. It is inevitable that there will be grey areas in every practice setting, where an intervention could be carried out by a number of different professionals. Having the confidence to trust another individual to fulfil the task can reduce the need for boundaries which can hamper patients' progression. Additionally, staff who tend towards perfectionism can find it difficult to delegate tasks to others, which could lead individuals to feel less trusted and respected as well as overloading the perfectionist staff member. Perfectionist behaviours can be barriers to interprofessional working, however, individuals can (and should) make changes to their behaviours to prevent this.

Ideally individual teams should regularly seek to check out and confirm roles to prevent confusion and to create an environment of open communication and trust. This is especially necessary when a new staff member joins a team and should be part of induction programmes as an essential requirement. Teams should review roles periodically to enable changes, improvements and to allow new staff to feel able to offer a contribution in areas where they feel they have strengths. With negotiation and trust, roles can change smoothly and have positive outcomes for patients.

Peer pressure within teams may be a reason for not working together. There is no simple explanation for this. Perhaps an individual has had a previous poor experience working when trust and respect were lost. This one incident can sometimes then be used to prejudice similar situations. Additionally, gossip and idle chat, negative opinions and historical grievances can affect partnership working. Professional stereotypes can also be problematic. Most training establishments are now engaging in interprofessional learning during professional training programmes to try to prevent these stereotypes from occurring before the students arrive in practice (Centre for the Advancement in Interprofessional Education, 2008). It is then down to teams to refrain from participating in behaviours that might affect another person's opinion or endorse stereotyped thinking. It is hard to stand up to this kind of peer pressure. Learning to be assertive and retaining your personal integrity is not only important for individuals, but can also help over time to change the way others work.

Perhaps the way towards interprofessional working is for individuals to reassess why they wanted to work in their chosen profession (see Exercise 19.1). They may then try to find intrinsic pleasure from doing that job for the benefit of the recipient rather than needing to be seen as an elite professional. Individuals could choose to work in this way and as all those individuals make the conscious choice this way of working will become the norm. Humility rather than power could be the key.

Rather than considering how occupational therapists work in an interprofessional way in different clinical specialties, we will now consider how different spheres of occupational therapy can benefit from this model and the skills that an individual may benefit from developing in order to be successful.

Interprofessional working in rural settings

Lessons can be learned from the professionals who strive to develop and maintain interprofessional working when they may only meet up in person on a rare occasion. The barriers of distance have been minimised in the recent past, through the improvement in technology. Telephone calls can now be replaced by video conferencing and Skype, both less expensive than a team's travel expenditure and inclusive for our clients, so client-centred care can be maintained. Additionally, improvements in electronic patient records have enabled timely communication, prevented duplication and can follow the client to all of the services they rely upon.

So do professionals need any particular skills to enable them to work in an interprofessional way in a rural setting? Patience and determination may come in handy, as well as a willingness to learn new IT skills and keep updating them. The ability to prioritise would also be a useful practical skill. From a communication point of view, professionals will need more than ever to work on their listening skills, be able to express information in a concise manner and be able to work on occasions without the non-verbal cue that can be picked up on during face-to-face interaction. These skills involve developing left and right brain competencies and professionals could look to learn these skills from people who have everyday practical experience of complex communication – people with sight loss will have expertise to share.

Interprofessional working in independent practice

With current traditional practice moving forward into new ways of working, occupational therapists may find themselves working within their own business, within the private or third sector, voluntary or charitable organisation. The interprofessional team develops a different dimension and individuals may find themselves needing to work alongside accountants, business managers, non-health and social care staff and other unregulated staff, who may have different values and priorities. Here, the traditionally valued communication skills of rapport building, reflecting and validating will need to be added to, with the ability to convey instructions, explain tasks, verbalise objectives and evaluate critically. The occupational therapist needs to understand how the same information can be communicated in different ways to ensure the receiver is engaged and hears the content in the most appropriate way.

Interprofessional working in specialist teams

There will be different experiences for practitioners working in specialist teams. Although the team role is much more focused, with clear lines of responsibility, the close-knit nature of the specialist team offers greater opportunity for understanding other roles and ensuring the team meets all the needs of the client. This leads to a potential blurring of roles with uncertain consequences.

Interprofessional working in academia

There are two distinct areas of interprofessional working in academia – educating the students in this area and developing programmes and modules with colleagues. Both are intertwined in that unless the modules and programmes are carefully considered, the student experience could be superficial.

A closer look

Independent sector perspectives

Based on my experience, it is more important to have the right people, at the right time, in the right place rather than what it says on their badge or the colour of their trousers!

Opportunities for genuine partnership with the person, their family and others are enhanced due to the way in which therapy is structured as well as the longer period of involvement that often occurs. Collaboration and communication ensures that everyone involved is working towards the same goals and evidences how these have been achieved. The potential for innovation and hypothesis testing is high as skills, knowledge and experience are shared across the whole team leading to sustainable outcomes.

Rachel Charles, Occupational Therapist

A closer look

Specialist teams

On joining the team, it felt like the roles of the different professionals were more blurred than in teams I had worked with previously and it felt less 'black and white' and more 'shades of grey'. For example, the specialist nurses in the team offer front-line advice about managing fatigue and energy conservation. It was really important to me to understand the various team members' roles and establish when it was appropriate to offer advice and when to refer on to another specialist and also for other team members to be fully aware of my role. Initial uncertainty about these things caused me to question my role in the team and to undermine my own confidence. By discussing this fully, spending time with other professionals in the team and educating them about the service I can provide, I was able to resolve things.

Nicola Simpson, MacMillan Occupational Therapist

Interprofessional learning needs to promote a shared active and deep learning experience. Just putting different disciplines in a room to learn a subject together does not necessarily mean they will learn to work with each other. Academic staff must act as positive role models, highlighting the need to seek out the knowledge and support of the other available professions.

Interprofessional working in the face of major change

Changes to health and social care over the last five years have been significant. It is apparent that this change will continue to happen. Engaging staff in interprofessional working while facilitating change management can be difficult, as individuals become protective of their professional roles which represent their livelihoods. The changes will continue to happen

and cannot be ignored. A sound understanding of communication skills is invaluable in these situations and, although many individuals will perceive their skills to be good, spending time as an individual or as a team to review communication may prove to be invaluable.

One way to establish your own communication style is to consider the Whole Brain Model, previously the Hermann Whole Brain Dominance Instrument (Hermann, 1994). Here it is possible to see how you (and others) best receive information and how you might be perceived by others. This is a very important skill in interprofessional working and could be used not only to improve individual's abilities, but additionally to reflect on teams where there is conflict and less observable collaboration to meet the shared goals.

A closer look

The academic view

Integration of interprofessional education (IPE) into the curricula of undergraduate health care programmes encourages a collaborative working culture which creates opportunities for students to 'learn with, from and about each other' (CAIPE, 2006). Through IPE, students gain real experience of working alongside other health care professionals at various stages of learning. Introducing this early in the curricula prevents negative stereotypes from developing, and enables health care practitioners to work more effectively together, to deliver high-quality care and meet the needs of their patients and clients. Activities involving students from various professional programmes 'talking to' each other rather than 'talking about' each other provide insightful learning experiences. In the delivery of IPE and the creation of a collaborative culture, academic staff members must serve as good role models, demonstrating respect for other colleagues' professional knowledge, and modelling good interprofessional working, in the delivery of teaching sessions and the facilitation of learning.

Dr Patricia McClure, Associate Head of School, School of Health Sciences University of Ulster

A closer look

Managing change

Initially there appeared to be reluctance/wariness from team members being removed from the security of their well established teams through a management restructure.

Some staff of my own profession also demonstrated reluctance to accept new members from a different profession, while at the same time struggling to 'let go' of staff from our own profession as they moved into different teams. Tensions can break over small things – like 'invading' the space of our small department – changing area, office space and storage for equipment. At times it felt a bit like a battle ground – resentment all round.

It was a steep learning curve – although both professions involved were therapies, working patterns were different, departmental structure and attitudes were very different.

Benefits over time have included influencing joint working on the wards – more so with new staff coming into the team who do not have knowledge of the previous structure. Support staff in particular can work more generically and the benefits for the patient journey are apparent.

Judith Metcalfe, Team Leader and Occupational Therapist

Conclusion

It is important to reflect on the enhancements that interprofessional working can bring to service users, carers, individual staff members, teams and organizations. It is essential that interprofessional working is incorporated and valued in undergraduate professional learning programmes as well as in in-house development within organizations. In developing the understanding of other roles there will be a better foundation for practice, with shared responsibility, delegation of tasks, improved communication and better use of scarce resources. The quality of services can be enhanced leading to greater satisfaction for all.

In conclusion, the value of interprofessional working for service users and carers is indisputable. Drawing on its diverse heritage, **the occupational therapy philosophy is instrumental in directing occupational therapists to practice holistically as part of an interprofessional team**.

Competent and insightful occupational therapists will actively engage in interprofessional working, through understanding their own practical, technical and interpersonal skills and the skills of others. They will **actively try to build trust and mutual respect and will communicate in an open and honest way**. Any challenges to interprofessional working can be overcome with humility, and it is up to individuals to ensure their part in this is fulfilled.

Further reading

College of Occupational Therapists (2010) *Code of Ethics and Professional Conduct*, London: College of Occupational Therapists.

Health Professions Council (2007) *Standards of Proficiency – Occupational Therapists*, London: Health Professions Council.

World Health Organization (2010) *Framework for Action on Interprofessional Education and Collaborative Practice*, Geneva: WHO.

References

Bristol Royal Infirmary Inquiry (2001) *Learning from Bristol: The Report of The Public Inquiry into Children's Heart Surgery at the Bristol Royal Infirmary 1984–1995*, London: Bristol Royal Infirmary Inquiry.

Cass, E., Robbins, D., and Richardson A. (2009) *Think Child, Think Parent, Think Family: A Guide to Parental Mental Health and Child Welfare*, London: Social Care Institute for Excellence.

College of Occupational Therapists (2006) *Recovering Ordinary Lives: The Strategy for Occupational Therapy in Mental Health Services 2007–2017, Results from Service User and Carer Focus Groups* (Core), London: College of Occupational Therapists.

College of Occupational Therapists (2008) *Pre-Registration Education Standards,* 3rd edn, London: College of Occupational Therapists.

College of Occupational Therapists (2010) *Code of Ethics and Professional Conduct,* London: College of Occupational Therapists.

Covey, S. R. (2004) *The 7 Habits of Highly Effective People*, London: Simon and Schuster.

Curtin, M., Molineux, M. and Supyk, J. (2009) *Occupational Therapy and Physical Dysfunction: Enabling Occupation*, 6th edn, Sydney: Churchill Livingstone.

Department of Health (2000) Care Standards Act, London: HMSO.

Department of Health (2002) NHS Reform and Health Care Professions Act, London: HMSO.

Department of Health (2008) Health and Social Care Act, London: HMSO.

Department of Health (2009) Health Act, London: HMSO.

Duncan, E. (ed.) (2006) *Foundations for Practice in Occupational Therapy*, 4th edn, Edinburgh: Churchill Livingstone.

Health Professions Council (2007) *Standards of Proficiency – Occupational Therapists,* London: Health Professions Council.

Health Professions Council (2008) *Standards of Conduct, Performance and Ethics,* London: Health Professions Council.

Hermann, N. (1994) *The Creative Brain*, Tennessee: Quebecor Printing.

Joice, A. and Coia, D. (1989) A discussion on the skills of the occupational therapist working within a multidisciplinary team, *BJOT* 52 (12), 466–8.

Kelley, K. J. and Van Vlaenderen, H. (1996) Dynamics of participation in a community mental health project, *Social Science and Medicine* 42 (9), 1235–46.

Kielhofner, G. (2009) *Conceptual Foundations of Occupational Therapy Practice,* 4th edn, Philadelphia, PA: F. A. Davis.

Low, H. and Barr, H. (2008) *Practice Learning for Interpro-fessional Collaboration: Perspectives from Programmes Leading to the Social Work Degree,* London: Centre for the Advancement of Interprofessional Education.

Low, H., Barr, H. (2008) *Practice Learning for Interprofession-al Collaboration: Perspectives from Programmes Leading to the Social Work Degree.* London: CAIPE. http://www.caipe.org.uk/resources/practice-learning-for-interpro-fessional-collaboration-perspectives-from-programmes-leading-to-the-social-work-degree-low-h-barr-h-2008/

Mayers, C. A. (1990) A philosophy unique to occupational therapy, *British Journal of Occupational Therapy* 53 (9), 379–380.

Parker, D. (2006) Implementing client-centred practice, in T. Sumsion *Client-centred Practice in Occupational Ther-apy,* Edinburgh: Churchill Livingstone.

Reilly, M. (1962) Occupational therapy can be one of the great ideas of 20th century medicine, *American Journal of Occupational Therapy* 16, 2–9.

Sealey, C. (1999) Clinical governance: an information guide for occupational therapists, *The British Journal of Occu-pational Therapy* 62 (6), 263–8.

SEU (Social Exclusion Unit) Taskforce (2009) *Think Child, Think Parent, Think Family: A Guide to Parental Mental Health and Child Welfare,* London: Cabinet Office.

Van den Hove, S. (2004) Between consensus and compro-mise: acknowledging the negotiation dimension in par-ticipatory approaches, *Land Use Policy* 23 (1), 10–17.

Yerxa, E. J. (1994) Dreams, dilemmas, and decisions for occupational therapy practice in a new millennium: an American perspective, *American Journal of Occupational Therapy* 48(7), 586–9.

Chapter 20
Social workers

Steve J. Hothersall

Chapter summary

In order to appreciate the issues relating to collaboration with other professions and agencies from the perspective of social work, it is first necessary to consider the issue of need followed by a consideration of the purpose of social work. This chapter will address issues of collaboration between social workers and other professionals, and in doing so will refer to a set of practices designed to more effectively and efficiently meet human need in its various guises. It is therefore important for us in this chapter to understand the issue of need, in order to place collaboration in a real context rather than to talk about a set of practices in a somewhat disembodied way, as well as having a clear sense of what social work *qua* social work is all about as distinct from other professions and/or disciplines with the wide variety of service-user groups it works with.

Issues about the role of social work in relation to areas such as the protection of vulnerable people, managing the risks to such people and the holistic approach of social work based upon skills and values which emphasise respect for, and interpersonal skills used with, service users and carers are examined. This chapter also examines how the needs of such groups are assessed in relation to how social workers address these issues with the other professions and agencies involved in providing services for such groups.

Learning objectives

This chapter will cover:

- how the social work profession promotes social change, problem-solving in human relationships and the empowerment and liberation of people to enhance well-being. Social work intervenes at the points where people interact with their environments
- how social work as a profession plays a pivotal role in the lives of those individuals in need of advice, guidance and assistance, and how in attempting to achieve this, working closely with other professionals and agencies is a necessity
- how social work is fundamentally about relationships between people, and assessment and intervention from perspectives of vulnerability, risk and protection

▶

- how in social work, people skills are paramount; if social workers are unable to engage with another human being at the level of their meanings, then their plans and interventions are likely to be less than effective

- how, for effective interprofessional practice, it is important that all those concerned are reflective and reflexive in relation to their practices, thereby functioning as both technical experts and reflective practitioners.

Exercise 20.1

What is social work all about?

It is important that as a social worker (or as a nurse, occupational therapist, physiotherapist etc.) you know what your role and task is all about. Look at the website address given here (http://www.ifsw.org/), compile a list of the main purposes of social work and think about what such things mean in terms of what social workers actually do. You might also want to look at either of the following publications:

General Social Care Council (GSCC) (2008): *Social Work at Its Best: A Statement of Social Work Roles and Tasks for the 21st Century*, London: GSCC, available at http://www.gscc.org.uk/cmsFiles/Policy/Roles%20 solid-and%20Tasks.PDF.

Scottish Executive (2006) *Changing Lives. Report of the 21st Century Social Work Review*, Edinburgh: Scottish Executive, available at http://www.scotland.gov.uk/Resource/Doc/91931/0021949.pdf.

Let me first state the obvious: life can be complex and complicated and the type and range of human need almost immeasurable. It was T. H. Marshall who said that welfare (in the sense of meeting need) was 'a compound of material means and immaterial ends' (Timms and Watson, 1976, pp. 51–2). Notions of human need have become much more sophisticated and societal and state responses to it more diverse and more *costly* in both the economic and the human senses of this word (Department of Health and Social Security, 1974; Laming, 2003, 2009; Scottish Executive, 2004). This being the case, it should come as no surprise to learn that it is becoming increasingly difficult, if not impossible, for one profession or agency to meet all aspects of need effectively and efficiently, and that includes social work. As a result, we have seen governmental exhortations and increasing swathes of legislation and policy emphasising that agencies and associated professionals must collaborate in the design, delivery and evaluation of services across all human service areas, and recent reports highlight the continuing centrality of interprofessional collaboration in achieving such aims (General Social Care Council, 2008; Northern Ireland Social Care Council, 2011; Scottish Executive, 2006).

Human need

As a social worker, the issue of need is something she or he will be dealing with every day. It is related to other important issues such as vulnerability, risk and protection (Hothersall and Maas-Lowit, 2010) and arises in many different ways, affecting all of us to a greater or lesser extent at some time in our lives. According to Maslow (1970), as humans we all have the same range of (universal) needs that are ranked hierarchically, with basic needs like food and shelter being more fundamental to our existence and survival than needs involving love and belongingness, which in their turn are more essential than the need to 'self-actualise' and achieve our potential in more 'esoteric' realms and endeavours. Needs are also to be seen as distinct from 'wants'. This is a very different conception of need and raises the issue of preference (Doyal and Gough, 1991). I may think I *need* a 56" flat-screen HD TV, but by recourse to general standards about what is generally seen as being *necessary and sufficient* for a reasonable standard and quality of life, this would be regarded as a *want*. However, given the relative nature of conceptions of need, often depending on who has the power to define it and pay for it to be met (Bradshaw, 1972), the issue of preference is highly relevant and with the emergence of the personalisation agenda (HM Government, 2007) this theme has taken on a new meaning and is one likely to generate some interesting debate over its interpretation (Ferguson, 2007). Clearly, however, social work has an important role in terms of defining need, determining who is in need and delivering services in some shape or form to meet need on behalf of the state. This might be in the form of statutory social work services delivered to children and their families, including child protection services (Frost and Parton, 2009; Hothersall, 2008), services to those with a mental disorder and those vulnerable and in need because of incapacity (Gould, 2009; Hothersall, Mass-Lowit and Golightley, 2008; Maas-Lowit, 2010;) and services for those people with other forms of disability or impairment (Bigby and Frawley, 2009; Kristiansen, Vehmas and Shakespeare, 2008; Oliver, 2009) or because of their particular stage of life (Clark and Lynch, 2010) and they may be delivered by private and/or third sector organisations or some combination thereof. Some services would be seen as being focused upon individual need, whereas others would have a focus on the needs of the wider community and the general populace, such as criminal justice services.

The essential issue here is to recognise that because need takes many forms, it is essential that professions and the agencies within which they operate provide coherent and collective responses to it, and such a statement in my view is one predicated less on governmental or other dictates to do this than it is on the moral imperative to do what it takes to get it right.

Key learning points

- Need is something we all experience, but it is a contested notion, particularly in relation to welfare.
- There are differing conceptions of need depending upon who is experiencing it, defining it, meeting it or paying for it.
- Needs and wants are different things but as notions of need alter, so do the categorisations, i.e. what may once have been defined as a need may now be seen as a want, particularly in challenging economic climates.

Any account of social work must (re-)consider the realities of its task, and the definition by International Federation of Social Work (IFSW) is a useful reminder of the nature, scale and inherent complexity of this when it reminds us that

> The social work profession promotes social change, problem solving in human relationships and the empowerment and liberation of people to enhance well-being. Utilising theories of human behaviour and social systems, social work intervenes at the points where people interact with their environments. Principles of human rights and social justice are fundamental to social work.
>
> (International Federation of Social Workers, 2004)

This gives us a clear sense of the centrality of social work as a profession and its pivotal role in the lives of those individuals in need of advice, guidance and assistance, and largely because of the sheer scale of its task, working with other professionals within whichever agency or organisational context they happen to be is now a necessity, therefore, social work, like other professions, has to think about how it can do this.

However, it must be said that social work is fundamentally about *relationships* between people.

What is collaboration all about anyway?

Although this book will have already provided several definitions and interpretations of collaboration, my focus here is to highlight those that have a particular resonance for social work, even though much of the literature on the theme of collaboration is written from a range of professional perspectives. What should be clear to you by now is that many of the themes and issues within collaborative working are applicable to all professions to greater or lesser extents depending on the particular context, so be open to these commentaries wherever they may arise.

So what does collaboration mean when thinking about it in relation to the social work task? I use the term to include the notion of a partnership between people (professionals, agencies and/or their organisations and service users) within the context of working towards shared and mutually defined goals, involving the sharing of resources, human and material, to achieve desirable outcomes. That joint working, collaboration, interdisciplinary practice etc. is a ubiquitous requirement is now unquestionable: Hudson (2002) notes that partnership working 'is now a central plank of public policy in the UK especially in the fields of health and social care' (p. 7), while Pollard, Sellman and Senior (2005) talk of 'interprofessional working to mean collaborative practice: that is, the process whereby members of different professions and/or agencies work together to provide integrated health and/or social care for the benefit of service users' (p. 10). Bronstein (2003) states that interdisciplinary collaboration is 'an effective interpersonal process that facilitates the achievement of goals that cannot be reached when independent professions act on their own' (p. 229), although Cameron (2011) notes incisively that 'Central to these initiatives is an assumption that the professions will be willing and able to adapt their professional practice' (p. 53).

These comments reflect the growing realities of the need for collaboration by social workers, as well as providing a cautionary note to remind us that collaborative activity is complex and that it can challenge professional identities and particular ways of practising. It is therefore important that all those concerned are reflective and reflexive in relation to these ways of working, thereby functioning as both *technical experts* and *reflective practitioners* (Jones and Joss, 1995).

What is the rationale for this emphasis on collaboration? Fundamentally, the main drivers regarding collaboration arose from the confluence of a number of factors: the changing nature of need and the way it is defined, and by whom; changing and ever-increasing demands upon human services and increasing service specialisation within a context of decreasing resources (Cameron, 2011); the impact of 'near misses', child fatalities (Laming, 2003, 2009; Hammond, 2001) and other serious incidents and the subsequent inquiries into these (Sinclair and Bullock, 2002); an increasing recognition of the need to address the whole person in terms of how services are designed and delivered (HM Government, 2007; Bronfenbrenner, 1989); service-user perspectives (Beresford, 2002; Dale, 2004); the emergence of 'New Public Management' and the need

---

Exercise 20.2

Skills for collaboration

Think about the types of *skills* or *competences* that might be useful for you to develop and possess in relation to working alongside other professionals, either if you are social worker, or what you might expect from social workers if you are another professional working with them. These could range from quite personal attributes like patience and tenacity, to more specialised things like effective communication skills, good teamworking skills and leadership skills. Barr (1998) suggested that there were three areas of competence essential for any professional:

- *Common competencies* – those held in common between all professions

- *Complementary competencies* – those that distinguish one profession from another

- *Collaborative competencies* – those necessary to work effectively with others.

Think back to other chapters you have read and see if you can identify what some of these might look like for a social worker.

---

for increased transparency and accountability; issues concerning the nature of professional identity, training and development and the boundaries between individuals, professionals, agencies and organisations including communication issues (Baxter and Brumfitt, 2008; Reder and Duncan, 2003; Suter *et al.*, 2009; Woodhouse and Pengelly, 1991; World Health Organization, 2010); awareness of organisational influences (Feilberg, 2007; Hudson, 1987) and the nature of working in groups (teams) (McLean, 2007; Øvretveit, Mathias and Thompson, 1997; Payne, 2000).

Thus, collaborative activity can be seen to have emerged as the result of a number of interrelated and sometimes *competing* factors from within and across a range of contexts. Sadly, some of the drivers have arisen because of the pain and suffering of others, and it has to be acknowledged that poor and ineffective communication between professionals has often been at the centre of these tragedies (Reder and Duncan, 2003). As a result, governments and policy-makers have sought to develop more and more sophisticated systems in an attempt to remedy the apparent shortcomings in collaborative practice, taking it as a given that if you regulate and prescribe how to do something, when, where and with whom, things are less likely to go 'wrong'. Unfortunately, more recent events testify to the fact that this has not worked as well as people would have hoped (Laming, 2009). These systems of recording, reporting and assessing will not, in isolation, protect or support anyone. These are nothing more than socially constructed entities and as such should be regarded as *tools*, used to assist professionals in exercising their professional judgements in discharging their duties. People protect people; systems can help to organise, coordinate and provide frameworks for action, but whether a response happens when it ought to and the form that response takes is fundamentally down to people and their actions (Keenan, 2007). Frost and Parton (2009) suggest that many of the changes introduced over the past few years across England and Wales in relation to children and young people, although it is arguable that the same point can be made across the whole of the UK and across all client-groupings, appear to 'have substituted *confidence* in systems in place of *trust* in individual professional practice' (p. 161: emphasis in original). This is a somewhat incongruous position to be in when, according to a number of governmental missives, the professional autonomy of social workers is in fact something to be promoted and regarded as fundamental to the promotion of well-being.

From the perspective of social work, and largely because of the breadth of its remit and the extent of its expertise, social work per se will often have a central and pivotal role in terms of collaborative activity. In childcare services for example, it is the social worker that is generally seen to be the professional who will act as the lead professional and take on a coordinating role. Similarly, where there are complex mental health issues, specialist social workers acting as approved mental health professionals/mental health officers will often be called upon to direct the collaborative endeavour and share their expertise and understanding of complex situations and the workings of the law, with other professionals.

Take a look at the case studies below.

In these situations, effective collaboration is essential. However, what is the role of the social worker here? It is important to think about the *overall context* in order to understand the issues relating to roles and responsibilities.

In relation to Alison, the health visitor contacted you because it was identified that there were things that needed responding to which were out of her sphere of knowledge and expertise at that time. Once

Case study 1

Alison has three children aged 2, 6 and 12 years and is now a single parent. The health visitor rang you to say that Alison does not appear to be coping very well at the moment. You arrange to visit her and on your arrival you discover the following:

- Alison does not work and has a very low income and recently her child benefit was suspended.
- Alison's mother has recently been admitted to hospital after suffering a fall. Alison is worried about her mother's increasing frailty, particularly as she lives alone.
- Alison appears to be very low and describes occasions when she has felt unable to get out of bed in the mornings and she has thought about ending her life.
- The two older children are having difficulties at school arising in large part from problems with reading and doing homework, and the six-year-old has recently been reported as having increasingly serious headaches.
- The flat is very cold and damp.
- Alison is very anxious because her ex-partner has threatened to report her to social services and 'have the children taken off her' and to 'do her in'. She receives no financial support from the children's father. Her anxieties increase when you arrive despite reassurances from the health visitor about the reason for your visit.

Case study 2

Sarah was born prematurely with a progressive neurological disorder, which meant that as she grew she became less and less mobile. She also has learning disability and grand mal epilepsy. At times, she is aggressive and has self-harmed on several occasions. Within the family setting there have been a number of historical concerns surrounding the quality of care afforded to Sarah's siblings over the years, which had resulted in several of them being placed on the child protection register and accommodated by the local authority for varying periods. The following professionals and agencies were involved with Sarah over a period of years:

Social worker (children and families team)   Residential school staff
Social worker (learning disabilities team)   Family centre staff
Health visitor   Benefits agency
Midwife   Housing department
District nurse   Child Support Agency
Physiotherapist   Voluntary organisation
GP   Community psychiatric nurse
Neurologist   Fostering services
Occupational therapist   Respite care services
Paediatrician   Reflexologist
Pharmacist   Herbal therapist
Family court   Massage therapist
Clinical psychologist   Speech and language therapist
Educational psychologist   Psychotherapist
Police   Homestart worker
Hospital staff   Surestart worker
Advocacy services   Psychiatrist

you have assessed the situation, you may well do the following:

- contact the housing department in order that they can respond to the issue of cold and damp
- contact the Benefits Agency and the Child Benefit Department to clarify and hopefully rectify issues concerning income
- offer advice on how Alison might contact the hospital to check on her mother. It might be possible to arrange for some financial assistance in relation to travel costs so that she can go and visit. You might also arrange for some childminding if it is not possible or appropriate for the children to accompany their mother to the hospital to see their grandmother
- liaise with the children's school. This may lead to a referral to an educational psychologist who might wish to assess the children in order that targeted assistance concerning their reading can be given. You

might suggest that the children go to the after-school club where they could get help with their homework
- support Alison in taking the six-year-old to the GP/opticians to get the headaches investigated
- offer advice concerning the threats from her ex-partner and liaise with the social worker in the domestic violence team based within the police
- arrange for Alison to see her GP concerning her depression, who may then refer her to a community psychiatric nurse or a social worker within the mental health team
- arrange for a worker from the local family centre to discuss strategies to deal with the children's behaviour
- arrange to see Alison again to talk about how she's feeling.

Here, the social worker collaborates and liaises with other professionals and agencies while aiming to empower Alison and having an eye on the identification and management of particular risks. As Payne (2005) reminds us, empowerment is about helping people 'to gain power of decision and action over their own lives' (p. 295). In this situation there is a clear sense of empowerment mixed with the worker 'taking the load' in relation to other areas. Collaboration in this situation has resulted in services being provided which could improve the family's situation while recognising that there are some risks that need to be managed effectively.

In relation to Sarah, the situation is clearly much more complex, as is the rationale for collaboration. This is because there is a clear *context for concern*. At one level the need for collaboration and liaison is obvious given the sheer number of services involved. It is likely that there would be some form of social work involvement in Sarah's situation even in the absence of childcare concerns. The level of need is significant and it would be crucial to ensure that service delivery is well coordinated. The social worker is likely to be the lead professional here, acting as the link between the service providers. At another level, the presence of particular concerns regarding Sarah's well-being above and beyond those attributable to her developmental needs makes the need for effective collaboration all the more acute. The social worker's remit is to ensure that Sarah's welfare is everyone's paramount consideration while providing support to the family in terms of dealing with the range of issues inherent within the situation, not the least of which is the sheer number of people involved and the magnitude of Sarah's difficulties.

Key learning points

- Collaboration and partnership are key features within contemporary social work practice.
- Effective collaboration and partnership must involve the service user and their families.
- Collaborative practice requires that social workers develop important skills to facilitate this aspect of practice.
- Social work is likely to be seen by many other professionals as the 'lead profession' in many situations.
- Effective social work practice cannot take place without some form of collaboration.

Regulating practice and delivering collaborative services

As a social worker in the twenty-first century their skills are as much about direct work *with other professionals, their agencies and organisations* as they are about direct work with service users. They must be able to make effective use of their communication and interpersonal skills in order to work effectively and efficiently with a wide range of other professionals whose own knowledge, values and skills are crucial to achieving the shared task. With ever-changing conceptions of need and increasingly complex demands upon services, achieving this should no longer be seen as the sole preserve of social work, although there are a number of important (reserved) functions which social workers are still best placed to carry out and as such, the title 'social worker' is now protected (see s. 61 Care Standards Act 2000 and s. 52 of Regulation of Care (Scotland) Act 2001), recognising that:

> those functions which require to be designated as reserved to social workers is to safeguard people in certain circumstances and to protect their rights. A clear articulation of what it is only a social worker should do will also bring greater clarity to the roles they carry, particularly in integrated services.
>
> (Scottish Executive, 2005, p. 4)

In terms of working together, each professional, agency and organisation is largely responsible for its own practice. All professionals deliver services in line with their own professional, agency and organisational standards, rules and protocols and regulate their practice by reference to particular ethical codes of conduct and practice standards, and these exist for social workers in different professional bodies across the four countries of the UK (General Social Care Council, 2010; Northern Ireland Social Care Council, 2002; Scottish Social Services Council, 2009; Wales Social Services Council, undated), nurses and midwives, doctors, psychologists, teachers and most other professional groupings. Such codes are integral to the professional identity of each grouping, to some extent they inevitably reflect professional self-interest and represent one means through which professions formally articulate their particular characteristics and expertise. What we see here, however, is the potential for the creation of *barriers* in respect of effective collaboration. Hall (2005) and Cameron (2011) argue that while the regulation of the professional workforce is clearly advantageous in many respects, from the perspective of collaborative working, distinctive processes of professional regulation also pose problems for workers who feel they cannot actually work beyond regulated professional 'boundaries', reinforced as they are by the presence of such codes and expectations, as well as the effects of primary professional socialisation via prequalifying and other forms of education and training. D'Amour *et al.* (2005) note that professionals

are socialized to adopt a discipline-based vision of their clientele and the services they offer. Each

discipline develops strong theoretical and discipline-based frameworks that give access to professional jurisdictions that are often rigidly circumscribed. This constitutes the essence of the professional system.

(2005, p. 117)

Collaborative practice implies an increased need for flexibility, and somewhat paradoxically perhaps, professional regulation may serve to diminish the likelihood of this (Lahey and Currie, 2005). This is where it is important to recognise and act upon the fact that collaboration is essentially a set of *interpersonal processes* and that an awareness of the issues of group dynamics can assist in the development of effective collaboration, although a clear appreciation of one's own distinctive role is in this author's view essential, even though this may be seen by some as counterproductive. In this

A closer look

The social worker's role: a tiered approach

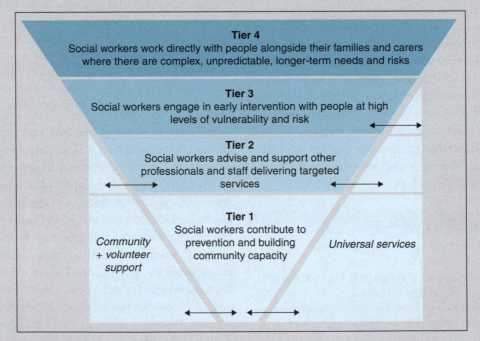

Figure 20.1

From Scottish Executive (2006) *Changing Lives: Summary Report of the 21st Century Social Work Review*, p. 16. Edinburgh, Scottish Executive. Available at **http://www.scotland.gov.uk/Resource/Doc/91949/0021950.pdf**.

(Reproduced under the terms of Crown Copyright Policy Guidance issued by HMSO).

respect, the Figure 20.1 in 'A closer look' box locates the role of the social worker within the broader remit of service provision from and with other professional groupings, recognising within this the particular knowledge and skills possessed and used by social workers in working with some of the most vulnerable (and sometimes, dangerous) individuals within society.

The same approach is now being planned (in 2011) for England, as a result of the work of the Social Work Reform Board (SWRB), with different levels of knowledge and skills proposed at different stages of social workers' careers and responsibilities (see www.education.gov.uk/swrb).

The context of and for collaborative practice

From our discussions so far, we can begin to appreciate that while there are many drivers and rationales for collaboration, we also have to take account of the various contexts that influence collaborative practice. These include, but are not necessarily restricted to:

- the legal and policy context
- the organisational and agency context
- the personal and professional context
- the practice context
- the higher education and learning context
- the service user and carer context.

The legal and policy context

The current legislative and policy context is one that has collaboration as a key theme. This emphasis on collaborative practice recognises that no one organisation or agency or any one professional group or discipline is able to successfully deliver the range of services required in the twenty-first century. Legislation and policy is now designed to facilitate collaborative working by providing a legally mandated framework within which this can take place and within which accountability issues can be made explicit.

Across the UK, legislation specific to particular client-based groupings as well more broad-based

statute law provide a range of 'platforms' upon and from which collaborative activity can and should take place. In general terms, these statutes place duties upon local authorities, health authorities and any other person or body authorised by the Secretary of State to provide help in the exercise of [their] functions, meaning that all of these bodies are required to collaborate with each other where it is clear that this is required in order to provide and deliver services. These requirements, variously phrased, form the legal basis for collaborative working between professionals, agencies and organisations and when such a request is articulated those so commissioned have a duty to comply. However, there is a caveat which refers to those requested as having to comply only if the request made is compatible with their own statutory or other duties and obligations. This of course makes perfect sense in most cases; for example, it would be inappropriate for a local authority to request that the health board provide a family with a house. However, what about those situations where a local authority social services department requests of the education department (another 'branch' of the local authority) that a specialist school place be provided for a child, and education say they do not have such a place available? Should the education department create a new resource? And what if they feel they can't because there is no money? These and other ethical dilemmas are very real and are likely to be faced by social workers and their colleagues at some point.

The organisational and agency context

As a social worker (or teacher, nurse, psychologist etc.) we work within an organisational context. Organisations have their own rules and regulations that govern their functioning and are designed primarily to ensure their continued existence. Social work operates within a range of different organisational contexts that may or may not be fully aligned to the value base of social work as a profession. For example, as a social worker you may be employed by an organisation that is profit-driven. A situation may arise where you feel, as a professional social worker, that a particular course of action is necessary. The organisation, on the other hand, believes that this will be too costly and affect profits. You are therefore prevented from undertaking this piece of work. In a local authority social work department, you may similarly believe that a child requires a particular resource but are told that this is not available as the budget is overspent. Another example may be where an external organisation to which your agency relates in a professional context requires that you produce reports for them within certain specified timescales. Your professional view may be that such a timescale is impossible to meet because any report produced in that time would not be sufficiently detailed to do full justice to what may well be a very complex situation. The era of performance management is upon us, and many workers are heard across the country bemoaning the fact that quantity appears to be what managers and policy-makers are interested in, rather than quality. These are the kinds of conflicts that can arise when the organisational and professional contexts appear to clash, and such concerns and the need to address them is clearly exemplified at the moment by the review of child protection in England and Wales, headed by Eileen Munro of the London School of Economics (see http://www.education.gov.uk/munro-review/index.shtml). In the wake of the tragic events surrounding the deaths of baby P and Victoria Climbié (amongst others), concerns regarding the degree of fit between professional and organisational values and practice within child care services have led to this systemic review of such services. One of the key assumptions being challenged here is the view that complex management and performance systems equate with effective service delivery and protection. It appears to many, however, that latterly, human services in general have had too much of a focus on systems and performance and too little focus on people.

The issue to recognise is that organisations have their own 'rules of engagement' and these may not always appear to be synchronous with the values of the profession in terms of ongoing practice. The social worker in these situations will have to utilise their own communication and interpersonal skills to the full and engage with the organisation on behalf of their client in an advocacy role. Thompson (2005) makes the point

that most social workers have as their practice focus direct work with individuals, but what is not so readily acknowledged, nor indeed readily attended to, is that an increasing amount of time is spent in direct work with organisations, agencies and other professionals. Thus, the needs of the organisation and its service delivery networks demand a significant amount of effort on the part of the individual professional. These skills we shall consider below. However, what does need to be acknowledged is that the organisational context has a pervasive influence on the practice of professionals and as such must be accounted for in relation to conceptions of day-to-day social work practice.

Hudson (1987) notes that there are two main difficulties for organisations when faced with the need to collaborate. Firstly, the organisation faces the loss of its freedom to act independently, having to relinquish control over its own domain. Secondly, and very importantly in relation to the current welfare climate, it has to invest scarce resources into developing and maintaining collaborative relationships. From an organisational perspective, the investment in collaboration may in fact not yield any future benefits. However, it is also the case that just such an investment may in fact increase the capacity for the organisation to achieve its goals, because it can utilise the resources of the other organisation(s) and thereby achieve a state of interdependence. Unfortunately, however, there is no guarantee that this will happen so, in tense economic climates, decisions which involve speculation may be avoided in order to ensure that scarce resources are directed at what the organisation considers as its 'core business', which may result in collaboration and other developmental activities being seen as less of a priority.

The personal and professional context

At the individual level there are a number of issues to consider which relate to the whole area of collaborative activity. Motivation is a key factor in terms of how well people work, both alone and as part of a team. Being part of a team implies many things, not the least of which is that the team will function effectively. Notions of teams and teamworking are contested issues and some of these will have been referred to throughout this book. Whatever the particular arrangement it is important to realise that teams are subject to particular dynamics and go through a number of processes in their development. These reflect human capabilities and concerns and can determine whether the group will function effectively or not at all. Tuckman and Jensen (1977) describe a four-stage process of forming (socialisation), storming (conflict), norming (rule setting) and performing (doing). Each of these stages are important to the formation and functioning of groups and governments, and policy-makers and managers would do well to recognise that if these processes are ignored, avoided or in any way circumvented, difficulties are *more likely* to emerge, particularly when in the face of political pressure to collaborate, more and more groups or teams are formed on a frequent basis and are often relatively short-lived, reflecting changing political and organisational priorities rather than professional ones. Group dynamics play a central role in determining how likely effective collaboration will be, so it is important that attention is paid to this aspect of practice (Molyneux, 2001).

Having a clear sense of professional identity is generally regarded as a vital ingredient of effective practice, irrespective of the discipline concerned or its location within a particular agency or organisational context (Fournier, 2000). Knowing what it is you do as a social worker, a nurse, a teacher, a doctor or a physiotherapist is pretty important to service users. This identity will reflect differing knowledge bases, theoretical orientations, value bases, skill levels and a range of other factors often unique to that profession. These differences must be seen constructively and recognition given to the value of professional diversity (Reynolds, 2007; White and Featherstone, 2005) while recognising that this may not be an easy task.

The practice context

By far the most important aspect of collaboration is that between the worker(s) and those with whom they have contact in terms of delivering services. It is important to recognise that the very nature of the intervention itself may help or hinder the sense of collaboration, cooperation and partnership experienced. Therefore, people skills are paramount; if you are unable to engage with another human being at what we might call the level of meanings, then your plans and interventions are likely to be less than effective. In all practice encounters, the service user must perceive that the service(s) being delivered are provided by a professional group that care, are coherent in relation to their stated aims, consistent in the way in which they approach the task(s), competent in how they do what they do, confident in relation to their role, and who are able to communicate with the service user(s) and their own colleagues.

From the perspective of what inquiries and reports have told us, there are a number of issues that appear to emerge time after time which relate to the whole issue of collaboration and why at times it appears to be problematic. These include but are not restricted to issues of communication, the sharing of information, the accuracy of recording information, the quality of analysis of information, an understanding of roles and responsibilities, clear time frames, effective decision making and access to and use of relevant resources. The nature of collaborative practice has therefore to include these things as well as the human elements referred to above.

The educational context and interprofessional education

In relation to the educational context, I refer specifically to the need for those institutions of higher education which provide pre- and post-qualifying training for social work and social care staff, as well as continuous professional and employee development courses, to actively include reference to collaborative working within the curriculum. UK-wide curriculum guidance makes repeated reference to the need for students of social work to be able to work effectively within a range of differing organisations and with a range of other professionals and related disciplines.

Developments relating to interprofessional education (IPE) (Miller, Freeman and Ross, 2001; Whittington, 2003), which recognise the need for students in a range of professions to learn together with other professionals from the very start of their careers and also while in practice, are still in their infancy and the results of research into IPE programmes are still ambiguous regarding its effectiveness (McFadyen *et al.*, 2010; Reeves *et al.*, 2010). Nonetheless, these developments are important in helping us to understand what some of the core, common, complementary and collaborative competencies are that contribute to effective practice and whether changes to the education of professionals are required (see also Chapter 21 by Patricia White).

The service user and carer context

There has been an increasing recognition of the need to actively involve those who use services and their carers in discussions concerning the quality of services they receive and their experiences of them. This also extends to their active involvement in pre- and post-qualifying training (Cooper and Spenser-Dawe, 2006).

The main principle here is that those who experience services have something valuable to say about them, and this is a trend that has a long but rather chequered history. This has rightly continued to develop and now represents an important dimension in all areas of social work and social care practice (Branfield *et al.*, 2006).

Conclusion

This chapter has considered the issue of social work's key roles and functions, how these fit with the work of other professionals, agencies and organisations in order to ensure that services and interventions are delivered fairly and effectively, and the place of social work within these processes. **Collaboration** is no longer something we might just think about doing if we have the time; **it is central to the social work task** and its relationships with other professionals and agencies,

and good communication and interpersonal skills, along with an understanding of the nature of group dynamics, are important functional prerequisites.

Knowledge of how people interact with their environments, and then basing assessments and interventions around this knowledge, are key features in social work practice, as is the ability to appreciate the perspectives of service users and carers in meeting their perceived needs and enabling their part in designing and determining their services as far as possible.

Social workers are often seen as taking the lead in certain areas of work, such as child protection, and particularly in such circumstances the social work role requires a wide range of skills and knowledge. Some of these are personal attributes like patience and tenacity, whilst others are skills-based, such as effective communication skills, good teamworking skills and leadership skills. These in turn are **based within the values of person-centred and holistic approaches to service users and carers** who are in need of advice, guidance and assistance. The social work task often involves work with such service users and carers from perspectives of vulnerability, risk and protection, which can be difficult to balance between the different interests involved in a situation.

Further reading

The Journal of Interprofessional Care is a good resource with papers covering all aspects of this area.

Useful websites

www.policypress.co.uk

The Policy Press, in partnership with *Community Care* magazine, have a series of short books with a focus on many aspects of partnership working. Their 'Better Partnership Series' can be found on their website.

http://www.scie.org.uk/publications/elearning/ipiac/index.asp

The SCIE website has a special section on interprofessional and interagency collaboration.

References

Barr, H. (1998) Competent to collaborate: towards a competency-based model for interprofessional education, *Journal of Interprofessional Care* 12 (2), 181–8.

Baxter, S. K. and Brumfitt, S. M. (2008) Professional differences in interprofessional working, *Journal of Interprofessional Care* 22 (3), 239–51.

Beresford, P. (2002) Making user involvement real, *Professional Social Work* June, 16–17.

Bigby, C. and Frawley, P. (2009) *Social Work Practice and Intellectual Disability*, BASW Practical Social Work Series, Basingstoke: Palgrave Macmillan.

Bradshaw, J. (1972) A Taxonomy of social need, in G. McLachlan (ed) *Problems and Progress in Medical Care.* Seventh series. Oxford: Oxford University Press, 71–82.

Branfield, F., Beresford, P., Chambers, P., Staddon, P., Wise, G., Findlay-Williams, B. and Andrews, E. (2006) *Making User Involvement Work: Supporting Service User Networking and Knowledge*, York: Joseph Rowntree Foundation.

Bronfenbrenner, U. (1989) Ecological systems theory, in *Annals of Child Development* 6, Greenwich, CT: JAI Press, 187–249.

Bronstein, L. (2003) A model for interdisciplinary practice, *Social Work* 48 (3), 297–306.

Cameron, A. (2011) Impermeable boundaries? Developments in professional and interprofessional practice, *Journal of Interprofessional Care* 25, 53–8.

Care Standards Act. (2000) www.legislation.gov.uk/ukpga/2000/14/contents (last accessed 2 February 2012).

Clark, A. and Lynch, R. (2010) Older people, in S. J. Hothersall and M. Maas-Lowit (eds) *Need, Risk and Protection in Social Work Practice*, Exeter: Learning Matters.

Cooper, H. and Spencer-Dawe, E. (2006) Involving service users in interprofessional education: narrowing the gap between theory and practice, *Journal of Interprofessional Care* 20 (6), 603–17.

Dale, P. (2004) Like a fish in a bowl': parents' perceptions of child protection services, *Child Abuse Review* 13, 137–57.

D'Amour, D., Ferrada-Videla, M., Rodriguez, L. and Beaulieu, M. D. (2005) The conceptual basis for interprofessional collaboration: core concepts and theoretical frameworks, *Journal of Interprofessional Care* May (Supplement 1), 116–31.

Department of Health and Social Security (1974) *Report of the Committee of Inquiry into the Care and Supervision Provided in Relation to Maria Colwell*, London: DHSS.

Doyal, L. and Gough, I. (1984) A theory of human needs, *Critical Social Policy* 4 (1), 6–38.

Doyal, L. and Gough, I. (1991) *A Theory of Human Need*, Basingstoke: Macmillan.

Feilberg, F. (2007) Working within the organizational context of dynamic change, in J. Lishman (ed) *Handbook for Practice Learning in Social Work and Social Care*, 2nd edn, London: Jessica Kingsley Publishers.

Ferguson, I. (2007) Increasing user choice or privatizing risk? The antinomies of personalization, *British Journal of Social Work* 37, 387–403.

Fournier, V. (2000) Boundary work and the (un)making of the professions, in N. Malin (ed) *Professions, Boundaries and the Workplace*, London: Routledge.

Frost, N. and Parton, N. (2009) *Understanding Children's Social Care: Policy, Politics and Practice*, London: Sage.

General Social Care Council (2008) *Social Work at Its Best: A Statement of Social Work Roles and Tasks for the 21st Century*, London: GSCC.

General Social Care Council (2010) *Codes of Practice for Social Care Workers*, London: GSCC.

Gould, N. (2009) *Mental Health Social Work in Context*, London: Routledge.

Hall, P. (2005) Interprofessional teamwork: professional cultures as barriers, *Journal of Interprofessional Care* May (Supplement 1), 188–96.

Hammond, H. (2001) *Child Protection Inquiry into the Circumstances Surrounding the Death of Kennedy McFarlane (17/4/97)*, Dumfries: Dumfries and Galloway Child Protection Committee.

HM Government (2007) *Putting People First: A Shared Vision and Commitment to the Transformation of Adult Social Care*, London: HM Government.

Hothersall, S. J. (2008) *Social Work with Children, Young People and Their Families in Scotland*, revised 2nd edn, Exeter: Learning Matters.

Hothersall, S. J. and Maas-Lowit, M. (eds) (2010) *Need, Risk and Protection in Social Work Practice*, Exeter: Learning Matters.

Hothersall, S. J., Maas-Lowit, M. and Golightley, M. (2008) *Social Work and Mental Health in Scotland*, Exeter: Learning Matters.

Hudson, B. (1987) Collaboration in social welfare: a framework for analysis, *Policy and Politics* 15 (3), 175–82.

Hudson, B. (2002) Interprofessionality in health and social care: the Achilles' heel of partnership? *Journal of Interprofessional Care* 16 (1), 7–17.

International Federation of Social Workers (2004) Ethics in Social Work, Statement of Principles, available at www.ifsw.org/f38000027.html, last accessed 2 February 2012.

Jones, J. and Joss, R. (1995) Models of professionalism, in M. Yelloly and M. Henkel (eds) *Learning and Teaching in Social Work*, London: Jessica Kingsley Publishers.

Keenan, E. K. (2007) Patterns of interaction: conceptualising the cross-roads between social structures, interpersonal actions and psychological well-being, *Smith College Studies in Social Work* 77 (1), 69–88.

Kristiansen, K., Vehmas, S. and Shakespeare, T. (eds) (2008) *Arguing about Disability: Philosophical Perspectives 1*, London: Routledge.

Lahey, W. and Currie, R. (2005) Regulatory and medico-legal barriers to interprofessional practice, *Journal of Interprofessional Care* 19 (Supplement), 197–223.

Laming, H. (2003) *The Victoria Climbié Inquiry*, London: The Stationery Office.

Laming, H. (2009) *The Protection of Children in England: A Progress Report*, London: The Stationery Office.

Maas-Lowit, M. (2010) Capacity and incapacity, in S. J. Hothersall and M. Maas-Lowit (eds) *Need, Risk and Protection in Social Work Practice*, Exeter: Learning Matters.

Maslow, A. (1970) *Motivation and Personality*, 2nd edn, New York: Harper and Row.

McFadyen, A. K., Webster, V. S., MacLaren, W. M. and O'Neill, M. A. (2010) Interprofessional attitudes and perceptions: results from a longitudinal controlled trial of pre-registration health and social care students in Scotland, *Journal of Interprofessional Care* 24 (5), 549–64.

McLean, T. (2007) Interdisciplinary practice, in J. Lishman (ed.) *Handbook for Practice Learning in Social Work and Social Care*, 2nd edn, London: Jessica Kingsley Publishers.

Miller, C., Freeman, M. and Ross, N. (2001) *Interprofessional Practice in Health and Social Care*, London: Arnold.

Molyneux, J. (2001) Interprofessional teamworking: what makes teams work well? *Journal of Interprofessional Care* 15 (1), 29–35.

Northern Ireland Social Care Council (2002) *Codes of Practice for Social Care Workers and Employers of Social Care Workers*, Belfast: NISCC.

Northern Ireland Social Care Council (2011) *Regulating Training: Roles and Tasks of Social Work*, available at http://www.niscc.info/roles_and_tasks_of_social_work-115.aspx, accessed 6 March 2011.

Oliver, M. (2009) *Understanding Disability: From Theory to Practice*, 2nd revised edn, Basingstoke: Palgrave Macmillan.

Øvretveit, J., Mathias, P. and Thompson, T. (eds) (1997) *Interprofessional Working for Health and Social Care*, London: Macmillan.

Payne, M. (2000) *Teamwork in Multiprofessional Care*, Basingstoke: Palgrave Macmillan.

Payne, M. (2005) *Modern Social Work Theory*, 3rd edn, Basingstoke: Palgrave Macmillan.

Pollard, K., Sellman, D. and Senior, B. (2005) The need for interprofessional working, in G. Barrett, D. Sellman and J. Thomas (eds) *Interprofessional Working in Health and Social Care: Professional Perspectives*, Basingstoke: Palgrave Macmillan.

Reder, P. and Duncan, S. (2003) Understanding communication in child protection networks, *Child Abuse Review* 12, 82–100.

Reeves, S., Zwarenstein, M., Goldman, J., Barr, H., Freeth, D., Koppel, I. and Hammick, M. (2010) The effectiveness of interprofessional education: key findings from a new systematic review, *Journal of Interprofessional Care* 24 (3), 230–41.

Regulation of Care (Scotland) Act (2001) available at www.legislation.gov.uk/asp/2001/8/contents, last accessed 2 February 2012.

Reynolds, J. (2007) Discourses of interprofessionalism, *British Journal of Social Work* 37 (3), 441–57.

Scottish Executive (2004) *Investigations into Scottish Borders Council and NHS Borders Services for People with Learning Disabilities: Joint Statement from the Mental Welfare Commission and the Social Work Services Inspectorate*, Edinburgh: Scottish Executive, available at http://www.scotland.gov.uk/Publications/2004/05/19333/36718.

Scottish Executive (2005) *Reserved Functions of the Social Worker*, Edinburgh: Scottish Executive.

Scottish Executive (2006) *Changing Lives. Report of the 21st Century Social Work Review*, Edinburgh: Scottish Executive, available at http://www.scotland.gov.uk/Resource/Doc/91931/0021949.pdf.

Scottish Social Services Council (2009) *Codes of Practice for Social Service Workers and Employers*, Dundee: SSSC.

Sinclair, R. and Bullock, R. (2002) *Learning from Past Experience: A Review of Serious Case Reviews*, London: Department of Health.

Suter, E., Arndt, J., Arthur, N., Parboosingh, J., Taylor, E. and Deutschlander, S. (2009) Role understanding and effective communication as core competencies for collaborative practice, *Journal of Interprofessional Care* 23 (1), 41–51.

Thompson, N. (2005) *Understanding Social Work: Preparing for Practice*, 2nd edn, Basingstoke: Palgrave Macmillan.

Timms, N. and Watson, D. (eds) (1976) *Talking about Welfare: Readings in Philosophy and Social Welfare*, London: Routledge.

Tuckman, B. W. and Jensen, M. C. (1977) Stages of small group development revisited, *Group and Organisational Studies* 2, 419–427.

Wales Social Services Council (undated) *Code of Practice for Social Care Workers*, available at www.ccwales.org.uk

White, S. and Featherstone, B. (2005) Communicating misunderstandings: multi-agency work as social practice, *Child and Family Social Work* 10 (3), 207–16.

Whittington, C. (2003) Collaboration and partnership in context, in J. Weinstein, C. Whittington and T. Leiba (eds) *Collaboration in Social Work Practice*, London: Jessica Kingsley Publishers.

Woodhouse, D. and Pengelly, P. (1991) *Anxiety and the Dynamics of Collaboration*, Aberdeen: Aberdeen University Press.

World Health Organization (2010) *Framework for Action on Interprofessional Education and Collaborative Practice*, Geneva: WHO.

Chapter 21
Physiotherapists

Patricia White

Chapter summary

This chapter will examine the physiotherapy profession's history, development and physiotherapeutic roles in various settings, and present a case study of a patient/client to illustrate the roles of different professionals and agencies involved in heath and social care provision.

It discusses the ways in which physiotherapy has become a profession in its own right and has moved from being under the direction of medicine to clinical independence, touching on issues of power and status.

Additionally, in an extended case study, it examines the issues that arose in the planning, implementing and refining of interprofessional education (IPE) at the University of the West of England Bristol (UWE) in order to highlight the kinds of issues and challenges of this undertaking and how they might be addressed most effectively. It reviews how IPE set out to prepare students for interprofessional working in practice (IPW). Significantly, while the focus is on implementing IPE at qualifying level, the issues highlighted are also informative for post-qualifying education and when considering key working relationships in interprofessional teams, explicitly serving the key prerequisite of working together when qualified. Such IPE and IPW intentions or opportunities can be summarised as:

> occasions that occur when two or more professions learn with, from and about each other to improve collaboration and the quality of care . . . and includes all such learning in academic and work-based settings before and after qualification, adopting an inclusive view of 'professional'. (CAIPE, 2006)

Learning objectives

This chapter will cover:

- whom physiotherapists work with in terms of their patients/clients and their areas of treatment
- examples of the types of work they do with other professional groupings and the key roles and types of work physiotherapists undertake in these situations

▶

- how knowledge of the history and development of professions, such as physiotherapy, is essential when considering the future of health and social care provision and the profession's roles and further development

- how interprofessional education can prepare practitioners for interprofessional working, not just at undergraduate level but also as part of considerations in work practice settings and continued professional development (CPD)

- how interprofessional working requires practitioners to be aware of the roles of others – as presented in the case of physiotherapy in this chapter – in addition to being highly skilled and aware of their own professional role, i.e. that they learn with, from and about each other to improve collaboration and the quality of care (CAIPE, 2006).

A brief introduction to the physiotherapy profession

The Chartered Society of Physiotherapy Curriculum Framework (2002) states that physiotherapy is a health care profession concerned with human function and movement and maximising potential:

- It uses physical approaches to promote, maintain and restore physical, psychological and social well-being, taking account of variations in health status.
- It is science-based, committed to extending, applying, evaluating and reviewing the evidence that underpins and informs its practice and delivery.
- It is reliant on clinical judgement and informed interpretation is at its core. (http://www.csp.org.uk)

The following section will review the history and development of physiotherapy and how physiotherapists have utilised what D'eon (2005) calls the five elements of best practice in cooperative learning: positive independence, face-to-face promotional interaction, individual accountability, interpersonal and small group skills and group processing.

The 'Society' of Physiotherapy was founded in 1890 by masseuses who sought to protect their reputation amid the 'massage scandals' of the 1890s when 'medical rubbing' became associated with deviant sexual practices. The founders used the term 'profession', which is defined as 'a vocation or calling, especially one that involves some branch of advanced learning or science' (Concise Oxford Dictionary, 2010). The professions had been divided into divinity, law and medicine, and physiotherapy was dependent on medical direction until 1974, when the by-law relating to working under the direction of a medical practitioner was amended. This decade saw a rationalisation of training schools, with several being transferred to the then polytechnics. In 1995 a modern curriculum was introduced. Teacher training was brought into line with general education by means of a Certificate of Education, and physiotherapy was subsequently made a graduate profession. Physiotherapy became an autonomous profession, wherein practitioners make their own clinical judgements and treatment choices and practice reflection (reviewing their own behaviour and success in their work and taking action as appropriate to solve problems they identify in themselves, i.e. diagnose and prescribe), in 1974.

Physiotherapy is a health care profession with a science foundation. The physiotherapist's range of work is very broad and involves working with people to promote their health and well-being in addition to managing their ill health. Physiotherapy helps restore movement and function to as near normal as possible after injury, illness, developmental or other disability that might impair an individual's function. Physiotherapy is, as has already been mentioned, a science-based profession which is committed to extending, applying, evaluating and reviewing the evidence that underpins and informs its practice and delivery. The exercise of clinical judgement and informed interpretation is at its core because physiotherapists are concerned with human function and movement and maximising an individual's potential.

Physiotherapists work in a wide variety of health settings which include intensive care, orthopaedics, outpatients, sports medicine, mental health, stroke recovery, paediatrics, occupational health, women's health, ergonomics, care of the elderly and general musculoskeletal treatment in hospitals, in general practitioner settings and in private practice.

A formal definition of physiotherapy states that physiotherapy is a physical approach which aims to 'promote, maintain and restore physical, psychological and social well-being taking account of variations in health status' (Chartered Society of Physiotherapy, 2002).

Physiotherapists aim to identify and make the most of movement by health promotion, preventative advice, treatment and rehabilitation. Core skills used by chartered physiotherapists include manual therapy, therapeutic exercise and the application of electrophysical modalities. In addition physiotherapists believe that it is important to appreciate the psychological, cultural and social factors that influence physiotherapy patient/clients and so have utilised a biopsychosocial approach, which looks at the patient/client holistically.

This holistic approach requires that all aspects of people's needs – psychological, physical and social and mental – should be taken into account and seen as a whole. In addition the patient/client is placed at the centre of this process because it is important that the patients have an active role in their rehabilitation in order to maximise both their independence and function.

Physiotherapy is an autonomous profession (practitioners make their own clinical judgements and treatment choices) and utilise systematic clinical reasoning in a problem-solving manner to identify and address patient issues. In applying a holistic approach to patient-centred care, both the mental and social aspects relating to the patient/client are considered along with the physical. Physiotherapists also practice reflection (reviewing their own behaviour and success in their work and taking appropriate action to solve problems they identify in themselves). Jarvis (1992) states that 'Reflective practice is something more than thoughtful practice': it is that form of practice which seeks to problematise

many situations of professional performance so that they can become potential learning situations in which the practitioners can continue to learn, grow and develop in, and through, practice. Donaghy and Morss refer to this as

> the higher order intellectual and effective activities in which physiotherapists engage to critically analyse and evaluate their experiences in order to lead to new understanding and the critical appreciation of the way they think and operate in the clinical setting. (2000, p. 13)

Chartered physiotherapists undertake three years of undergraduate training (which includes 1,000 clinical hours) and work with a broad variety of physical problems, especially those associated with the neuromuscular, musculoskeletal, cardiovascular and respiratory systems. The students work alongside physiotherapy colleagues in interprofessional and multi-professional teams. Physiotherapy practice is characterised by reflective behaviour and systematic clinical reasoning, both contributing to and underpinning a problem-solving approach to patient-centred care. Training to become a physiotherapist and working as a qualified physiotherapist is challenging, especially in the present economic climate, but there is a rich and rewarding variety of work available to qualified physiotherapists and opportunities, within the profession, in the UK and internationally. Chartered physiotherapists combine their knowledge and skills to improve a broad range of physical problems associated with different 'systems' of the body. In particular, physiotherapists treat neuromuscular (brain and nervous system), musculoskeletal (soft tissues, joints and bones), cardiovascular and respiratory systems (heart and lungs and associated physiology) in addition to physical problems that stem from mental ill heath and/or dementia.

People are often referred for physiotherapy by doctors or other health and social care professionals; however, as a result of changes in health care, people are now referring themselves directly to physiotherapists without previously seeing any other health care professional.

The next A closer look box demonstrates the roles of physiotherapists within different specialities.

A closer look

Specialities in which physiotherapist work

- **Outpatients.** *Treating musculoskeletal and biomechanical dysfunction, e.g. spinal and joint problems, accidents and sports injuries, repetitive strain injuries*
- **Intensive care units.** *Maintenance of limb mobility and ensuring that chests are kept clear of sputum*
- **Women's health.** *Ante- and postnatal care advice, exercise and posture, managing continence and post-gynaecological operations*
- **Care of elderly.** *Maintaining mobility and independence, rehabilitation after falls, treatment of arthritis, Parkinson's disease and other neurological conditions, chest conditions, mental health etc.*
- **Dementia.** *Maintain functional ability, reduce the risk of falls and improve muscle strength and coordination*
- **Neurology.** *Helping people restore normal movement and function in stroke, multiple sclerosis and other conditions*
- **Orthopaedics and trauma.** *Restoring mobility after hip and knee replacements and spinal operations, treating patients after accidents*
- **Mental health.** *Taking classes in relaxation and body awareness, improving confidence and self-esteem through exercise and relaxation*

- **People with learning difficulties.** *Using sport and recreation to develop people, assessing and providing specialist footwear, seating and equipment*
- **Occupational health.** *Treating employees in small to large organisations and companies, looking at work habits to prevent physical problems such as repetitive strain injury*
- **Terminally ill (palliative care).** *Working in the community or in hospices, treating patients with cancer and AIDS*
- **Paediatrics.** *Treating sick and injured children, those with severe mental and physical disabilities, and conditions such as cerebral palsy and spina bifida*
- **Community.** *Treating a wide variety of patients at home and giving advice to carers*
- **Private sector.** *Working independently in private practice, clinics, hospitals, and GP surgeries, treating a wide range of conditions*
- **Education and health promotion.** *Teaching people about many conditions and lifestyle choices. This may include back care, ergonomics, taking exercise classes and cardiac rehabilitation groups*
- **Sports clinics.** *Treating injuries in sportsmen and women, advising on recovering fitness and avoiding repeated injury*
- **Voluntary organisations.** *Advising and consulting for organisations supporting and caring for people with multiple sclerosis and Parkinson's disease*

Policy changes relating to interprofessional education and interprofessional working: their advantages and disadvantages

Recent policies have put people in more control of their own health and care.

- *Personalisation.* Personalisation, for example, places service users at the heart of interprofessional working (IPW) (Department of Health, 2005, 2006) and operates across the boundaries of social care, health, housing, voluntary, community,

benefits, leisure and transport. Furthermore, this policy drive has been endorsed by professional bodies and the Quality Assurance Agency (QAA) which, in 2006, published a statement of common purpose for health and social care emphasising the importance of cooperation and collaboration (Quality Assurance Agency, 2006). Indeed, Miers and colleagues (2009) state that 'quality of care is interprofessional care'.

- *Communication.* Breen and colleagues (2010) believe that good communication between professions is the key to patients receiving quality care. However, Hammick and colleagues (2009) warn that, while communication is a vital part of inter-

Key learning points

- Originally professions were divided into divinity, law and medicine.
- Physiotherapy was dependent on medical direction until 1974.
- Physiotherapy can be defined as a physical approach which aims to 'promote, maintain and restore physical, psychological and social well-being' taking account of variations in health status (Chartered Society of Physiotherapy, 2002).
- Physiotherapy is an autonomous profession (practitioners make their own clinical judgements and treatment choices) and utilises systematic clinical reasoning in a problem-solving manner to identify and address patient issues.
- People are often referred for physiotherapy by doctors or other health and social care professionals; however, as a result of changes in health care, people are now referring themselves directly to physiotherapists without previously seeing any other health care professional.

professional working (with a wide range of methods that could be utilised, i.e. verbal, non-verbal, written etc.) all types of communication have their advantages and disadvantages. Within an educational context, and illustrated in this chapter's extended complex case study, one advantage of teaching the relevance and importance of communication in IPE is that it assists students in learning about other professions and professional roles while learning about their own. On the other hand, a disadvantage of focusing on communication in IPE is the paucity of published evidence supporting the claim that if individuals from different professions learn together they, and their agencies, will work better together to improve care and the delivery of service.

So the challenge is to conduct more research within the fields of interprofessional education and working because, in general, assessing the positive and negative impacts of interprofessional learning (IPL) remains a highly contested area. Studies by Dienst and Byl (1981) and Reeves and Freeth (2002) have reviewed the impact of IPL on patient care and highlight the difficulty of demonstrating any impact of IPL on service delivery and patient care. Bjørke

and Haavie (2006) did report positively on student assessment in IPL covered in years 1, 2 and 3 of their qualifying degrees but their work gave little information about the students' learning experience. Despite this, a review of 21 of the strongest evaluations of IPE conducted by Hammick and colleagues (2007) evaluated contemporary evidence and showed that IPE initiatives delivered internationally continue to 'evolve towards a robust science' (p. 749) and so have helped to shape future interprofessional education.

Historically and culturally it is not surprising that collaborative working can meet resistance as it can challenge and criticise existing practice. Baxter and Brumfitt (2008) note that the 'call for change' to health care service delivery has been 'resounding', in the last few years with the attention being paid to training, employment and working together while it has also been recognised that, unlike in business and industry, health care workers have 'professional groupings and different allegiances' (Firth-Cozens, 2001). Baxter and Brumfitt's (2008) findings, from semi-structured interviews and fieldwork observation, highlight the influence of professional differences and significant elements of professional groupings in IPW which are knowledge and skills, professional role and identity along with power and status. Reeves et al. (2010) show why individual professions have developed on the basis of their separateness rather than their togetherness, which 'creates a severe headache for those trying to effectively lead teams constituted of two or more professional groups'.

Professional and other perspectives

Hammick et al. (2009) recognise that being interprofessional is not a simple way of working, especially as different public service professionals came into being in different ways and so have their own histories, professional cultures, ethical and value bases and training and career trajectories (p. 25). In addition to this, professional groups have had to relate to the tradition of being educated separately and to the dominance of the medical profession. Today nursing and allied health professionals are independent, but for many years the medical profession exercised control over the curricula, examinations and professional registration. The benefits of IPE are increasingly important as the roles of health and social care practitioners undergo fundamental change, e.g. old nursing roles are becoming increasingly redundant as nurses admit and discharge their own patients, prescribe medication, monitor long-term conditions and arrange diagnostic tests (Clifton *et al.*, 2006). However, Hammick *et al.* (2007) found only two studies (Dienst and Byl, 1981; Reeves and Freeth, 2002) which were able to demonstrate any impact of interprofessional learning on patient care. Hammick *et al.* (2007) report on seven studies that provide evidence of the effectiveness of postqualifying interprofessional learning initiatives.

Pollard *et al.* (2008) found that qualified practitioners with interprofessional learning (IPL) were more positive about their interprofessional relationships than practitioners on uni-professional curricula courses and deduced that 'experience of IPL appeared to produce and sustain positive attitudes towards collaborative working' (p. 86). Durrell (1996) noted that physiotherapists are also breaking down old barriers of medical practice, expanding their scope of practice and forging new roles within outpatient clinics and that reforms in the health service have contributed to the changing professional boundaries. In addition, Kersten *et al.* (2007) note that many drivers for workforce configurations are driven by politics and economics and state that there is an urgent need for robust research in physiotherapy to evaluate the role of the 'extended scope practitioner'.

Key learning points

- As stated by Lumague *et al.* (2006), student physiotherapists and other health and social care disciplines need to be provided with opportunities enabling them to develop the skills, behaviours and attitudes required for interprofessional collaboration (pp. 246–53).
- There is a paucity of published evidence to support the claim that when different professions learn together they, and their agencies, will work better together, thus improving care and the delivery of service.

The development of interprofessional education at the University of the West of England (UWE): a case study

The following section gives a critically reflective account of the development of IPE at the UWE; which also highlights issues of IPW in postqualifying work practice.

In 2000 IPE in health and social care was championed by the Department of Health (DOH, 2000a, 2001a) after the National Health Service (NHS) plan (DOH 2000b) clearly indicated that better teamworking and collaboration was needed to produce a workforce that is 'fit for purpose'. Similarly, the Centre for the Advancement of Interprofessional Education (CAIPE) has defined multi-professional education as 'occasions when two or more professions learn together for whatever reason' and state that IPE is distinguished by its purpose and so is a subset of multi-professional education. IPE is therefore defined by CAIPE as 'occasions when two or more professions learn together with the object of cultivating collaborative practice' (CAIPE, 1997).

It can be argued therefore that the emphasis and time given to IPE is essential because, with the pressure of work, practitioners have limited time to systematically reflect upon and develop their understanding and skills in IPW. From an educational perspective UWE therefore recognised the need to promote IPE at undergraduate level to ensure best IPW practice for the service user and that the delivery and development of IPE needs to be always evolving and developing. Broadly the approach at UWE has been to encourage students to analyse and reflect on their own learning as advocated by D'eon (2005) that relates to 'an experiential learning framework cycling through the four stage model of planning, doing, observing and reflecting' (p. 49).

The development of undergraduate IPE at the UWE began in 1999 after four years of working to promote shared learning in a number of level one first-year modules. By 2002, UWE had developed an IPE curriculum framework at levels one, two and three on its professional degree courses which developed the skills required for IPW and interagency collaboration whilst retaining uni-professional education which was taught alongside it (Barrett *et al.* 2003). The framework incorporated key elements identified by Miller and Freeman (1999) to ensure that the interprofessional strand of the faculty's programme was developed while also incorporating interprofessional learning outcomes within the 'uni-professional' modules and within supervised clinical practice.

Students from ten professional awards undertook this programme. The Faculty of Health and Social care has an annual intake of approximately 1,000 students to ten prequalifying programmes, i.e. four nursing pathways, midwifery, social work, diagnostic imaging, radiotherapy, physiotherapy and occupational therapy. Initially both first and second year IPE were delivered over a period of six weeks at the commencement of each year, and then level two was subsequently delivered as a two-day IPE conference and included second year medical students from the University of Bristol. Level three was designed as an online module in which students met face-to-face for up to three hours during the introduction to the module and subsequently worked solely online.

Each level IPE module at UWE had its own Internet site which provided students with an individual group bulletin board through which they communicate with one another and submit small sections of their assignment which they can all read online.

A closer look

Key elements for interprofessional practice identified by Miller *et al.* (2001)

Interprofessional:

- *learning* is ongoing throughout the educational experience
- *delivery* develops the prerequisites for teamwork
- *curricula* are patient/client-focused
- *curricula* are interactive
- *learning* is case/scenario-based
- *learning* is built on a model of student development.

This complies with the interprofessional aim of learning from and about one another (CAIPE, 1997). The level one IPE module mirrored the design of the level three IPE module in its patchwork assessment and also changed its delivery from two hours per week, for the first pre-clinical six weeks of the first year, to a three-day delivery during the pre-clinical period. After the final face-to-face day students were asked to write an essay explaining their experience and understanding of interprofessional working.

A scenario enquiry-based learning (EBL) approach was used in which academic staff acted as facilitators, rather than tutors. Their role was to support students in their enquiry into scenarios and subsequent discussions rather than to act as didactic 'teachers'. It was thought that EBL, and the patchwork delivery of this module, helped students develop their writing and referencing skills while they also learnt with and from one another – also as advocated by CAIPE (1997). In addition they were given a hard copy of relevant interprofessional publications in a reader that was provided to ease congestion when they required relevant documentation from the library to support their work.

EBL is a student-centred approach and each student is responsible not only for their own learning, but also for the learning of other group members – the group's effectiveness is dependent upon everyone's attendance and full participation. Past student evaluation of IPE year one has highlighted the negative impact of poor attendance on learning and on relationships within the group. EBL requires that students work interactively and cooperatively as a team, which reflects the necessity for this in professional practice (Pollard *et al.,* 2005). Collaborative working has been promoted by the government via policy documents, such as the *National Service Framework for Older People* (Department of Health, 2001b) – one of the many frameworks which set measurable goals, within specific time frames, to improve standards and the quality of health and social care.

In the initial 1999 implementation of IPE level one, the development of user-centred scenarios proved to be difficult. The team reviewed a number of text-based scenarios and mapped the learning generated by these against both subject-based and interprofessional learning outcomes. Staff representing all 10 professional awards scrutinised the scenarios but there was some disagreement regarding the eventual choice (Barrett *et al.*, 2003). The final scenario resulted in specific professional groups identifying the fact that certain issues raised in them were not relevant to their own professional discipline, e.g. one scenario related to a young homeless girl begging outside a well-known retail shop in a busy shopping centre and, although all students could understand the predicament the young girl was in, they found it difficult to relate her problems to their own professional contribution to her care as the midwives knew she was not pregnant; the learning disabilities students knew that she did not have an obvious learning disability; the child nurses appreciated that she was not a child; the physiotherapists were not aware of her having a respiratory or musculoskeletal or neurological problem nor were the mental health students aware of her having any mental health problems while the radiotherapists and radiographers assumed, as they had not been informed, that she did not require an X-ray or that she had cancer.

Subsequent scenarios, as discussed below, were designed to be applied more effectively to all the health and social care disciplines. These scenarios can also be considered by different professionals in their personal and/or group considerations of their possible work with physiotherapists from their own work role.

Examples of 'level one' EBL scenarios

Scenario one

The health and social care needs of patients/clients are often complex and require effective collaboration between health and social care professionals. Recommendations from a number of high-profile inquiries highlighted the need for effective interprofessional working (IPW) (Kennedy, 2001; Laming, 2003).

Government policies now recognise this need and have placed increasing emphasis on IPW, within the context of health and social care, with initiatives such as *Modernizing social services: promoting*

independence, improving protection (Department of Health, 1998a); *National Service Framework for Mental Health: Modern Standards and Service Models* (Department of Health, 1999) and *The NHS Plan* (Department of Health, 2000b).

Other policies, such as *The new NHS: modern, dependable* (Department of Health, 1998b) and *A first class service: quality in the new NHS* (Department of Health, 1998c), have also sought to improve the quality of care, but Barrett *et al.* (2005) recognise that policy directives alone cannot ensure effective IPW and interagency working. They state that health and social care professionals require a range of interpersonal and interprofessional skills, in addition to a depth of professional knowledge, to equip them to engage in complex relationships and to prevent, or overcome, difficulties that are often associated with collaborative practice.

Barr *et al.* (2000) assert that IPW can be enhanced through IPE by enabling those involved to develop the knowledge and skills that are required for collaborative practice.

Aims To explore Department of Health legislation and to discuss its relevance to the service users and service providers.

Scenario two

'Consider what health and/or social care services you, a member of your family or close acquaintance has recently required and/or used. This may have involved primary, secondary or tertiary health care or the person in question may have sought assistance from social services in relation to home care, family support, residential care, respite care, child protection, adoption and fostering etc'.

Aims To use the shared knowledge and experience of the group to explore health and social care needs and the demands these put upon the subsequent provision of services. Please only discuss issues that you feel comfortable in sharing and be sensitive to one another.

Scenario three

Behan (2006) considered that the challenge of delivering personalised care cannot be met by simply bringing organisations together: it can only be met by changing the nature of the relationship between those who commission and provide care and those who receive care. Having defined what he called the inter-professional workforce perspective the author then stated that 'the delivery of innovative personalised services will require partnerships between health, councils, housing and others' thus signalling the Government's continuing commitment to a widening Interprofessional interagency care model.' Discuss.

Aims To explore Department of Health initiatives and to discuss its relevance to the service users and service providers.

Case study

The patient

- A heavily pregnant 41-year-old woman has been admitted to an intensive care unit after being hit by a car.
- She has multiple injuries, goes into premature labour and is subsequently delivered of a Down's syndrome daughter.

Past medical history

- She has been a recipient of primary, secondary and tertiary medical care for her mental health since her late teenage years.
- Her physical health and ability to cope with life was good until she had a relationship with an abusive partner three years ago.
- She is currently unemployed but used to work as a secretary.
- She is an only child.
- Both parents are deceased.

Task 1

Consider what your own profession's professional role will be for this 41-year-old patient's management at all stages of her care and after discharge.

Task 2

Consider other professions professional roles and their interventions.

Task 3

Reflect on what you have learnt and consider areas you need to explore more fully and topics for further research:

- At this stage of this patient's recovery
- At discharge from hospital stage
- When she is in the community.

Task 4

Interprofessional working will be vital throughout the management of this complex case, and communication, in all of its forms, will be key:

- Team meetings to discuss the patient – who will lead these?
- Who will take part in them?
- What problems might these meetings reveal?
- How might these problems be overcome?
- What services will be required?
- What role will you play in the above?

The EBL method was chosen to assist students to meet the learning outcomes for the interprofessional modules and to assist in the development of transferable teamwork skills which Miller and Freeman (1999) and Russell and Hymans (1999) consider essential to collaborative approaches to care. After 11 years, and in response to students' feedback, it was decided that introducing IPE within the first six weeks of training, before any of the students had placements in clinical or social work practice, was too early, and so as of 2011 it would be delivered after, and not before, all students have had at least one placement experience, i.e. in levels two and three. Students would continue to work face-to-face with other multi-professional students, at the commencement and end of the module, to develop a clear understanding of IPW issues, to apply effective IPW thinking and to reflect on IPW principles which would enhance their clinical practice and improve the care of their patients/service users.

Students were expected to present or submit a 'blended' piece of coursework that reflects their interaction with other health and social care students and what they have learnt from the module. In order to do this they are delegated to specific interprofessional education groups and work alongside a facilitator member of staff. The aim of this new module is to use clinical practice as a base for some of the assessment points, but in addition IPE will be supported by the introduction of a virtual reality 'Second Life' hospital and rehabilitation setting in which students will direct their own avatar and engage in interprofessional practice related to the service user/patient/carer scenarios.

With regard to assessing the effectiveness of the interprofessional curricula and mixed discipline groups, Clarke *et al.* (2007) noted that most early studies into IPE focused on issues affecting students' interactions with one another which included participation, group roles, tasks and cohesion and a tendency to avoid conflict. Mandy *et al.* (2004) also reported on first-year prequalifying initiatives and noted that demographic, cultural, academic and ethnic differences within the professional groups added complexity to the group process. Miller *et al.* (2006) considered these factors and concluded that the 'diversity within the group served to exacerbate negative stereotyping'. Clarke *et al.* (2007) suggested that

Exercise 21.1

Consider the patient in the above case study's condition and list possible injuries sustained in order to establish the care she will require from the interprofessional and multidisciplinary teams from day one to her being discharged into the community.

Points for the team to take into account:

- this 41-year-old woman sustained head injury fractured ribs, pneumothorax, fractured fibula and clavicle, possible internal injuries and superficial skin abrasions
- she is heavily pregnant with her first child
- she lives in a refuge having been abused by her partner
- she has had mental health problems but has been stable for many years
- she is unemployed but used to work as a secretary until two years ago
- she is an only child and both parents are deceased.

Exercise 21.2

Consider the roles of the following in caring for this patient and how these roles might best be coordinated to work interprofessionally.

At the accident site

Police
Ambulance
Fire services
General public

Casualty

Nurses
Doctors
Registrar
Consultant
Radiographer
Obstetrician
Physiotherapist
Social worker

Premature labour and birth of child

Midwife
Obstetrician
Paediatrician
Psychiatrist
Psychologist
Nurses

1) While in hospital
2) While in the community

such forms of stereotyping added social and psychological factors to the challenges of interprofessional relationships, and it was this finding that prompted them to examine the experience of students engaged in such face-to-face learning. They concluded that overall students 'were positive about their experiences of interprofessional learning and reported increased awareness of the need for, and skills associated with, Interprofessional learning and working' (p. 211).

Research conducted by Thomas *et al.* (2007) at UWE confirmed that expert facilitation was paramount in supporting groups to resolve difficulties which, Miller *et al.* (2006) consider, are all too easily exaggerated by negative stereotyping.

The case study on p.283 was presented in order to highlight and investigate some of the issues that need to be considered in relation to both IPE and IPW, in order to develop knowledge of how to make IPW between physiotherapists and other professions more effective.

Enquiry-based learning (EBL), as set out in Appendix 1, Figure 21.1, is based on the resolution of problems but is more challenging than problem-based learning because students utilise their own existing knowledge and experience and generate their own 'problems', namely areas for further development, by responding to the scenario and developing interprofessional understanding and professional skills.

Conclusion

This chapter has considered the development of the physiotherapy profession, who physiotherapists work with in terms of patients/clients, and gives examples of the types of work they do with other professional groupings, setting out the key roles and types of work physiotherapists will undertake in these situations. In exploring the types of issues that arise for physiotherapists (and all other professionals) in learning to work together as students and in practice settings, the chapter has critically evaluated how UWE has embraced interprofessional education and utilised EBL in preparing students for interprofessional working in practice – as undergraduate students and also when qualified practitioners. It has also highlighted the need to further develop IPE in order to support and improve IPW.

Further reading

Journal of Interprofessional Care www.policypress.co.uk.

Kersten, A., McPherson, K., Lattimer, V., George, S., Breton, A. and Ellis, B. (2007) Physiotherapy extended scope of practice – who is doing what and why? *Physiotherapy* 93, 235–42.

Useful websites

www.csp.org.uk
Chartered Society of Physiotheraphy

References

Barr, H., Freeth, D., Hammick, M., Koppel, I. and Reeves, S. (2000) *Evaluations of Interprofessional Education: A United Kingdom Review for Health and Social Care*. Fareham: The United Kingdom Centre for the Advancement of Interprofessional Education with The British Educational Research Association.

Barrett, G., Greenwood, R. and Ross, K. (2003) Integrating interprofessional education into ten health and social care programmes, *Journal of Interprofessional Care*, 17 (3), 393–301.

Barrett, G., Selman, D. and Thomas, J. (2005) *Interprofessional Working in Health and Social Care: Professional Perspectives*, Basingstoke: Palgrave Macmillan.

Baxter, S. K. and Brumfitt, S. M. (2008) Professional differences in interprofessional working, *Journal of Interprofessional Care* 22 (3), 239–51.

Behan, D. (2006) Key note speech to Care and Health Conference 19 April 2006 Civil Partnerships: Joint Commissioning for the Individual – Implementing the Health and Care White Paper.

Bjørke, G. and Haavie, N. E. (2006) Crossing boundaries: implementing an interprofessional module into uniprofessional bachelor programmes, *Journal of Interprofessional Care* 20 (6), 641–53.

Breen, K. J., Cordner, S. M., Thompson, C. J. H. and Plueckhahan, V. D. (2010) *Good Medical Practice: Professionalism, Ethics and Law,* New York: Cambridge University Press.

CAIPE (1997) *Interprofessional Education – A Definition*, London: CAIPE Bulletin 13, 19.

CAIPE (2006). *Interprofessional Education – A Definition*, London: CAIPE.

Chartered Society of Physiotherapy (2002) Curriculum Framework January 2002, see the society's website for details, http:www.csp.org.uk

Chartered Society of Physiotherapy Bulletin http://www.csp.org.uk

Clarke, B., Miers, M., Pollard, C. and Thomas, J. (2007) Complexities of learning together; students' experience of face-to-face interprofessional groups, *Learning in Health and Social Care* 6 (4), 202–12.

Clifton, M., Dale, C. and Bradshaw, C. (2006) The impact and effectiveness of interprofessional education in primary care: a Royal College of Nursing literature review, http://www.rcn.org.uk/_data/assets/pdf_file/0004/78718/003091.pdf

Concise Oxford Dictionary (2010) Oxford: Oxford University Press.

D'eon, M. (2005) A blueprint for interprofessional learning, *Journal of Interprofessional Care* Supplement 1949–59.

Department of Health (1998a) *Modernising Social Services,* London: Department of Health.

Department of Health (1998b) *The New NHS, Modern and Dependable: A National Framework for Assessing Performance – Consultation Document* , London: Department of Health.

Department of Health (1998c) *A First Class Service: Quality in the New NHS,* London: Department of Health.

Department of Health (1999) *National Service Framework for Mental Health: Modern Standards and Service Models,* London: Department of Health.

Department of Health (2000a) *A Health Service of all the Talents: Developing the NHS Workforce,* London: Department of Health.

Department of Health (2000b) *The NHS Plan: A Plan for Investment, A Plan for Reform*, London: Department of Health.

Department of Health (2001a) *Investment and Reform for NHS Staff – Taking Forward the NHS Plan*, London: Department of Health.

Department of Health (2001b) *National Service Framework for Older People,* London: Department of Health.

Department of Health (2005) *Independence, Well-being and Choice: Our Vision for the Future of Social Care for Adults in England,* London: HMSO

Department of Health (2006) *Our Health, Our Care, Our Say: A New Direction for Community Services,* London: The Stationery Office.

Dienst, E. R. and Byl, N. (1981) Evaluation of an educational program in health care teams, *Journal of Community Health* 6 (4), 282–298.

Donaghy, M. and Morss, K. (2000) Guided reflection: a framework to facilitate and assess reflective practice within the discipline of physiotherapy, *Physiotherapy Theory and Practice* 16 (1), 3–14.

Durrell, S. (1996) Extending the scope of physiotherapy: clinical physiotherapy specialists in consultants' clinics, *Manual Therapy* 1 (4), 210–13.

Firth-Cozens, J. (2001) Multidisciplinary teamwork: the good, bad and everything in between, *Quality in Health Care* 10, 65–9.

Hammick, M., Freeth, D. S., Goodsman, D. and Copperman, J. (2009) *Being Interprofessional*, Cambridge: Polity Press.

Hammick, M., Freeth, D., Koppel, I., Reeves, S. and Barr, H. (2007) A best evidence systematic review of interprofessional education. *Medical Teacher* 29(8), 735–751.

Jarvis, P. (1992) Reflective practice and nursing, *Nurse Education Today* 12, 174–81.

Kennedy, I. (2001) *Learning from Bristol: The Report of the Public Inquiry into Children's Heart Surgery at the Bristol Royal Infirmary 1984–1995.* CM 5207 (1), London: The Stationery Office.

Laming, Lord (2003) *The Victoria Climbié Inquiry,* CM5720. London: HM Government.

Lumague, M., Morgan, A., Mak, D., Hanna, M., Kwong, J., Cameron, C., Zener, D. and Sinclair, L. (2006) Interprofessional education: The student perspective. *Journal of Interprofessional Care*, 20(3), 246–253.

Mandy, A., Milton, C. and Mandy, P. (2004). Professional stereotyping and interprofessional education. *Learning in Health and Social Care* 3 (3), 154–170.

Miers, M., Rickaby, C. and Clarke, B. (2009) Learning to work together: health and social care students' learning from interprofessional modules, *Assessment and Evaluation in Higher Education* 34 (6), 673–91.

Miller, C. and Freeman, M. (1999) Lessons in teamwork, *Nursing Standard*, 14 (9), 33, available from http://gateway.ovid.com/athens/ovidweb.cgi?T=JS&NEWS=N&PAGE=fulltext&AN=00002311-199911170-00047&LSLINK=80&D=ovft, accessed 28 October 2010.

Miller, C., Freeman, M. and Ross, N. (2001) *Interprofessional Practice in Health and Social Care: Challenging the Shared Learning Agenda*, London: Arnold.

Miller, C., Woolf, C. and Mackintosh, N. (2006) *Evaluation of Common Learning Pilots and Allied Health Professions First Wave Sites: Final Report*, London: Department of Health, http://www.cipw.org.uk/index.php?p=pubrep&m=October-2006

Pollard, K., Miers, M. and Gilchrist, M. (2005) Second year scepticism: pre-qualifying health and social care students' midpoint self-assessment, attitudes and perceptions concerning interprofessional learning and working, *Journal of Interprofessional Care* 19 (3), 251–68, available from http://www.ncbi.nlm.nih.gov/pubmed/16029979, accessed 29 October 2010.

Pollard, K., Miers, M., and Thomas, J. (2008) *Understanding Interprofesional Working in Health and Social Care. Theory and Practice*. Palgrave: Macmillan.

Quality Assurance Agency (2006) *Statement of Common Purpose for Subject Benchmarks for Health and Social Care*, Gloucester: QAA: Agency for Higher Education in England.

Reeves, S. and Freeth, D. (2002) The London training ward: an innovative interprofessional initiative, *Journal of Interprofessional Care* 16 (1), 41–52.

Reeves, S., Macmillan, K. and Van Soeren, M. (2010) Leadership of interprofessional health and social care teams: a socio-historical analysis, *Journal of Nursing Management* 18, 258–64. Doi: 10.1111/j.1365-2834.2010.01077.

Russell, K. and Hymans, D. (1999) Interprofessional education for undergraduate students, *Public Health Nursing* 16 (4), 254–62, available from http://www.blackwell-synergy.com/doi/pdf/10.1046/j.1525-1446.1999.00254.x, accessed 28 October 2010.

Thomas, J., Clarke, B., Pollard, K. and Miers, M. (2007) Facilitating interprofessional enquiry-based learning: dilemmas and strategies, *Journal of Interprofessional Care* 21, 463–5.

Appendix 1

The process of enquiry-based learning (EBL) and the iterative cycle

Read and discuss the trigger(s) (issues/case scenarios presented to the group) and complete the following cycle to clarify terms, answer questions and to identify new learning issues:

1. Read and discuss the trigger.
2. Wordstorm. Identify learning issues. Allocate tasks.
3. Research and learn via individual study and enquiry (homework).
4. Feedback to the group and share findings.
5. Revisit trigger and identify any new learning issues.

Repeat the cycle to address these new issues until no more questions are generated.

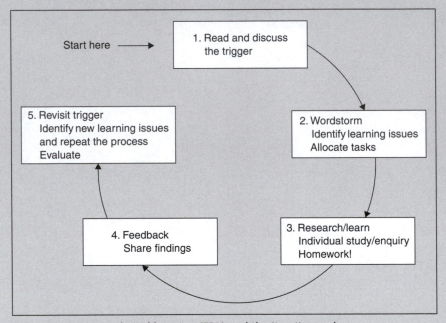

Figure 21.1 Enquiry-based learning (EBL) and the iterative cycle

Chapter 22
Nursing interprofessionally

Paul Illingworth

Chapter summary

This chapter will explore the roles nurses undertake when contributing to the modern health, social and wider care sectors in the twenty-first century. It defines the profession of nursing and describes the broad role of the nurse before discussing the development of interprofessional practice. Nurses association with other professions/agencies relating to interprofessional working is discussed together with the tensions these associations can raise. Case scenarios are then provided which demonstrate these issues in the context of different fields of nursing: adult, child, mental health and learning disabilities. Each scenario has a brief section afterwards which highlights actual and/or interprofessional involvement.

Learning objectives

This chapter will cover:

- Exploring the roles nurses undertake when contributing to the health, social and wider care sectors
- Defining the profession of nursing and describing the broad role of the nurse before discussing the development of interprofessional practice
- Presenting case scenarios to demonstrate interprofessional issues in the context of the different fields of nursing: adult, child, mental health and learning disabilities.

Introduction

The Nursing and Midwifery Council's (NMC) Code (NMC, 2008, p. 5) states that nurses must 'Work with others to protect and promote the health and wellbeing of those in your care, their families and carers, and the wider community.'

Nurses are independent practitioners and many have had their roles and responsibilities enhanced by gaining approval to undertake non-medical prescribing, and some have become nurse consultants. Nevertheless, nursing is about working with others by respecting their skills, expertise and contribution and giving other professions/agencies the benefit of their own skills and expertise for greater benefit to service users.[1] By valuing others, service users' needs are best addressed; however, service users are by definition 'experts' and have to be central in their own care (see Chapter 14 by Peter Beresford, and Chapter 15 by Carmel Byers and the Creating Links group, as partners in collaborative interprofessional working). Indeed this is another central theme of the above *Code*:

Collaborate with those in your care

You must listen to the people in your care and respond to their concerns and preferences.

You must support people in caring for themselves to improve and maintain their health.

You must recognise and respect the contribution that people make to their own care and wellbeing.

You must make arrangements to meet people's language and communication needs.

You must share with people, in a way they can understand, the information they want or need to know about their health. (NMC, 2008, p. 3)

It is also worth noting that towards the end of the *Code*, the following statement is included as a footnote:

Healthcare professionals have a shared set of values, which find their expression in this code for nurses and midwives. These values are also reflected in the different codes of each of the UK's healthcare regulators.

(NMC, 2008, p. 8)

Not surprisingly the Quality Assurance Agency (QAA), which has responsibility for ensuring the quality assurance of higher education (universities), benchmark statements include the statement that an award holder should *'contribute with skill and confidence to effective multi-professional/multi-agency working'* (QAA, 2001, p. 16). The NMC Standards for pre-registration nurse education (NMC, 2010) have also emphasised the need for interprofessional working and stressed the need for interprofessional learning which they defined as

An interactive process of learning which is undertaken with students or registered professionals from a range of health and social care professions who learn with and from each other.

(NMC, 2010)

Clearly then nurses, working in whichever field, do not work in isolation. The health and social care sector is becoming increasingly complex, and therefore mutual working practices are vital. Nurses are employed in a wide variety of contexts, in many different and diverse sectors and not always within health and social care settings; for example many work within prisons, schools and industry. They also work on advice lines, in private practice and care homes and in individual service users' homes. Each of this wide variety of settings requires an ability to work with others, not all from a health or social care professional background, such as housing, education or leisure.

This chapter will help you to understand nurse contribution to interprofessional practice. Many of the different roles nurses undertake will be mentioned but this will not be an exhaustive list. Through case studies, you will be encouraged to explore nurses' interprofessional roles.

Nursing: a definition

To fully understand nursing in an interprofessional context, it is important to appreciate the nursing role. The definition most often quoted is that of Virginia Henderson (1966, p. 6):

---

[1]Service user encompasses terms that include patient or client, and will be the term used throughout the chapter, unless another term is used within a direct quote.

The unique function of the nurse is to assist the individual, sick or well, in the performance of those activities contributing to health or its recovery (or to peaceful death) that he would perform unaided if he had the necessary strength, will or knowledge. And to do this in such a way as to help gain independence as rapidly as possible.

While this broad definition does, to an extent, apply to nursing today, in contemporary health and social care this definition is perhaps lacking. Since this was first offered as a definition, many professions have developed their roles and that of nurses has also changed very substantially. Yet even within nursing there has never been a fully consensual definition of 'a nurse'. In part this stems from the diverse nature of nursing. Not only are there four fields of nursing, as mentioned above, but also there are multiple roles within each field; for example, in mental health nursing work in hospital and community settings. Within hospitals mental health nurses work in acute and older people wards, and there are also psychiatric intensive care units, amongst others. In the community, some of the areas mental health nurses work within include community mental health teams, crisis and home treatment teams, assertive outreach and in-reach teams (going into prisons to work with offenders who have mental health problems). The other three fields incorporate a variety of specialisms also. Because of this, agreement upon one succinct definition is difficult to arrive at.

The QAA, in order to develop benchmarks, described nursing as a discipline that

> Focuses on promoting health and helping individuals, families and groups to meet their health needs. Nursing work involves assisting people whose autonomy is impaired, who may present with a range of disabilities or health related problems; to perform a range of activities, sometimes acting for, or on behalf of the patient. A definition featuring nursing is that it provides twenty-four hour care with a focus on meeting people's intimate needs.
>
> (QAA, 2001, p. 6)

Both the QAA and Henderson's definitions have limitations, but what both claim is that nurses do what is required whenever it is needed. They suggest that the role of the nurse does not have clear boundaries. In the widest sense that is perhaps true, yet within the fields of nursing and between specialists within those fields, boundaries do exist. What the nurse will do is work with any professionals or agencies appropriate to the service user's needs. Whatever a nurse does, and whoever they work with, service-user needs remain pivotal to nursing practice. It is this characteristic of nursing which potentially places the profession at the heart of effective collaborative practice, given the continuity and immediacy of practitioners' involvement in a wide range of aspects of health and social care on behalf of the service user.

It is perhaps useful here to make use of the reflections of Henderson (2006) on Florence Nightingale. Nightingale has often been considered one of the founders of professional nursing. Nightingale believed that in the end only nature cured; doctors can remove some of the underlying problems with their medicine or surgery but that is all they could do. Once they had done that they would rely on nature and it would be the nurse who could do most to support nature by putting the patient in the 'best condition for nature to act upon him'. The nurse would ensure the required cleanliness, nutrition, elimination and comfort that put the body in the best position to heal itself. Without these vital, but often little acclaimed, skills the efforts of other professionals would often be in vain.

In today's modern health and social care services it is not only nature that can cure. It is not only doctors who remove obstructions and it is not only nurses who can do most to support recovery. Hospital-acquired infections, poor nutrition and other failings have shown that this does not always happen. Indeed there have been many instances where nurses (and other professionals) have altered the course of nature – for example, Beverley Allot and Ann Gregg.

As this book is being written the deaths in Salford have just occurred, where a nurse was alleged to have injected insulin into saline drips. This allegation was later withdrawn, but it is a striking example where professionals may no longer be seen as 'naturally' having the best interest of the service user at heart. There are also the deaths caused by the GP Harold Shipman, not to mention failings of other professions, notably social services. No individual or professional group is immune to allegations of failure. Virtually any inquiry into such failings has cited poor communication as the single most important factor; Richie (1994) and Capon (2005) are two examples. To address such failings, interprofessional working has been seen as one of the most important factors in improving health and social care.

Silo-professional

Historically, different professional groups have been either trained or educated within their own professional group, what Boon *et al.* (2004, p. 3) termed parallel practice. Indeed what are now known as the four 'fields' of nursing trained separately, each having their own unique syllabus. In previous eras, having trained in schools of nursing attached to hospitals and therefore mainly gaining practice experience in the same hospital or related community settings, nurses were then expected to work with other members of the health care team (most often doctors, physiotherapists, clinical or educational psychologists, occupational therapists) and would occasionally liaise with other professions/agencies such as social workers. Little or no preparation was given to any professional group for this situation. There was

Key learning points

- As nurses' roles change and develop, an understanding of each other's developing professional roles, ways of working and objectives become key in their relationships with other professionals.
- Nursing is not just about meeting physical needs of those with a particular health need, but also the wellbeing and capacity of the service user, family and other carers where this is indicated for that individual.
- Nurses are numerically one of the largest professional groups of staff in health and social care field, having numerous daily interactions relating to the short- and long-term needs of service users.

generally an expectation that everyone knew what the other profession did. This reflected attitudes of health professionals at the time, that is, 'You do your job, and I'll do mine' – the inference being that somehow all the professionals' practices and beliefs will naturally and without special effort become integrated into an effective team approach to care.

However, multi-agency working, instead of improving working practices, can encourage or sustain a 'silo approach' to care. Therefore it could increase working in isolation, resulting in a sense of protecting 'professional boundaries'. In theory, interprofessional education, training and working should offer the chance for equality and knowledge between professionals.

Key to the success or failure of professionals working together is communication. Ritchie (1994) and Capon (2005) were both critical of individual and organisational communication failure that brought about a lack of coordinated care. With the increasing number of professional groups and specialists within professions, never has effective communication played such an important role in the care of service users.

Interprofessional

In the 1990s and the advent of what became known as the 'Project 2000' curriculum for nursing, the four what were then called branches of nursing came under one educational programme. Initially involving an 18-month 'common foundation programme' which all four branches undertook there followed an 18-month 'branch programme' where they specialised in their chosen branch prior to qualifying. This programme later became a 12-month common foundation programme and two-year branch programme. This effectively runs today, although approvals of such programmes by the Nursing and Midwifery Council are no longer undertaken and those still approved are being discontinued as the new all-graduate nurse education programmes are coming on stream in response to new nursing standards produced by the NMC (2010).

Throughout the 1990s there was a growing interest in joint working, although there have been various terms used to cover this practice (Illingworth, 2006, p. 31); the preferred term currently is interprofessional. Nursing saw itself as pivotal to this activity. Traditionally nurses had worked on the wards for 24-hour periods and as such felt/believed they were in a better position to understand and know the needs of service users. Identifying themselves as 'patient advocates', nurses saw themselves as standing up for the rights of the people they cared for. However, in mental health, social workers were also promoting their role as advocates and the service-user movement was building momentum and beginning to use independent advocates or advocating for themselves.

Additionally the medical model had been challenged for a number of years, in both learning disability and mental health provision in particular, with the psychological and social care models growing in strength. Traditionally nurses had worked more closely with medical doctors but a new breed of nurses, many graduates and some with doctorates, began to champion nursing as a unique discipline that should be on a par with other professions within the multidisciplinary team. Nurse education had not only taken the step towards an all-graduate profession, it had also made the wholehearted move into higher education.

The interprofessional nature of health and social care working remained 'added-on' to professional education for some time, apart from a few areas across the UK. The World Health Organization (WHO 1988) had originally stated that interprofessional learning was critical for achieving holistic care. More recently, emphasis has been placed on education and training to achieve effective interprofessional practice. The Department of Health (2003) required health and social services to provide effective interprofessional education in undergraduate programmes and within work settings and interprofessional education became compulsory for health staff. The WHO (2010, p. 10) talked of students being 'collaborative practice ready' when they qualified and an 'Interprofessional Capability Framework' was produced through the higher education authority (Interprofessional Education Team, 2010) which provided a guide to enable understanding of how collaborative workers could be developed.

Twenty-first-century nursing

In the current health, social and economic climate, health providers are examining traditional working practices and workforce configuration is central to many health care managers' current focus. But nurses see that they have a large part to play in any such changes. New roles within nursing have emerged: clinical nurse specialists, advanced nurse practitioners and nurse consultants. As mentioned, all are graduates, many have doctorates and they are now working alongside medical doctors, no longer as their handmaidens or just helping nature do the healing. Their expertise and knowledge allows them to challenge practices on an equal status with other graduate professionals. However, not all nurses currently are graduates, but with the profession having now commenced with a graduate entry to nursing and universities supplying 'top-up' degrees for nurses who have a diploma, it should not be many more years before the all-graduate status is reached.

Yet in the context of workforce changes, with health care workers developing their knowledge and skills through academic courses and many then continuing into education to become a nurse or another profession, the roles will continue to evolve. If that is the case will not more of the nurses' role be eroded? Will even more blurring of roles occur? And will there be a time when non-nurses challenge whether the professional term 'nurse', which can only be used by someone who has successfully undertaken an approved nursing education programme and become registered as a nurse, should be a prerequisite for the duties they currently carry out.

Additionally the major shake-up of the NHS which is being driven through by the UK Coalition Government on the grounds of needing to make the NHS more effective and efficient will have a significant impact on professional practice. The wage bill for the NHS is a major drain on resources and government policy to freeze salaries, increase pension contribution, extend the age of retirement and reduce pension payouts is likely to 'encourage' a significant number of more senior and experienced professionals to retire early. These may not all be replaced like for like. Roles are likely to be reviewed, with less experienced staff taking on roles previously undertaken by the more senior professionals and the knock-on effect of passing tasks down to less qualified health care staff.

The move to an all-graduate nursing workforce and the likely reduction in qualified nurses entering the profession will also result in empowering health care assistants and others to take on the roles graduate nurses may no longer want to undertake. But this need not be counterproductive. To an extent this has been the case for many years. Doctors have relinquished some of their roles to nurses. Nurses have relinquished some of their roles to others and as new professions have emerged and developed, more specialists are now part of the health care team.

Interprofessional practice

The following case studies give examples of service users who are cared for within the separate fields of nursing. Each of the examples highlights problems

Key learning points

- Nurses have much the same developing issues as others in the multi-professional field, with an emphasis of moving away from a silo-professional model, working in parallel to other professions, to a model of collaborative working with them.
- Nurses have taken on new and more complex roles as their profession has developed, affecting the nature and content of their working relationships with other professionals.
- As from 2012, nurses will only be able to register on qualifying programmes at universities which will be at Bachelor's degree level, and no longer on sub-degree programmes.
- Health care assistants may come to take on more of the current roles of professionally qualified nurses.

which can be encountered by nurses working in that field. After reading all the scenarios, or an individual scenario, reflect on the professions/agencies that are or could be needed to help in the care of the service user. You should be mindful though, that not all service users are alike. You could have three people all with an identical medical diagnosis, but each one may need a different combination of health and social care professionals, depending on their individual circumstances. Even a relatively straightforward health problem, for example in the child field scenario below, needs several professionals' involvement. Communication is vital for successful care delivery but also key is the need to involve the service user and/or their carer(s) in any assessment, plan and implementation of care.

Exercise 22.1

- How many times have you/your family or friends received a service from a nurse?
- What was this for?
- What were the main functions/activities/aims of the nurse's assessment and intervention?
- What other professionals did they work with, and to what purpose?

In the following case studies, the other professional role(s) in providing a service for the service user alongside and with the nurse has/have been briefly described and some have links to websites for further information about that role more generally.

Exercise 22.2

How does the role of the nurse differ from that of the other professionals involved in the following case study? What were the main functions/activities/aims of the nurse's assessment and intervention?

What will be the role of the nurse in this case study? What are the main functions/activities/aims of the nurse's assessment and intervention?

Case study

Adult

Eileen is 85 years old. She lives on her own in a warden-controlled flat but has remained fairly independent and relatively active. She has two children: Barbara aged 60 years old who has been widowed for two years and lives three miles away (Barbara has two grown-up children who live nearby, they are both married and have young children); her other child is Lee who is 55 years old and lives over 150 miles away with his wife and three children.

Four years ago Eileen had laser surgery on a cataract that was partially successful and she has partial vision in the other eye. Apart from childhood illnesses she remained in relative good health although she has had increasing difficulty mobilising in the last three years. She can climb into her bath but due to the positioning of the handle she is unable to climb out. Consequently she has been unable to have a bath or shower for over two years.

This situation was reported to the local council, who run the home and she had 'someone from social services' come to the flat to assess the situation two years ago. She is still waiting for the bath to be replaced.

Due to some changes to her bowel functioning she went to see her GP who referred Eileen to the colorectal surgeon and she was diagnosed with bowel cancer in the ascending colon. Eileen was admitted for laparoscopic surgery to remove a part of the large intestine where the cancer was situated. The surgery was successful and she did not require chemotherapy. While in hospital she was assessed by an occupational therapist to see if she was able to manage by herself when she went home. The assessment involved seeing whether she was able to cook a light meal and make a drink.

Eileen's daughter had brought up the issue of the bath with the medical and nursing staff while still in hospital, they then referred her to social services. Prior to discharge back to her flat no one had contacted her about it. Two days after she had been discharged she was rung and told someone would be coming to assess her situation regards the bath the following week. Eileen informed them that she had already been assessed two years ago, the person on the phone said 'oh well in that case there's no point me assessing you again'.

Interprofessional involvement

GP (a medical practitioner who specialises in treating acute and chronic illnesses and provides preventive care and health education in community settings).

Housing (see http://www.direct.gov.uk/en/HomeAndCommunity/Councilandhousingassociationhomes/Councilhousing/index.htm).

Social Services/Adult Social Care. There are a range of local authority services available, although not always sharing the same title. For more information visit http://www.direct.gov.uk/en/index.htm.

Ophthalmic surgeon (medical practitioner who specialises in surgery of the eye).

Colorectal surgeon (medical practitioner who specialises in surgery of the large bowel).

Anaesthetist (qualified doctors who specialise in pain management, anaesthesia and intensive care medicine. They often deal with emergency situations by providing advanced life support, the ability to breathe and resuscitation to the heart and lungs).

Colorectal nurse specialist (registered nurse who specialises in working with people and their families who have had cancer of the bowel).

Operating department practitioner (works with surgeons, anaesthetists and theatre nurses to ensure every operation is as safe and effective as possible).

Recovery nurse (monitors patients when they are still under the effects of anesthesia. They are registered nurses who have had additional professional development in critical care).

Hospital porters are responsible for moving frail and often very ill patients between different departments and wards. They also transport complex and valuable equipment around the hospitals.

Inpatient nursing staff (registered nurses working on wards within hospitals).

Occupational therapist helps people with their physical, mental or social problems which have resulted from an accident, illness or ageing to do what they want to do. These include daily activities, to more complex activities such as caring for children, or maintaining a healthy social life. See also Chapter 19 in this book.

Pharmacist (pharmacists are, in broad terms, experts in medicines. They work in a number of settings: community, hospital, primary care, academia, amongst others). For more information visit http://www .rpharms.com/careers-in-pharmacy/pharmacy-roles.asp. See also Chapter 23 in this book.

Had Eileen required chemotherapy she would have also had a consultant specialising in this together with further nursing staff. She may have also needed radiotherapy, in which case she would have also needed a radiation oncology medical specialist.

Case study

Child

Claire is an eight-year-old child with a younger five-year-old sister. Both her parents work full time and both children are often picked up from school by their mothers' parents, who live close by. While at school Claire complained of lower abdominal pain, she is taken to the school nurse who informs her parents and advises them to take their child to their GP which they do. The practice nurse sees Claire before getting a second opinion from the GP who reviews the child and believes the cause of the pain to be appendicitis. Claire is sent to the children's hospital via the accident and emergency department. She sees a doctor who requests a surgical opinion. A surgeon then sees Claire and arranges an ultrasound and blood tests before admitting her to the surgical ward for emergency appendectomy. On arrival to the ward Claire is initially greeted, admitted and settled onto the ward by the nurses, she is soon seen by an anaesthetist and anaesthetic nurse prior to surgery. Following the surgery Claire comes round in the recovery suite where she is looked after by the recovery nurses, she is later taken back to the ward.

Over the next few days Claire makes a good recovery from the operation but needs to remain on the ward for a few days. A play specialist is involved in her care while in hospital, together with the other children, and a teacher attends the ward daily. Claire was also seen by specialists from the pain team (postoperative pain management). She is eventually discharged from the ward back to her parents' home. A district nurse reviews her when she is at home and her parents take her back to hospital 10 days later for follow-up with the clinic nurse and doctor.

Interprofessional involvement

School nurse (provides an assortment of services such as health and sex education within schools, running developmental screening, undertaking health interviews and administering immunisation programmes).

GP (previously cited above).

Practice nurse, works in GP surgeries. They can be involved in most facets of patient care, such as treating small injuries, helping with minor operations, health screening, family planning, vaccination programmes (e.g. flu), and running stopping smoking programmes.

Accident and Emergency medical and nursing staff.

Surgeon (medical practitioner who specialises in surgery).

Radiographer (two types of radiography, diagnostic and therapeutic. Both need considerable knowledge of technology, anatomy and physiology and pathology to carry out their work. In this case it would have been a diagnostic radiographer. For more information visit http://www.nhscareers.nhs.uk/details/default.aspx?id=189).

Phlebotomist (specialised clinical support workers who collects blood from patients for examination in laboratories, to assist in diagnosing illness. For more information visit http://www.nhscareers.nhs.uk/details/Default.aspx?Id=252).

Anaesthetist (cited above)

Hospital porters (cited above)

Operating department practitioner (cited above)

Recovery nurse (cited above)

Children's nurse (Registered Nurse from the child field)

Hospital play specialist (use their understanding of child development and therapeutic play activities to facilitate children to cope with pain, anxiety or fear they might experience during their time in hospital).

Teacher (help students keep up on their school work while recovering from whatever illness they have had/have). (See also Chapter 17 in this book).

District nurse (a registered nurse who has undertaken specialist practitioner programmes at degree level. They visit people in their own homes or in residential care homes, providing care for patients and supporting family members).

Specialist nurse in pain management (Registered Nurse who has undertaken an advanced practitioner educational programme in pain management).

Exercise 22.3

How does the role of the nurse differ from that of the other professionals involved in this case study? What were the main functions/activities/aims of the nurse's assessment and intervention?

What will be the role of the nurse in this case study? What are the main functions/activities/aims of the nurse's assessment and intervention?

Case study

Learning disability field

Michael is a young man with severe autistic spectrum condition with some challenging behaviour, for example, he hits his own head when upset, and lashes out at siblings. Michael lacks understanding and has no awareness of other family members' emotions and feelings. Initiating or being involved in conversations with others is an area he has problems with. He is 21years old and about to leave special school.

He lives at home with his parents and two siblings who are all struggling to cope with Michael's behaviour. He is 6ft tall and becoming overweight; he will only eat savoury snacks and biscuits. Michael has some respite/short break care each month (two nights) but the family needs more help.

Michael is very structured in his behaviour and tied very much to his routines. One such behaviour is when he takes a bath. He must have the same amount of water and same temperature of the water, each time he bathes. Similarly he requires the same amount of soap to be in the same place and he must have the same towel, placed in the exact same place.

His parents are especially concerned about his longer-term care as he is not likely to be able to function independently as he gets older. His siblings are also concerned in that they may have to care for him long term.

Interprofessional involvement

Social worker (see Chapter 20)

Community learning disability nurse (Registered Nurse from the learning disability field working in community settings).

Dietician (qualified health professional who assesses, diagnoses and treats diet and nutrition problems). For further information visit http://www.bda.uk.com/careers/index.html).

GP (cited above)

Speech and language therapist (SALT) (allied health professionals and work with children and adults with disorders of speech, language, communication and swallowing. For further information visit http://www.rcslt.org/speech_and_language_therapy/what_is_an_slt).

Clinical psychologists (work with individuals/families to reduce psychological distress and to enhance and promote psychological well-being). For further information visit http://www.bps.org.uk/psychology-public/how-can-psychology-help-you/how-can-psychology-help-you).

Educational psychologists (work with children or young people who experience problems within an educational setting. Their aim is to improve the learning of the individual. For further information visit http://www.aep.org.uk/home).

Respite care staff/short breaks coordinator (social services). (Respite care is any sort of help and support that enables a person to take a break from the responsibility of caring for somebody else.)

Teaching staff (cited above).

Exercise 22.4

How does the role of the nurse differ from that of the other professionals involved in this case study? What were the main functions/activities/aims of the nurse's assessment and intervention?

What will be the role of the nurse in this case study? What are the main functions/activities/aims of the nurse's assessment and intervention?

Case study

Mental health field

David is 35 years old, weighs 19 stone and lives with his mother on the tenth floor of a tower block, with a lift that rarely works. His mother has managed to bring him up on her own, by holding two, sometimes three, part-time jobs. His father and mother split when David was seven years old and has no direct contact with either David or his former wife and has never contributed financially to David's upkeep. David's mother has had some relationships with other men but they always end the relationship, often stating that David was the cause. David had been expelled from two schools for disruptive behaviour and had on one occasion physically attacked a teacher who had tried to stop him repeatedly opening and closing a cupboard door. He had been arrested by the police on several occasions for anti-social behaviour, usually involving him swearing and verbally abusing people and sometimes physically attacking them. On each occasion his behaviour had been unprovoked. David had also been arrested twice for walking into a local shop and stealing cola and sweets and threatening staff if they tried to stop him. On the second occasion he was given a six-month sentence in a prison several miles from home. This meant his mother was unable to visit him. David's sentence was extended by six months due to him being involved in fights with other prisoners. While in prison David was considered a suicide risk by the prison officers.

While at school David had no friends, played on his own mainly and disliked taking part in any physical activity. He was often mocked by other pupils, however, due to David's size; he had always been overweight and often got into fights for no apparent reason, so mocking of him was often done from a safe distance. On leaving school he had achieved no GCSEs and was unable to get a job. He spent most of his time at home watching television while drinking large quantities of cola and eating junk food. His mother had tried to improve his diet but he would become violent towards her and eventually she gave up trying.

He continued to put on weight and became less active. He became more and more isolated and the violence became more frequent and there appeared to be no apparent cause for it. His mother eventually told her GP after David had physically assaulted her causing a black eye, broken nose and knocking out three of her teeth. The GP referred David to a consultant psychiatrist who visited him at home to undertake an assessment. David, who had not been told by his mother the psychiatrist was coming to see him, or why, became verbally abusive to the consultant and started to attack his mother. The consultant called the police and arranged for David to be admitted to an acute inpatient unit under a section of the Mental Health Act. David was eventually diagnosed with schizophrenia. Other tests showed David was also suffering from Type II diabetes, chronic constipation and had a urine infection.

Interprofessional involvement

Educational psychologists (previously cited above).

Housing personnel (see http://www.direct.gov.uk/en/HomeAndCommunity/Councilandhousingassociationhomes/Councilhousing/index.htm).

Job Centre staff (staff working in such centres, which are executive agencies of the Department for Work and Pensions, are responsible for helping people of working age to find employment. They also have responsibility for administering some benefits for people of working age and for the administration of National Insurance numbers).

Community mental health nurse (possibly attached to a multidisciplinary mental health team including psychiatrist, social worker, psychologist and occupational therapist).

Probation officer (work to rehabilitate offenders by implementing the conditions of court orders and release licenses, conducting risk assessments to protect the public, and ensuring offenders' awareness of the impact of their crime on their victims and the public).

Prison officers (have the responsibility for the security, supervision, training and rehabilitation of people within prison. Additionally prison officers establish and maintain positive working relationships with offenders, in order to influence rehabilitation).

GP (cited above).

Dietician (cited above).

Diabetic nurse (similar to the role of any other registered nurse. However, diabetes specialist nurses work primarily with diabetic patients and their families, helping them to understand, control and manage their diabetes).

Inpatient mental health nurses.

Health care assistants (can work in community or hospital settings under the supervision of a qualified healthcare professional. For further information visit http://www.nhscareers.nhs.uk/details/Default.aspx?Id=485).

Consultant psychiatrist (medical practitioner who specialises in treating people with mental health problems in either community or inpatient settings).

Clinical psychologist (previously cited above).

It is possible David might have staff from a crisis and home treatment team should the situation occur. Such teams are interprofessional, usually consisting of mental health nurses, social workers, psychologists, psychiatrists, occupational therapists and Support Time & Recovery (STR) workers. Their main aim is to work with the service user and carer where appropriate, to get them through the immediate crisis, while keeping them in their home environment.

Exercise 22.5

How does the role of the nurse differ from that of the other professionals involved in this case study? What were the main functions/activities/aims of the nurse's assessment and intervention?

What will be the role of the nurse in this case study? What are the main functions/activities/aims of the nurse's assessment and intervention?

How can we ensure that the service user remains 'in control' with so many different professionals involved? What is the role of the nurse in supporting this aspect of the intervention?

Conclusion

Each scenario demonstrates a breadth of professional and agencies involvement. However, the examples can only ever give the tip of the iceberg in regards to the volume and breadth of health and social care professionals, together with criminal justice (police, probation officers, prison staff), people from the various faiths (the main ones being Buddhist, Christian, Hindu, Judaism, Islam). Additionally people working in the following areas often contribute: housing, education, leisure, voluntary, private and third sector organisations. Behind this wealth of groups of professionals/agencies are a multitude of administrators, managers, finance staff, domestics, catering staff, not to mention all those who maintain equipment, clean laundry and buildings and all those needed for the information technology (IT) which supports much of the working practices and record keeping. And most importantly the service user and their carer *must be central* to any care provided; indeed carers often contribute a significant amount of the care.

In the twenty-first century the unique function of the nurse, as Henderson asserted (Henderson, 1966), needs revisiting. Many of the functions nurses undertook have been taken on by others, while nurses, as advanced practitioners and consultant nurses, have taken on other roles. What has remained, and must continue for high-quality care to be achieved, are for nurses and others to understand each other's roles.

Increasing complexity of health and social care delivery and the need to look at the physical and mental health needs in combination, together with the increase in those professions and agencies involved in health and social care provision, are central to care delivery. As a consequence, never has the need for clear, accurate and effective communication been more important.

Nursing interprofessionally is not an option, it is a necessity. Nursing has moved from the role often portrayed as a handmaiden of doctors, to one who is now an independent nurse practitioner. But whatever the nurse's role, at whatever level and in whichever field of nursing, nurses communicate and work with a vast array of people. To that end, each and every nurse will 'work with others to protect and promote the health and wellbeing of those in your care, their families and carers, and the wider community' (NMC, 2008, p. 5).

Further reading

Goodman, B. and Clemow, R. (2010) *Nursing and Collaborative Practice. A Guide to Interprofessional Learning and Working*, Exeter: Learning Matters.

Reeves, S., Lewin, S., Espin, S. and Zwarenstein, M. (2010) *Interprofessional Teamwork for Health and Social Care*, Oxford: Wiley-Blackwell.

Useful websites

www.nmc-uk.org
NMC

References

Boon, H., Verhoef, M., O'Hara, D., and Findley, B. (2004) From parallel practice to integrative health care: a conceptual framework, *BMC Health Services Research*, http://www.biomedcentral.com/1472-6963/4/15 accessed 27 July 2011.

Capon, B. J. (2005) *Panel Report from the Inquiry into the Care and Treatment of Richard King*, Norwich: Norfolk and Waveney Mental Health Partnership NHS Trust.

Henderson, V. (1966) *The Nature of Nursing: A Definition and Its Implications for Practice, Research and Education*, New York: MacMillan.

Henderson, V. (2006) The concept of nursing, *Journal of Advanced Nursing*. 53 (1), 21–34.

Illingworth, P. (2006) Partnerships in mental health Care, in I. Peate and S. Chelvanayagam (eds) *Caring for Adults with Mental Health Problems,* Chichester: Wiley.

Interprofessional Education Team (2010) *Interprofessional Capability Framework 2010 Mini Guide*, Sheffield: HEA.

NMC (2008) *The Code: Standards of Conduct, Performance and Ethics for Nurses and Midwives*, London: Nursing and Midwifery Council.

NMC (2010) *Standards of Proficiency for Pre-Registration Nurse Education*, http://www.nmc-uk.org/Educators/Standards-for-education/Standards-of-proficiency-for-pre-registration-nursing-education/, accessed 27 July 2011.

QAA (2001) *Subject Benchmark Statement: Health Care Programmes – Nursing*, Gloucester: QAA.

Ritchie, J. (1994) *The Report of the Inquiry into the Care and Treatment of Christopher Clunis*, London: HMSO.

WHO (1988) *Learning Together to Work Together for Health. Report of a WHO Study Group on Multiprofessional Education of Health Personnel: The Team Approach*, World Health Organization Technical Report Series No. 769, Geneva: WHO.

WHO (2010) *Framework for Action on Interprofessional Education and Collaborative Practice*, Geneva: WHO.

Chapter 23
Learning to work together: Experience from pharmacy

Neena Lakhani and Brian Simon

Chapter summary

This chapter will focus on pharmacists in the interprofessional context. Like many others, pharmacy is a profession which has only recently been acknowledged as a 'player' in collaborative practice, and the profession has thus experienced a rapid growth in terms of guidance, policy and implementation frameworks to support this developing aspect of practice. The chapter will reflect on these recent developments, and offer some thoughts about the practical implications and challenges for pharmacy in coming to terms with contemporary expectations and ideas about its place alongside others concerned with working together in the best interests of patients/service users.

Learning objectives

This chapter will cover:

- the policy and organisational frameworks for pharmacy's role in interprofessional collaboration
- pharmacy's contribution to effective joint working in hospital settings
- pharmacy's contribution to effective joint working in community settings
- some of the challenges facing pharmacy as a relative newcomer to the interprofessional domain
- the benefits to be gained from effective collaboration
- the knowledge, skills and attitudes central to good teamworking from a pharmacy perspective.

Introduction

Within all health care settings, service users (also known as 'clients', 'patients', or 'people who use services', see Chapter 4) are cared for by multidisciplinary teams involving a wide range of health care regulated professionals and the voluntary sector. Hence it is essential that effective teamworking, collaboration and communication exist between all the people working with service users across all interfaces and, also, that it exists across practitioner boundaries. Interprofessional learning and interprofessional collaboration between different professions is a vital aspect of achieving such teamworking. In some instances cross-boundary working involves many other statutory organisations such as police, teachers and housing, and is always important to recognise service users and carers themselves as part of the 'team'.

It must be emphasised that interprofessional education (IPE) should not be confused with multi professional education, which involves two or more professions learning the same content side by side (see Chapter 3). IPE focuses on the way in which practitioners will learn together to work together to benefit the user. For pharmacists, it is important to develop respect for other professions who work in different ways, as well as trust and communication skills in working together to enhance and strengthen a diverse workforce. It is also useful to understand the contribution they can make in contributing to the principles required for collaborative working within the NHS (Lakhani and Anderson, 2008). This is particularly important for pharmacists because until recently their own role as potential members of collaborative teams has probably been under-recognised.

The General Pharmaceutical Council (GPhC) is the regulatory body for pharmacy in the United Kingdom. It defines the minimum standards of 'competencies' that a university-based pharmacy programme has to adhere to in order for the graduate and student to meet the requirements of the professional body. The following competencies relate to interprofessional practice:

The graduate. . .

. . . can communicate effectively, orally and in writing, with his/her teachers and peers, as a sound basis for future interaction with patients, carers and other healthcare professionals

. . . is able to interpret and evaluate, for safety, quality, efficacy and economy, prescriptions and other orders for medicines, and to advise patients and other healthcare professionals about medicines and their usage,

The student . . . gains first hand structured experience of practice, including contact with patients and practitioners of other healthcare professions.

> **GPhC website:** http://www.pharmacyregulation. org/sites/default/files/MPharm%20accreditation %20standards%20and%20indicative%20syllabus %20m.pdf, accessed 2 February 2012.

For pharmacy students to learn to practice effectively, efficiently and confidently they need to know about, understand and have the skills to operate within the healthcare systems, alongside and together with other health professionals and other scientists.

It is important that the principles behind IPE also translate into practice (Blenkinsopp and Bond, 2007). Pharmacy education programmes have undergraduate students working in 'placements' to get an experience of working alongside their peers in order to learn about how to apply their science-based training into practice-based skills. In order to practice as a pharmacist in the United Kingdom, the pharmacy student has to undergo a one-year period of 'pre-registration' as required by the GPhC. It is important that they continue their collaborative skills in practice and apply this to the concept of interprofessional practice-based learning.

Interprofessional practice-based learning (IPL) involves members (or students) of two or more professions associated with health or social care engaged in learning with, from and about each other during their practice placements (e.g. clinical placement, rotation, fieldwork placement) (Barr *et al.*, 2005).

Pharmacy undergraduates and postgraduate trainees will learn and practice in primary and secondary care. In primary care settings, most will practice as community pharmacists. Within secondary care, pharmacists will work in acute and community hospitals. A small percentage will work in the pharmaceutical industry and academic institutions. Within these settings, pharmacists can develop their roles further. Opportunities for such specialism include consultant pharmacists (specialising in certain therapeutic areas) and primary care pharmacists (working in Primary Care Trusts, Strategic Health Authorities or general practice surgeries). Many pharmacists may also progress to become supplementary prescribers or independent prescribers, which allows them to prescribe medication in their chosen therapeutic area.

Hospital pharmacists are already familiar with participating in multidisciplinary ward rounds and discussions around patient care. However, community pharmacists often find themselves working in isolation from other health care professionals, but in closer contact often with the public and people who use services. They are often asked by patients about social care problems, or where to go if they needed more specialist help. In this way they become part of the complex web of advisors who can help to ensure people's health care needs are met. It follows that community pharmacists need also to appreciate the roles of other health care professionals and refer appropriately (British Medical Association and National Pharmacy Association, 2009). However, communication between health and social care professionals in primary care seems to be fraught at the best of times. Professional prejudices are still rife, creating barriers that have long been impermeable with many still working in 'silos' (Lakhani and Anderson, 2008).

In 2006, the Department of Health announced some fairly radical changes of the ways in which pharmacy services should be configured to meet demands of patients, posing challenging problems for service delivery and pharmacy education (Department of Health, 2006). We believe that IPE has the potential to improve the effectiveness of teamworking between health and social care professionals and thus the quality of patient care in both the hospital and community setting. This has also been highlighted for 'preparing pharmacists for 2020' (Blenkinsopp and Bond, 2007) and by the Department of Health (2008). If this is successfully implemented, barriers between professions should be acknowledged and at least partially broken down.

Almost all service users who seek medical care interact with more than one health or social care professional. Figure 23.1 illustrates how many professionals a pharmacist is likely to work with in either the hospital or community setting.

Pharmacists need to broaden their vision of continuing education to include continuing professional development (CPD) in the context of interprofessional collaboration and practice improvement. This may help pharmacists and their professional partners find answers to the myriad of problems most important to the health of their service users and communities.

Professionals who communicate with pharmacists

For the pharmacist or pharmacy student, lack of interaction with other health professionals may have unfortunate consequences. At a time when pharmacy is asserting its clinical role, isolation can be particularly counterproductive. Pharmacy students may encounter future colleagues who characterise the pharmacist as a 'pill counter', working at the back of a high street store, a 'shopkeeper' who works in a lost corner of a chain chemist or a 'boffin' in the basement of a hospital. Such stereotypes may be exacerbated by the media and at best can put an unnecessary barrier to the integration of the pharmacist into the health care team in the eyes of both the public and other health care professionals.

The number of professionals involved and the importance of their ability to work collaboratively increases with the complexity of the patient's needs. New standards to improve management of diseases such as asthma, diabetes or congestive heart failure have been set in the NHS National Service Frameworks (NSFs) (http://www.nhs.uk/NHSEngland/NSF/Pages/Nationalserviceframeworks.aspx). The NSFs outline the importance of collaboration between health care professionals. The concept of 'medicines management' (MM) is highlighted in the NSFs. This is defined as the clinical, cost-effective and safe use of medicines to ensure that patients get the maximum benefit from the medicines they need, while at the same time minimising potential harm. This is a particularly

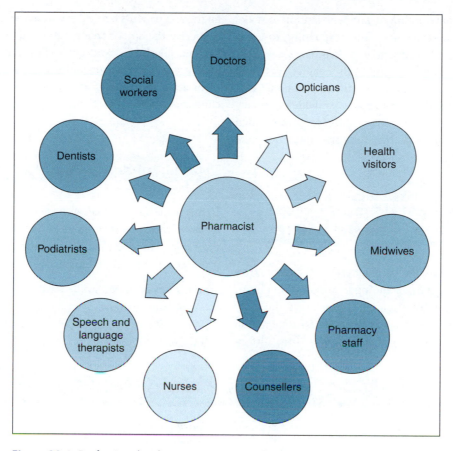

Figure 23.1 Professionals who communicate with pharmacists

A closer look

NICE guidance

The National Institute for Health and Clinical Excellence (NICE) provides patients, health care professionals and the public with authoritative and reliable guidance on current 'best practice' for some medicines and treatment modalities. NICE guidelines highlight a need for professional collaboration in order to implement their strategies. Health care professionals have a duty to help patients make informed decisions about treatment and use appropriately prescribed medicines to best effect. NICE has produced guidance about enabling patients to make informed choices by involving and supporting them in decisions about prescribed medicines (National Institute for Health and Clinical Excellence, 2009).

important aspect where pharmacists play a vital role to ensure that medicines are used correctly (Department of Health, 2004).

As pharmacists we play a significant part in supplying the right medicine to the right person at the appointed time. This is not simply a reactive responsibility, it requires good communication with a number of individuals within the pharmacy team as well as other health care professionals. Although there has been criticism of the pharmacist's contribution to the primary health care team, it is acknowledged that effective delivery of the pharmacists' roles may require a more significant move into the fold of the primary care team – possibly even abandoning the shopkeeper image – and learning new ways of interacting with patients and medical colleagues (Bradley, 2009). However, this very experience of working regularly with members of the community also suggests that pharmacists have an important contribution to make in terms of understanding and responding to commonly expressed needs and concerns.

As we progress through this chapter, you will become aware of some of the interprofessional collaboration which takes place as we provide pharmacy services to patients and some of the problems which may and do arise if this discourse does not take place.

Interprofessional practice-based learning in the hospital setting

There are a number of challenges of collaborative practice in hospitals, including the timings of a number of different ward rounds and 'handovers', difficulty in locating medical records, illegible documentation in patients' clinical notes, incomplete drug history taking and patients being away from the ward in order to receive therapy or treatment. In spite of these, the hospital pharmacist still gives clinical benefit to the patient when directly or indirectly modifying patient medication and by informing and educating other clinicians and the patient themselves.

The pharmacist's role

In this scenario, pharmacists have responsibilities and a duty of care in ensuring safe and effective medicinal provision. We will look at the hospital part of the processes in three time frames:

1. What has occurred in the past.
2. What happens now.
3. What takes place in planning for the immediate future.

Case study

Mr XX

As with any other health care profession, the patient is the focus of any interventions made. We will follow the care Mr XX receives as he moves through various settings, identifying opportunities for interprofessional collaboration and potential challenges along the way.

Mr XX is an 85-year-old man who lives at home. He is admitted to a hospital following a fall at home which has given rise to concerns over his medical well-being.

On admission to the hospital, he is 'clerked' by one of the on-call junior doctors and his admission details are as follows:

Presenting Complaint:
Fall
(Reason for admission)

History of Presenting Complaint:
Loss of Consciousness (LOC), trip fell/confused

Drug History:
Isosorbide mononitrate 20 bd
Blue inhaler

Brown inhaler
Blood pressure tablets??

Medical History:
Hypertension
Angina
COPD (chronic obstructive pulmonary disease)

Social History:
Lives at home with wife

Investigations:
Troponin I,
U&Es (urea and electrolytes)
FBC (full blood count)
MSU (mid-stream urine sample)

Plan:
Withhold anti-hypertensive
Treat ??UTI (Treat a suspected urinary tract infection)

The past

One of the first things we must do is establish the medication the patient was previously taking in order to ensure appropriate medical decisions can now be made once the confirmed drug history is brought to the attention of the physicians.

This drug history can be sought in a number of ways:

- from the patients themselves if they are sufficiently lucid
- from the patient's repeat medication prescription request sheet
- from the patient's own drugs if brought in
- from the carer's knowledge and recollection
- from the GP surgery.

To be able to do this seemingly small task requires the pharmacy practitioner to be able to communicate and share information with a wide range of individuals:

- the patient's named staff nurse may be approached to ascertain what medicines the patient has brought in on admission to the hospital
- the ward clerk may be approached for the contact details of the patient's GP if the details are not available
- when speaking to the GP surgery, the pharmacy staff member may have to discuss the need and details of the patient's drug history with receptionist staff, a GP practice nurse or the GP themselves in order to obtain the correct information
- the patient's hospital doctor would be informed of any amendments made to the drug history as part of the medicine reconciliation process
- if the patient is taking any specialised medication such as restricted psychiatric medicines, then the specialist pharmacist would need to be contacted in order establish the correct drug regime and obtain an appropriate drug supply
- the patient himself and his carer are also important potential sources of information, and can provide a more detailed account of his use of prescribed (and other) medication.

It is already clear that the critical process of obtaining accurate and potentially vital information is highly complex and depends on a willingness to communicate effectively with the time and skills (such as active listening) to support this. It is essential that we do not assume that some of those involved will automatically 'know better' than others.

After review, the list of medicines previously taken might be identified as follows:

Drug history

- Isosorbide mononitrate 20mg bd (twice a day)
- Salbutamol inhaler 2 puffs PRN (when required)
- Beclomethasone 200 inhaler 2 puffs bd
- Bendroflumethiazide 2.5mg om (in the mornings)
- Glyceryl trinitrate spray 1–2 sprays PRN
- Nitrazepam 5–10mg on PRN.

The present

Once the drug history is amended, this information is communicated to the patient's doctor so that therapy is prescribed or discontinued as appropriate. This is also a good point at which to perform a detailed clinical review of his medicines. This entails reviewing the patient's condition with regard to the medicines they are taking and deciding which drugs are useful and need to continue, which drugs are no longer necessary and can be stopped, and whether any other medication needs to be prescribed.

After differential diagnosis, drug history and medication review, Mr XX's medication list might show several changes:

Aspirin 75mg od

GTN spray 1–2 sprays when required for chest pain

Anti-hypertensive (bendroflumethiazide) discontinued

Benzodiazepines (Nitrazepam) changed to zopiclone (shorter acting with less 'hangover' effect)

Choice of inhalers/devices reviewed and administered using the appropriate spacer device (device used to aid inhaled drug delivery)

In complex exchanges, it is important to recognise who is taking responsibility for what aspect of the task, and to be explicit about who is taking the lead for which aspects of the process.

Discussion takes place with the junior doctor in suggesting the addition of omitted or necessary drugs and changing medicines to more suitable ones. A specialist respiratory nurse and Mr XX's named nurse would be spoken to when assessing which inhaler to use and the associated spacer device.

Professionals with whom the pharmacist has liaised:

- hospital doctor on drug recommendations
- respiratory specialist nurse
- ward nurse, choice of medicines, medicines management plan.

The well-being and medical management of the patient is continually assessed amongst professionals, and this multidisciplinary team enables the patient to be cared for in the best way possible while they are being treated in the hospital prior to being discharged. Clearly, too, a full explanation of any planned changes and the implications must be provided to the patient and where appropriate to his carer.

The future

Due to his circumstances and ability, Mr XX will be going to a residential home. In preparing his medication, the pharmacist checks the discharge letter containing the discharge plan and a list of the medicines, their doses and frequencies, which Mr XX is to take.

Discrepancies often occur at this stage. On identifying these, the pharmacist liaises with the prescribing doctor to ensure that medication is prescribed as intended.

Professionals with whom the pharmacist has liaised:

- doctor – discharge letter
- nurse – discharge letter
- residential home manager/matron – medicines available and advice as necessary
- technical/dispensing staff – medicine supply.

Asserting one's own professional skills and knowledge may be important at this point – it is not always best just to avoid conflict. Healthy disagreements are a positive feature of good collaborative practice.

Other health care professionals with who pharmacy staff may collaborate include physiotherapists, occupational therapists, speech and language therapists and dieticians, in order to ensure that there is a full understanding of the consequences of changes in medication within the wider 'team'.

Interprofessional practice-based learning in the community pharmacy

Mr XX was discharged and brought to a residential care home setting. A few weeks later, his wife comes to the pharmacy. She explains that Mr XX has had a fall and his leg is badly grazed. The residential home staff had informed the GP, who came out to see Mr XX. He prescribed some more medicines and left the prescription with the care home staff. She hands in the prescription for his drugs.

Mrs XX explains to the pharmacist that there were some medicines in the medicine cupboard at home and that she is not sure whether Mr XX still needs them. Mrs XX mentions that her husband is very confused about his medication and finds it difficult to remember taking his drugs. Mrs XX normally gives them to him and she is now finding things confusing and difficult. The GP had been to see Mr XX recently and he has been prescribed some more medicines. The GP had said what the new medicines were for, but Mr XX was very confused. She also explains that Mr XX's breathing is getting worse. Is there anything the community pharmacist can do to help?

The prescription is for the following medicines, dressings and appliances:

- Isosorbide mononitrate 20mg bd (twice a day)
- Glyceryl trinitrate spray 1–2 sprays PRN (2 sprays in bag)
- Aspirin 75mg once a day

- Lisinopril 10mg od (once a day): new drug
- Simvastatin 40mg on (at night): new drug
- Zopiclone 7.5mg at night (only when required)
- Metformin 500mg od (once a day): new drug
- Salbutamol CFC inhaler 2 puffs when required
- Beclomethasone 200 inhaler 2 puffs bd
- A spacer device
- Granuflex dressings (10cm × 10cm) × 30: new preparation
- Mepore dressings × 10 packs: new preparation

Mrs XX also hands in a bag containing the following medicines:

- Paracetamol 500mg tablets for pain
- Some cough syrup
- Multivitamin tablets
- Nitrazepam 10mg on (remember, this was taken off in the hospital)
- E45 cream

The pharmacist's role

This may seem a daunting task. In this scenario, community pharmacists, like hospital pharmacists, have responsibilities and a duty of care in ensuring safe and effective provision of medicines. However, there are no health care professionals to consult on site, unlike the hospital scenario above. The obvious challenge is that there are more drugs on the prescription now than when the patient was discharged. We can look at what processes the community pharmacist should follow in this scenario, and where there are opportunities for interprofessional skills and learning.

In this scenario, the immediate problems are:

- the drug nitrazepam was stopped by the hospital and this needs to be reviewed
- there are an excessive number of dressings prescribed
- Mr XX's breathing is getting worse. The dose of his inhaler medication needs to be checked, as well as confirming with the GP that there are no other causes of breathlessness (e.g. heart failure or a chest infection)
- new drugs have been started, and as there is a confused history from Mrs XX, the pharmacist must use due diligence and check if the medication was appropriately prescribed

- unlike the hospital scenario, community pharmacists do not have access to the patient clinical record in the pharmacy. The only record they keep is the patient's medication record (PMR).

The community pharmacist can be expected to follow these steps:

- make sure that the medication is clinically appropriate and safe for Mr XX
- consider what action should be taken before the prescription is dispensed
- make sure that the pharmacy support staff dispense the medication according to standard operating procedures
- ascertain that Mr XX understands how to use his medication
- consider what should now take place in planning for the immediate future
- consult with care staff (social worker, care manager, residential care workers) over the problems of confusion and apprehension.

The practice receptionist

The practice receptionist is normally the first port of call. The pharmacist will need to be clear about how to communicate with the receptionist. The receptionist can normally confirm if the items prescribed match the items.

The GP

The pharmacist will need to check that the nitrazepam was in fact stopped by the hospital. The quantities of dressings will also need to be checked. The pharmacist may wish to confirm the changes to Mr XX's condition and the additional medication prescribed. A more experienced pharmacist may ask if appropriate therapeutic tests have been performed in order that the medication is appropriate (e.g. renal and liver function tests, blood tests). The GP confirms that the nitrazepam should not be taken and needs to be disposed of. The GP comments that the pharmacist will need to contact the district nurse regarding the dressings as she recommended these to be prescribed. The GP also explained that

Mr XX would need to see the practice asthma nurse to do a spirometry reading to confirm if his breathlessness is due to the deterioration of his COPD before any changes can be made to his medication.

Actions

The pharmacist would need to speak to the district nurse and explain that the number of dressings prescribed may not be necessary. They may want to highlight the evidence base behind the recommendations.

The pharmacist may wish to contact the practice asthma nurse on Mr XX's behalf so that an appointment is arranged for Mr XX to have a spirometry reading. They may also decide to do a medication use review (MUR) and a prescription intervention (PSNC, 2004).

In the pharmacy, Mr XX's prescription would be dispensed and the pharmacist will liaise with the following:

- **Pharmacy technicians:** community pharmacists have support staff (like the hospital scenario) who deal with the dispensing and labelling of medication as one of their many roles.
- **Pharmacy counter assistants:** counter assistants are normally based in the front of the shop. They assist with many tasks, including the sale of 'counter' medicines (such as paracetamol, medicines for coughs and colds etc). Many of these medicines can only be sold under the supervision of the pharmacist. Whilst the pharmacist is busy dealing with the query, the counter assistants normally accept prescriptions and do vital safety checks to ensure that the prescription is for who it is intended, i.e. check the name and address of the patient and whether they pay for prescriptions.

It is significant here that the collaborative team incorporates not just those conventionally seen as 'professionals' who hold decision-making roles, but also those others who are inevitably involved in a sequence of activities which needs to be functioning well in order to ensure that the intended outcomes are delivered. Pharmacy staff, care home staff and practice administrators are all significant links in this very long chain.

The pharmacist may also need to consider their responsibility for taking proactive steps to involve other professionals, such as care providers or adult social services, when they do not appear to be fully engaged in provision of appropriate interventions.

Exercise 23.1

Draw a diagram of all those who might be part of the 'team around' a service user who is a chronic substance misuser, and the potential connections between them.

A closer look

Medicines Use Review (MUR) and prescription intervention service: an 'advanced' service by community pharmacists

The pharmacist conducts a concordance-centred medication review with the patient. The review assesses any problems with current medication and its administration. The patient's knowledge of their medication regimen is assessed and a report with the patient's consent fed back to the GP. The patient's knowledge of their medication and why they are taking it is increased; problems with their medication are identified and addressed. The MUR is conducted on a regular basis, e.g. every 12 months. The Prescription Intervention Service is in essence the same as the MUR service, but conducted on an ad hoc basis, when a significant problem with a patient's medication is highlighted during the dispensing process. With the patient's consent, the pharmacist will feed back suggestions and comments to the prescriber using standardised paperwork (eventually electronically). Reviews have to be conducted in a private consultation area, which ensures patient confidentiality. Pharmacists must successfully pass a competency assessment before they can provide 'advanced' services.

PSNC (2004) http://www.psnc.org.uk/data/files/PharmacyContract/pharmacy_contract_summary_dec_2004.pdf, accessed 2 November 2009.

The concept of a shared duty of care may be important in this context.

Intervention and follow-up for this scenario

The pharmacist invites Mr XX to the pharmacy for an MUR. Mr XX's permission must be obtained before the community pharmacist does the MUR. The pharmacist will also inform Mr XX that the MUR is confidential, and only Mr XX's GP will get a copy of the outcomes of the process and the recommendations.

The pharmacist goes through all medication with Mr XX, and his wife in her role as carer, including informing Mr XX that the drug nitrazepam has been discontinued and that the pharmacist will dispose of this medicine.

The quantities of the dressings could be reviewed and altered by the district nurse.

The pharmacist makes sure Mr XX has understood the instructions of all the newly started medication as well as the existing medication. In a multi-ethnic community, this may necessitate drawing on the services of professional interpreters, as well as those more conventionally viewed as part of the interagency team.

Mr XX's inhaler technique was checked by the pharmacist. The pharmacist found that Mr XX's technique was fine, but he was not getting optimum treatment because he was using two inhalers and used to forget which one he had used. The pharmacist suggested that Mr XX's COPD medication dosage should be reviewed by the GP and asthma nurse and offers to speak to the practice asthma nurse on Mr XX's behalf.

The pharmacist may offer Mr XX a medication compliance aid (e.g. a 'dosette' box) in order to help Mr XX remember to take his medication. A dosette box is a compartmentalised container, where Mr XX can clearly see when he needs to take his medication without getting confused. This will also help Mrs XX, as she finds bottles very difficult to open. The pharmacist would inform the matron and carers of the residential home that Mr XX was now having his medication from a dosette box, which had clear instructions of what medication was within the box and how the medicines were to be taken.

The pharmacist would also check all additional medicines used by Mr XX that were not prescribed by the doctor. This is to make sure that these medicines were safe and appropriate to use alongside the prescribed medication. Mr XX no longer needed the cough preparations he had bought and these would also be disposed of by the pharmacist.

All recommendations that the pharmacist makes are documented. Any potential clinical interventions should be made using appropriate evidence-based recommendations. In this case, a recommendation was made that Mr XX would benefit from the addition of an additional inhaled drug to control his breathing. A 'combination' inhaler (containing two medications) was suggested so that Mr XX could better comply with his medication regime.

Mr XX was given one copy of the review, and a copy sent to his GP. A third copy of the MUR was retained by the pharmacy. This would enable the GP to assess the intervention and enter these into Mr XX's clinical record.

The GP practice staff acknowledges the report, and invites the community pharmacist to a clinical meeting to discuss Mr XX's case. The pharmacist has the opportunity to inform the practice about the MUR processes. The pharmacist asked to observe an asthma clinic with the nurse. This would be an excellent opportunity for further professional development.

On reflection, the pharmacist's role takes on the aspect of leadership as a result of the intervention. This enhances the role of the pharmacist as an autonomous professional, thus challenging conventional assumptions that they are just 'subordinates' (Hughes and McCann, 2003). Interprofessional collaboration can enhance better understanding of these 'new' roles

Exercise 23.2

Why is leadership an important consideration for collaborative practice, especially in complex community settings where the pharmacist is at the interface between formal and informal members of collaborative teams?

A closer look

Using guidance

To improve medicines reconciliation at hospital admission NICE/National Patient Safety Agency has recommended that:

- all healthcare organisations that admit adult inpatients should make sure that they have policies in place for medicines reconciliation on admission. This includes mental health units, and applies to elective and emergency admissions.
- in addition to specifying standardised systems for collecting and documenting information about

current medications, policies for medicines reconciliation on admission should ensure that:

- pharmacists are involved in medicines reconciliation as soon as possible after admission
- the responsibilities of pharmacists and other staff in the medicines reconciliation process are clearly defined; these responsibilities may differ between clinical areas
- strategies are incorporated to obtain information about medications for people with communication difficulties (NPSA, 2007).

which envisaged the radical changes for service delivery within the NHS.

The future

The pharmacist could take the opportunity to inform Mr XX more about the management of his conditions. For example, to help the management of Mr XX's diabetes, he should be advised to have regular eye tests with an optician and to have his feet examined regularly by a podiatrist. Advice from a dietician would also help Mr XX. In this way, Mr XX and his informal carers are engaged as active members of the team.

This scenario illustrates the excellent opportunities that could enhance the community pharmacist's knowledge, competence, confidence and professionalism with the GP practice staff and service users like Mr XX. Figure 23.2 highlights the health and social care professionals who may be integral in ensuring Mr XX's effective care.

Case summary: key issues

In this chapter we have seen some of the results of professional collaboration from a pharmacy perspective. Mr XX's patient journey has been

smoother, safer and more cost-effective than would have been the case had the collaboration not taken place.

We can identify a number of the benefits of professional collaboration during the drug use review process:

Positive outcomes

The correct drugs prescribed for the patient once they have been admitted to the hospital ward.

- The appropriate medicines are used for the condition being treated. In communicating with one another, we can also ensure that other critical factors are also correct, such as the dose of each medicine; the right formulation (i.e. whether tablet, capsule, liquid); the correct container (whether child-resistant tops are needed or not, if the patient or carer can manage tablets which have to be popped out of blister packs, the use of medicine compliance aids (e.g. dosette boxes), the correct inhaler and spacer devices.
- Ensuring that drugs are prescribed in accordance with the local hospital and primary care drug formulary, this often a cost-saving in the drug budget.
- Adverse drug reactions are prevented as a result of obtaining a complete and accurate drug history and documenting any previous allergies to medicines.

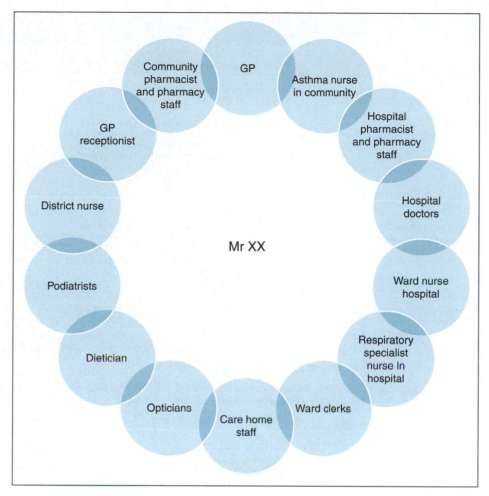

Figure 23.2 The professionals involved in Mr XX's case from the hospital into the community

- Where such problems do arise, the team around and including Mr XX are able to take action quickly and to address any concerns appropriately.
- Concordance may be improved when giving advice to patients having discussed the desired outcomes with their hospital doctor or general practitioner, who can be included in this conversation. Patients should have a better understanding of the medication process and any possible problems which might arise.

Conversely, we can identify a number of adverse results without professional collaboration during the drug use review process.

Negative outcomes without collaboration

Failure to ensure medicines reconciliation occurs meaning that an incomplete and/or inaccurate record of the patient's medication may be documented with associated adverse outcomes, such as wrong medication or doses being re-prescribed; inappropriate drugs being initiated as they may interact or counter act previous drug therapy. These may result in causing harm to the patient, and even if physical harm does not result, lack of clarity and anxiety for the patient may well ensue.

The NPSA has reported the number of incidents of medication errors involving admission and discharge

A closer look

How has IPL and a more positive orientation to collaborative practice made an impact on the service user and health care professionals in this case?

IPE/IPL competency	Scenario
Knowledge ‒ *the learning of specific facts*	Raising awareness of community pharmacist roles to patients and health care professionals, e.g. signposting patients to other health care professionals by pharmacists, the MUR service in community pharmacy, preventing waste due to over-prescribing, preventing harm due to inappropriate prescribing, safe disposal of unwanted medicines, drug formulary development
	Professional development, e.g. spirometry training for the community pharmacist, specialist clinical training for the hospital pharmacist
Skills ‒ *the practice of knowledge*	Ascertaining that the recommendations are based on sound evidence
	Effective documentation and communication of pharmacists recommendations and actions
	Using appropriate team working skills by the community pharmacist (e.g. with pharmacy staff, asthma nurse and GP and hospital doctors)
	Communication with residential home staff
Attitudes ‒ *the development of appropriate values demonstrated through professional behaviour*	Placing the patient centrally to the healthcare professional's work, and listening carefully to what they say
	The ability to resolve conflict (e.g. over-prescribing of dressings, inappropriate use of drugs)
	Assertive communication techniques by pharmacist
	Appreciation and respect for other health care professionals' roles and boundaries
	Value of skills of health care professional staff
	Appropriate professional values and upholding ethical behaviour as guided by the requirements of the RPSGB
	Recognising the need for professional development, e.g. spirometry training for the community pharmacist, leadership and management training

as 7070 with 2 fatalities and 30 that caused severe harm (figures from November 2003 and March 2007) (NPSA, 2007).

- Duplication of effort which wastes the resource of time.
- Time delays in initiating the correct drugs at the correct times to the length of stay in hospital, delay discharge and incurring additional expense per hospital stay. This in turn has a negative impact on the number of hospital admissions that can be made in a given time period, restricting the service as the bed is not available for another patient to use.
- Poor collaboration between pharmacy staff within the hospital and between community team members may also contribute to the hospital discharge being delayed if the result is a delay in the

dispensing of medicines which are not immediately available in the community setting.

Conclusion

Interprofessional collaboration is essential for pharmacy practice. To be successful, **traditional prejudices between pharmacists and other health and social care professionals must be broken down**. Shared goals around patients' needs, and an approach focus on processes that serve those needs, can help transcend traditional barriers. There must be willingness among all involved to engage in the process. The **challenge to become and remain truly interprofessional and collaborative remains not just for students** but also for professionals already in practice and throughout their careers.

Further reading

General Pharmaceutical Council (2010) *Standards of Conduct, Ethics and Performance,* http://www.pharmacyregulation.org/pdfs/other/gphcstandardsofconductethicsandper flo.pdf, accessed April 2011.

References

Barr, H., Koppel, I., Reeves, S., Hammick, M. and Freeth, D. (2005) *Effective Interprofessional Education: Argument, Assumption and Evidence,* Oxford: Blackwell Publishing, CAIPE.

Blenkinsopp, A. and Bond, E. (2007) Pharmacists must learn to play their part in multidisciplinary health teams, *Pharmaceutical Journal,* 279, 330–2.

Bradley, C. P. (2009) The future role of pharmacists in primary care, *British Journal of General Practice* 59, 891–2.

British Medical Association and National Pharmacy Association (2009) *Improving Communication: Between Community Pharmacy and General Practice,* London: BMA/NPA.

Department of Health (2004) *Management of Medicines – A Resource to Support Implementation of the Wider Aspects of Medicines Management for the National Service Frameworks for Diabetes Renal Services and Long-term Conditions,* London: The Stationery Office.

Department of Health (2006) *Our Health, Our Care, Our Say: A New Direction for Community Services. Health and Social Care Working Together in Partnership,* Cm 6737, London: The Stationery Office.

Department of Health (2008) *Pharmacy in England – Building on Strengths, Delivering the Future,* Cm7341, London: The Stationery Office.

Hughes, C. and McCann, S. (2003) Perceived interprofessional barriers between community pharmacists and general practitioners: a qualitative assessment, *British Journal of General Practice* 53 (493), 600–6.

Lakhani, N. and Anderson, E. (2008) Interprofessional education: preparing future pharmacists for 2020, *The Pharmaceutical Journal* 280, 571–2.

National Institute for Health and Clinical Excellence (2009) *Medicines Adherence: Involving Patients in Decisions about Prescribed Medicines and Supporting Adherence,* NICE Clinical guideline 76, London: National Institute for Health and Clinical Excellence. (http://www.nice.org.uk/nicemedia/live/11766/43042/43042.pdf, accessed 10th January 2012).

National Patient Safety Agency (2007) *Medication Errors and Medicines Reconciliation 2007,* http://www.npsa.nhs.uk/corporate/news/guidance-to-improve-medicines-reconciliation, accessed 9 December 2009.

PSNC (2004) *The New NHS Community Pharmacy Service,* The Pharmaceutical Services Negotiating Committee, http://www.psnc.org.uk/data/files/PharmacyContract/pharmacy_contract_summary_dec_2004.pdf, accessed 2 November 2009.

Chapter 24
Working together in dentistry: the key issues and challenges

Pamela Ward

Chapter summary

Like most other professionals, dentists find themselves working both in teams with other dental staff and engaging with other professions outside the 'dental family'. These two aspects of interprofessional practice in dentistry can be referred to as internal and external interprofessional working. The first aspect refers to the working of clinical dentists with their colleagues in the professions complementary to dentistry: oral health educators, dental nurses, dental therapists, hygienists and dental technicians. The second aspect relates to the interface of dentistry with other occupations, professions and their agencies, primarily medicine, education, pharmacy and social services. In the 'theoretical' part of this chapter, aspects of interprofessional working will be explored through the lens of the multi-professional dental team. Three aspects will be considered: firstly, the emergence of dental teamwork and its significance in contemporary dentistry; secondly, the resonance of the issues raised to other areas of interprofessional working; thirdly, the implications of the special factor within dentistry of different professional groups operating under a single regulatory body. Application of themes addressed to interprofessional working elsewhere in health and social care is provided through case examples.

Learning objectives

This chapter will cover:

- how dentistry has been a relatively recent addition to the interprofessional fold
- that policy and guidance has recently begun to acknowledge the collaborative potential of dentistry
- dentists are involved in both in-house treatment teams and with wider groupings of practitioners and others with a concern for personal health and well-being
- dentists need to be ready to take a proactive leadership role in initiating teamworking

▶

- other professionals may not readily see dentists as natural collaborators and may themselves need to be 'educated'
- dental patients themselves are key members of the care/treatment team.

Introduction

For most people dentistry is probably not an obvious medium through which to discuss interprofessional and interdisciplinary working. However, like most other professionals, dentists have come to find themselves working both in teams with other dental specialists and dental support workers and in engaging with other professions outside the 'dental family'.

The author's interest in interprofessional and interdisciplinary working arose as a result of experience gained when, in 2002, her practice was selected by and developed in collaboration with the Modernisation Agency to test out new ways of delivering dentistry. She came to appreciate, more consciously than perhaps had been the case previously, that there are two aspects of interprofessional practice in dentistry which could be referred to as internal and external interprofessional working. The first aspect refers to the working of clinical dentists with their colleagues in the professions complementary to dentistry: oral health educators, dental nurse, dental therapists, hygienists and dental technicians. The second aspect relates to the interface of dentistry with other occupations, professions and their agencies, primarily medicine, education, pharmacy and social services. Oral health interfaces with general health; dentists can be at the front line in dealing with the consequences of violence and abuse; they have an important role in the care of the elderly. Recently, there has been a publicised case involving a phobia in which the relationship between dentist and psychologist has been put under scrutiny.

In the 'theoretical' part of this chapter, aspects of interprofessional working will be explored through the lens of the multi-professional dental team. There are three main facets. Firstly, the emergence of the dental teamwork, at this level, is of great contemporary significance in dentistry. Secondly, the issues raised have resonance in other areas of interprofessional working. Thirdly, there is the special factor within dentistry of different professional groups operating under a single regulatory body, and the implications of this. Application of themes addressed to interprofessional working in the wider health and social care terrain will be provided through case examples.

Background

Dentistry originally broke away from medicine and became a separate discipline a century or two ago when the barber surgeons set up in business providing pain relief with extractions. Since then, as Sarah Nettleton (1992) illustrates so well in her study *Power, Pain and Dentistry*, it has 'expanded its gaze', moving from being totally tooth-focused, when dentists did little but count and treat teeth, to the profession having a more holistic view of the patient. Although many readers may still identify with the picture of a single-handed registered dentist supported by a solitary receptionist, dentistry has, over the years, evolved from being a solitary profession to becoming a team activity, providing services within a social context. As shown in the case examples, it is not uncommon for the dental team to reach out to provide care for people who are unable to access the surgery, for example, disabled people and the housebound elderly, to provide oral health education in schools and young people's recreational organisations, to contribute to the safeguarding of vulnerable children and to meet with other health care professionals in the planning and delivery of patient care. Peter Mossy (2004) emphasises the importance of interaction and reciprocation between those in the delivery of dental services and on focusing on the whole dental team as a multi-professional unit where professional issues involved in working together are addressed and where the benefits of working in a group are championed. These comments apply equally to dentists'

A closer look

Child caries

The dentist and the dental team regularly encounter children with grossly broken down teeth. These children are often irregular attenders, whose only contact with a dental practice is when in pain. Often they present with complex but under-resourced treatment needs. Many of the profession and the non-attending public are accepting of a culture of emergency attendance only to deal with immediate pain. In these circumstances the dental team has no opportunity to educate or to carry out preventive dentistry.

Acceptance of dental decay passes from parent to child so there are many children with grossly carious teeth, for whom their carers do not seek treatment and with whom dentists have no contact until an emergency arises. Such children, who are seen by the dental professionals often repeatedly fail appointments, fail to comply with planned treatment, return in pain at frequent intervals and require repeated general anaesthetics for dental extractions.

It has been reported anecdotally that other health care professionals who work regularly with children are shocked that the dental team often fails to follow up such children (COPDEND, 2006). However, dental practitioners are becoming much more aware that these indicators may be signposts for concern. Increasingly appropriate referral pathways are being developed through which dentists can raise concerns and liaise with other healthcare professionals in the interests of the child. At the Peninsula School of Dentistry students were given the following case scenario:

Jade Jackson is five years old. She is fit and well but the appearance of her front teeth is preventing Jade from interacting normally at school. The head teacher is concerned about Jade's shyness and behaviour in class.

Jade is a reticent child who is reluctant to be examined. When you, the dentist, examine her mouth you find that posteriorly all of the teeth have large carious cavities, while the upper anterior teeth are blackish brown in colour and are almost down to gum level.

Explain why Jade's teeth are like that and what you, the dentist intend to do about it.

The students discussed how they would liaise with the school and the possibility of the dental team going into the school and working with the teachers and becoming involved in dental education projects to increase awareness of oral health.

increasing involvement in wider health and social care provision.

The dental team as well as the dentist includes dental hygienists and dental therapists whose duties have been regulated by the General Dental Council since the Dentists Act in 1984. Since July 2008 dental nurses and dental technicians have also registered on a single Dental Care Professional (DCP) register, alongside the hygienists and therapists.

Originally the General Dental Council laid down a very prescriptive list of permitted duties for members of the dental team. This has moved to a *Scope of Practice* (General Dental Council, 2009) which describes what dentists and dental care professionals (DCPs) are trained and competent to do. It describes the areas in which they are expected to

have knowledge, skills and experience to practice safely and effectively in the best interests of patients. The GDC acknowledges that this 'scope of practice' is likely to change over the course of a practitioner's career, and that everyone has the potential to expand their scope by developing new skills or to narrow their scope but deepen their knowledge in a particular area by choosing more specialised practice.

Guidance provided by the General Dental Council sets out the skills and abilities which each registered group should have. It also describes additional skills that person might develop after registration to increase their scope of practice. The guidance lists reserve duties which they can only practice if they are registered in a particular group. So if someone wants to carry out these extra duties they would need to receive further training and gain a qualification which would allow them to register in a different registry group.

Clearly there are training issues here. Peter Catchpole, a lay member of the GDC, quoted by Mathewson and Rudkin (2008), emphasises that it is not just the tasks themselves that are relevant, the patient's whole oral health background matters. Catchpole is concerned that someone might learn the skills to clean someone's teeth but also needs to take into account the general health of the patient and to obtain consent. He argues that, for patient safety reasons, dental staff should not move from one professional title to another without undertaking a full programme or course. The patient's needs underpin everything: 'There is a need to ensure the patients in the dental chair are safe no matter who is treating them' (p. 572).

In an interview, Anthony Townsend (2005), former Registrar of the GDC, talked about commonalities in the building blocks such as in areas of science and issues to do with confidentiality and consent which would provide common ground across the curricula of DCPs and dentists. Suitable training modules for therapists alongside dental students and a transferable credit system would enable DCPs, using a skills escalator model, to progress into new areas of enhanced responsibility and even eventually become dentists if they wished. This would mean adopting more widely the modular approach to educational provision, which is now well established in other areas including those associated with health care. Such developments are more achievable where the different professions operate under a single regulatory umbrella than is likely to be the case where different regulatory bodies are involved, which is usually the position where professionals come together. In these latter circumstances, there is less likely to be mutual confidence and respect across professional boundaries.

However, as the case examples show, in reality much interprofessional working does take place outside this dental family and the issues which will now be considered, primarily, in the context of the inner (dental) ring apply substantially also to work in the outer ring, the wider health and social care field.

Collaboration

The distinctions of interprofessional, interdisciplinary, multi-professional and multidisciplinary working are not ones that have taxed writers in the dental field to date and the terms tend to be used interchangeably. For convenience the term interprofessional will be used in this chapter.

For dentistry, as in other service contexts, interprofessional working involves members of the dental practice team, each with a separate role but with shared ownership of the service's common purpose, having a planned team approach to delivering dental treatment. As Pirrie et al. (1998) argue, in order for this to work effectively the team must work together and learn together to fully understand each other's separate but interrelated roles and responsibilities, distinctive areas of competence and the contributions which each discipline makes. For example, in the surgery patients present with diverse dental needs and aspirations. Complex restorative work undertaken by the dentist or a specialist is only sustainable when underpinned by oral health education to ensure patient understanding and motivation. In the case of many young patients, who have been exposed to fluoride throughout their lives, there will be little need for invasive work and their needs can be managed by therapist, hygienist and oral health educator after assessment by the dentist.

Clearly, also, it is essential not to forget that patients are part of the team. In The doctor's communication handbook, Peter Tate (2002), in his discussion of patient relationships, emphasises the need to involve patients in decision making to foster patient autonomy and to increase patient self-reliance. He stresses the need for practitioners to be aware of their own power and to demonstrate understanding and empathy.

The importance of patient involvement, now a central agenda in all health and social care provision, has been given prominence in the GDC's standards guidance for dental professionals (General Dental Council, 2005). It states the need to:

- respect the patient's dignity and choices
- recognise patient's responsibility for making decisions about their bodies

319

Exercise 24.1

How would you go about helping the patient to feel part of the team when commencing assessment and treatment?

- treat patients fairly and in line with the law
- listen to patients and give them the information they need to make appropriate decisions.

The application of these principles by the dental team itself and in its collaborations with other health and social care professionals is shown in a range of practice settings in the case examples.

Possibilities for interprofessional working within dentistry

Over recent years there have been a number of changes to the regulatory framework, which means that there is less restriction on delivering dental care, providing opportunities to increase the range of dental professionals in the dental team. This has brought about a change of culture. However, other factors have also been instrumental in bringing about change:

- Interprofessional working, maximising the skills of the whole dental team, has been prompted by the projected demographic shift in the ageing population. Health needs and demand are outstripping the capacity of the established professions to provide full and responsive services in their traditional format. Attention has turned to the role of allied and complimentary professionals (see Ward, 2006).
- The advent of fluoride toothpaste and heightened awareness of the importance of diet and oral hygiene have meant that many of the population will be dentally fit. For these patients ongoing prevention and the use of simple protective techniques, along with regular screening by the dentist to discount any serious oral disease, will keep their mouths healthy. This section of the population could be serviced by suitably trained DCPs.

- The Darzi report (2008) included a quality agenda across the health service which had application to general dental practitioners in England. It advocates:
  - easier access to primary care
  - an increasingly multidisciplinary primary care workforce
  - an increased range of health care services provided by primary care practitioners in primary care settings
  - an independent review of NHS dental services.

The Steele report (Steele, 2009) highlighted the issues of interprofessional working within the dental team:

> Good oral health depends on more than just access: prevention and high-quality provision are also essential. These are related concepts which depend on the dental profession and the dental team working towards a common oral health goal. (p. 6) . . . Outstanding practices (are) led by exceptional people with a strong personal healthcare ethic. The services they provide are as good as you will find anywhere. The staff in such practices work together as a team, are well looked after and are very well supported to develop their careers (p. 27).
>
> [However] a frequently cited view is that the current contractual system does not support the use of an extended team business model. Dentists have mixed views about how or even whether to use this diverse workforce but some are doing so imaginatively and successfully (p. 31).

Furthermore, the General Dental Council has set out a statement outlining the principles of dental team working (2006):

- Good dental care is delivered by a dental team.
- The quality of teamwork is closely linked to the quality of care that the team provides.
- All members of the dental team contribute towards patient care.
- Effective communication is essential.
- All members of the dental team are individually responsible and accountable for their own actions and for the treatment and processes which they carry out.
- As a registered dental professional a member is also responsible for the actions of any member of

the team they lead or manage who delivers care to the patients.

- All members of the team should take part in continuing professional development to update their knowledge and skills.

These principles resonate closely with notions of interprofessional and interdisciplinary working as the following example, drawn from outside dentistry, illustrates. Parsloe (1981) sees advantage in the football team analogy in which members bring together differing experiences, qualifications and methods of working. In such a team, she argues, group members work together, are dependent on each other's skills and draw strength from their experiences within the group.

Returning to dentistry, Lambert-Humble, in Teamwork (2003) stresses that a dental team, to be successful, must be pulling in the same direction and be working for, as well as with, one another. Arjuna Aluwihare, Professor Emeritus, Sri Lanka, speaking to the Faculty of General Dental Practitioners in 2005, felt that a surgical team could take lessons from white-water rafting: they have to take responsibility for their colleagues, a member cannot bail out and duck responsibility halfway through and there must be lifejackets for safety (Alluwihare, 2006). Professor Aluwihare also added that an important lesson learned from working within a small clinical team is that there are dangers if one member tries to be duly prominent. Interestingly this was paralleled in the comments of de Ronde (2008) about the Oxford and Cambridge boat race, in which an Olympic rower was removed from one of the teams because his exceptional prowess meant that he did not sit comfortably with the other team members.

An example from within the author's experience was, as previously noted, the establishment of her practice as a field site piloting new ways of delivering dentistry under the aegis of the government's Modernisation Agency. One of the aims of the field site was to make maximum use of DCPs utilising the best skill mix available for routine care. A dental therapist successfully took over many of the routine tasks and responsibilities which had previously been undertaken by the dentists in order to free up the dentists' time for more technically demanding work. The therapist, newly out of dental school, was well trained in patient management and patient education and in using the least invasive techniques in restorative work. The dental therapist had previously worked as a dental nurse, oral health educator and practice manager which gave her the capacity to understand, empathise and relate to the work of the other DCPs.

As required by the GDC regulations, the dental therapist remained accountable to the dentist who continued to be responsible for diagnosis and treatment planning. Clearly the roles of dentist and dental therapist overlap and every member of the practice team was aware of which activities, be they hands on or about general health and consent, should be reserved for the dentist or could be taken on themselves.

Gains and losses

Reflecting on teamworking, Gratton makes an observation which could equally well be found in any discussion of interprofessional work:

> The creation of value and innovation rarely springs from personal individual endeavour. The productive capacity of the team reflects the competencies and skills of members to work together, learn about each other, resolve their conflicts and manage the rhythm and pacing of work.
>
> (Gratton, 2007)

In the opening chapter of this book the editor, Roger Smith, talks about improving the quality, productivity and efficiency of a process by breaking it down into smaller straightforward tasks. This process, described as 'commerce industrialisation', has been discussed in relation to dentistry (Cottingham and Toy, 2009) focusing on the apparent economic benefits of division of labour as posited by Adam Smith some 200 years ago. In dentistry many aspects involve carrying out relatively simple repetitive and time-consuming procedures and Bain (2003) argues that it is in everybody's interests that available time is used efficiently and, when a procedure can be effectively delegated to a DCP, this should be done.

However, this is not to devalue such tasks, which are necessary for the sustainability of more complex and technical work. Indeed, as Roger Smith states in his introduction, it would be seen as over-simplifying to transfer lessons simplistically from industry to health. This draws attention again to the significance, complexities and continuing debate about the processes of interprofessional working.

In his book *The Craftsman*, Sennett (2008) talks about the art of diagnosis and discusses practice wisdom. He argues that it is a very personal process and experience. He talks of the 'craftsmanship' involved in engaging with patients, driven by curiosity, retaining the ability to learn by ambiguity. He talks of the subtle and practiced interplay between tacit knowledge and self-conscious awareness. Perhaps an interprofessional teamwork approach to delivering health care carries a danger of diluting the unique patient–practitioner relationship and inhibiting the development of the skills to which Sennett refers. Certainly this would be the case if an industrial perspective prevailed. In turn this draws attention to team leadership and practice management skills which, until recently, have not been prominent in the dental curriculum.

Professional development for dentists has often been viewed as an individual personal responsibility and activity (Bruce, 2005). However, the professional role of dentist now involves cross-boundaries with responsibilities for the whole dental team and for colleagues in the local dental community. Team rather than individual training opportunities are becoming increasingly available. These may be formal and outside the practice, but can also include ongoing audit and governance activities. Demonstrating the continuing importance of interpersonal group learning, it can be taken as an opportunity for members to have the opportunity to discuss and learn together, cross boundaries and see the components of dental care from different perspectives. As it becomes established as a familiar and routine activity, it empowers both dentists and team members to shape collectively their future behaviour (Bruce, 2005, p. 141).

Routine opportunities arise in medical emergencies and cross-infection control training. In addition, in the author's own practice, the practice team worked together to achieve Investors in People accreditation

and to sustain the internal staff development processes to maintain the standard.

Such learning is grounded on social interaction and points towards the development of what have been conceptualised elsewhere as 'communities of practice' (Wenger (1999) in McHarg and Kay, 2008, p. 636). Here, in order to share knowledge and develop a working relationship with one's peers, trust is generated and the challenge of operating across boundaries is valued (Gratton, 2007).

Concerns for the future

However, even as interest in inter-and multi-professional working has increased in many areas of health service work, the emerging evidence suggests, in dentistry no less than other settings, that neither professional groups nor individual practitioners find this an easy task (Grace 2004). Difficulties arise in three areas of the practice landscape:

■ *The structural context:* existing professionals may fear the prospect of finding themselves with 'new' professionals in a marketplace and vying for the same resources. This leads to protectionism when sharing of resources is actually what is required. In the contract with the NHS, the financial reward system is tied into targets which only dentists can deliver. It has been suggested, therefore, that DCPs are not cost-effective (see Ward, 2006). However, concurring with Holt (2004), this results from assessing therapist activity quantitatively, an approach that does not value the whole therapist package which emphasises patient management and preventative education.

■ *The cultural context:* different interests, professional values and occupational cultures can militate against collaboration. As a result staff are reluctant to collaborate in the face of what can be perceived as challenges to their identity and sphere of exclusive activity. Historically the whole clinical experience for the patient has been in the hands of the dentist and few dentists have received the management training to involve DCPs in patient care. Many dentists, therefore, would in effect protect their territory by instinctively questioning the capacity of 'new' professionals to do the job to the same standard.

- *The skills context:* there has been little investment in developing the capacity of institutions or the skills, knowledge and attitudes needed among staff if they are to work collaboratively. Processes and skills for creating clarity, becoming explicit about roles and developing working arrangements are underdeveloped (Payne, 2005). Many providers of CPD are responding to dentist's own personal development plans. Interprofessional working does not currently feature high on the list of priorities. However, the picture is not altogether bleak. Teamwork and working with other health care professions are now included in undergraduate dental curricula and in compulsory training undertaken immediately after qualification.

Challenges for the future

Providing leadership

As clinicians with responsibility and professional and public accountability for patients, dentists find themselves as de facto leaders of multidisciplinary practice teams comprising dental nurses, hygienists, dental therapists, dental technicians and reception and administrative staff. With the extension of professional registration to nurses and other ancillary staff in the professions complementary to dentistry, members of these groups are becoming increasingly conscious of their own professional status and areas of expertise.

Leading such a team requires strong personal organisation, sound professional judgement and the ability to respond immediately to complex events – to think, act and communicate (Bruce, 2005; Dental Vocational Training Authority, 2003). Gratton (2007, p. 149) outlines the qualities she has recognised in leaders in successful private companies: courage and the confidence to ask the hard questions, to see old problems in new ways and to use discipline and rigour to get at the heart of issues; stimulating the creation of personal networks and friendships that encourage others to value the relational element of the

organisation and the maintenance of networks within and beyond it; the championing of practices that resonate with the values of the organisation and their own personal beliefs and vision. Hocken (2009), a dentist himself, describes such an approach as 'inspirational leadership', a method that blends the positive aspects of autocratic and democratic leadership and avoids the pitfalls of a laissez-faire style (Lewin *et al.*, 1939).

Applying these ideas to dentistry, it is possible to identify an agenda for developing competent and effective interprofessional leadership which applies to both the dental team and collaboration with colleagues in the wider health and social care field. However, besides the professionals, as the case examples show, there is also the question of effectively involving patients and their carers as committed partners if health, including dental health, objectives are to be achieved. In the author's practice, this entailed the collaboration described at the clinical level and, additionally, as an aspect of the Modernisation Project field site, instituting a patient consultative council and acquiring patient feedback through questionnaires and focus groups.

Role awareness

It is necessary to give dental teams the attitudes and managerial expertise to employ skill mix effectively and efficiently. Not only does the dentist need educating but also continuing professional development programmes need to be in place for the whole of the dental team to give opportunities for team members to enhance their skills, increase their awareness of the current best practice guidelines and to develop a culture of cross-boundary working.

Public protection measures

Greater teamwork and interprofessional working has implications for registration and indemnification.

Exercise 24.2

Dentists may not be viewed as a natural part of the collaborative team by other professionals. In what ways might you go about challenging this kind of implicit assumption?

A team member registered with the General Dental Council is responsible for their own acts and omissions. However, there is always a concern to the dentist who can be held vicariously liable for treatment provided by DCPs. Indemnification is required through the Dental Protection Societies but clearly this comes at a cost. Protecting patients in line with the GDC's guidance increases the costs of oral health. As a *British Dental Journal* editorial states (Hancocks, 2009, p. 301) having skilled, knowledgeable and experienced individuals does not come cheap.

The patient experience

Conventionally, patients have had a unique relationship with a single practitioner. Many will have developed confidence and trust in their 'own' dentist: someone they are happy to communicate with; from whom they are confident to receive treatment and to whom they will look for continuing aftercare. To move from this to a more dispersed team-based approach is likely to be a surprise at least, perhaps alarming, for some (Bakewell, 2006, p. 34).

A closer look

Elderly patients and continuing care

Demographic shifts mean that there are a lot more elderly people in the community. This has a significant effect on dentistry. People who were young adults at the inception of health service dentistry after the Second World War are now in their seventies and eighties and provide huge challenges to the dental profession (McHarg and Kay, 2009). Many continue to be dentate with the result that the dentist has to deal with restorations of huge complexity but, as they become more frail, there is a reduction in the ability to self-care. Very elderly people might be resident in sheltered accommodation, residential homes or nursing homes and there is a variety of levels of independence for the individual which can affect their oral hygiene, denture hygiene and their food choices (Preston, 2010).

There are many diseases that become more prevalent as people get older, some of which can directly or indirectly affect oral health. Dentists will increasingly find themselves treating older patients with complex medical histories which may include autoimmune diseases, cancers, coronary heart disease, stroke, the dementias, Parkinson's disease, Alzheimer's disease, chronic obstructive airways disease and diabetes mellitus, to mention but a few. When the history is unclear it may be necessary for the dental practitioner communicate with the doctor.

Other reasons for contacting the medical practitioner might be when the patient is unable to complete medical history; the patient cannot provide the name of a prescription drug they are taking; when the dentist identifies something that needs medical attention; when the patient presents a medical situation that might need special treatment considerations or when it is unclear if the patient is fit for elective surgical procedures (Bain, 2003).

Patients of advancing years require special care when prescribing medicines (Department of Health, 2001). Elderly patients often receive multiple drugs for multiple conditions: polypharmacy. Not only does this affect the way the dentist manages the patient but many of the drugs cause reduced salivary flow which can be very distressing to the patient and which, together with the sugar in many medications, affects the tooth decay process. Communicating with the pharmacist is an essential part of a dentist's practising life.

There are times where it is necessary for the dentist to liaise with a dietician to ensure that the old person who probably has fewer teeth and reduced chewing capacity receives the easier to eat foods necessary for good health.

The ability of the salivary glands to keep the mouth moist decreases with age and this, combined with the medicines mentioned above, can produce a problem for an older patient. Occasionally radiotherapy regimes can also effect the oral environment.

The dental team often feel that it is necessary to involve a carer, either formerly or informally, in the supervision and ultimately the provision of oral hygiene for the older patient. When this stage occurs the dentist or oral health educator has an important role in educating the carer in the most appropriate strategies for the provision of oral health care to another. Unfortunately there may be a problem with acceptance among old people as the provision of personal oral health care by another can be seen as yet another aspect of failing health and loss of autonomy.

In such circumstances, the importance of effective communication both with the patient, in explaining any new arrangements, and the consistency of messages from across the team, cannot be underestimated. Patients are likely to have at least one of three areas of concern: quality of treatment and pain control, timeliness and sequencing of appointments and financial costs. It is important that all team members can deal with these consistently and accurately face-to-face. In support of this personal rapport, the author, when introducing an interprofessional approach to her practice under the Modernisation Agency pilot project, produced a leaflet for patients of the practice and an explanatory video which played in the waiting room. In addition, all staff attended away-days at various points in the implementation of the project and, indeed, as an interprofessional team, presented the project to wider audiences at national conferences. The belief was that buy-in and satisfaction among patients would be best ensured if mirrored by effective communication and strong commitment among the team.

Clearly, to protect patients and to provide a good experience, as discussed already, it is crucial to ensure consistency in the quality of care delivered across the members of the interprofessional team. All team members must be confident about their own role and the role of their colleagues. Not everyone may have the same motivation for crossing boundaries and challenges may arise, particularly when integrating newcomers to the team. These are common challenges in all interprofessional working.

NHS funding systems within dentistry

The funding system needs to encourage the greater use of other professionals. This is one of two fundamental problems with the use of DCPs currently. Unlike the situation in general medical practice, where incentives exist both to employ and to refer to other health care professionals, currently there is a financial disincentive for general dental practitioners to refer any work to their DCP. The second difficulty

to greater use of DCP is the size of the workforce: are there enough DCPs to go around? According to the Workforce Numbers Advisory Board, in November 2004, there were 348 dental therapists on the register although, at the present time, there is very little information on how many are in general practice.

Registering the whole dental team

There is a need to clarify for all members what the ground rules are. The outgoing chairman of the GDC acknowledges the need to define roles clearly and explore dental relationships both within the dental team and outside of dental care (Mathewson and Rudkin, 2008). Within dental care, the General Dental Council has moved from providing a list of permitted duties to stating that DCPs could work within the limits of their competence, thus regulating through ethical guidance and curricula, to the current *Scope of practice*. This identifies core skills and abilities for each group but acknowledges that 'registrants might expand their scope by developing new skills' (General Dental Council, 2009, p. 3). There was a concern that the original position stunted innovation, the next was vague and unclear. The current statement has provided greater clarity.

Conclusion

Thirty years ago the majority of patients had dental health problems which were middling in their complexity, and culturally it was acceptable for people to lose teeth and wear dentures in middle age. This state of affairs has long gone. In the next 30 years patients will have very different dental needs from those of today. Those who were middle-aged in the 1970s and 1980s, with healthy heavily restored mouths, will have become elderly and are likely to have retained their teeth. Dentistry has never before had to face the prospect of a large cohort of people who are likely to live to extreme old age and to be dentate. This group of people have extremely complicated oral health needs and require complex restorative techniques. Making space for use of the skills of the dental team in terms of prevention and carrying out the simpler dentistry will free up the dentists to undertake the complex restorative work they will require.

Although it is clear that different procedures can be delivered by different members of the dental team with different levels of training, it is necessary that **all members of the team should have acquired the knowledge, skills and attitudes to manage a complex cohort of patients**. However, the horizon stretches beyond the dental team. There is the wider canvas upon which patient's needs and services to meet them exist. In a world where there is greater integration between health and social services planning and provision, who will be our colleagues and how do we interact with them in addressing this task? What are our responsibilities? What is the expectation of a dental care professional in assessing, monitoring and coordinating patient need in partnership with other professionals, service users and carers?

In this expanded world, **each team member will need a high level of communication skills, verbal, non-verbal and written. They will need to appreciate the social environment of their patients**. They will require knowledge of medicine and pharmacy and the ability to deal with medical emergencies and to manage complex drug interactions. They will be involved in designing packages of care and managing the implementation of those packages in association with both clinical staff – the dental specialists, medical practitioner, pharmacist, the dental technician and the dietician, with non-clinical staff: the social worker, care home staff, the learning disability team and, crucially, with the patients themselves and their carers.

Dental practitioners in this new world will need to show respect for the individual, to demonstrate sound judgement and to deal with differences in opinion and, above all, to have a realisation that the patient is centre-stage. They will need the skills to review and monitor service delivery. They will need to participate in teamworking and team training. They will require an interprofessional perspective, skills and mentality.

In an editorial in the *British Dental Journal*, Hancocks (2009, p. 301) argues that, if the true status of the dental team is to be apparent, extolled and appreciated it also has to have investment, a degree of openness and greater acknowledgement than has been fully forthcoming to date.

Finally, it seems that a number of recent developments have begun to transform relationships between dentistry and the wider professional environment. For instance, although dentistry has been thought of traditionally as a solitary occupation, modern dentists are increasingly thinking and working 'outside the box'. **Interprofessional work in dentistry takes place both within the dental family and with other health and social care professionals**. So, in the latter case, dentists find themselves dealing directly with the consequences of violence and abuse; they have an important role in the care of the elderly.

Contemporary dentistry also involves managing both an ageing population that presents increasingly complex needs and a younger group who predominantly require monitoring and often very little dental intervention. Using a team approach ensures equal emphasis is given to prevention of dental disease and maintenance of oral health while freeing up the dentist's time to deal with the more technically demanding work. **To achieve effective interprofessional working, attention must be given to the development of competent and effective interprofessional leadership.** This applies to the contexts of both the dental team itself and to that of collaboration with colleagues in the wider health and social care field.

Further reading

General Dental Council (2006) *Standards Guidance: Principles of Dental Team Working*, London: GDC.

Gratton, L. (2007) *Hot Spots: Why Some Companies Buzz with Energy and Innovation and – Others Don't*. Harlow: Pearson Education. Although not directly on the topics of dentistry or inter professional working, I found this book thought-provoking, inspirational and applicable to my thinking on these issues.

Lambert-Humble, S. (2003) Teamwork, in P. Rothwell (ed.) *Pathways in Practice, volume 2,* London: Faculty of General Dental Practitioners (UK).

Ward, P. (2006) The changing skill-mix – experiences on the introduction of the dental therapist into general dental practice, *British Dental Journal* 200, 93–197.

References

Alluwihare, A. (2006) Teams and surgery, *Bulletin of the Royal College of Surgeons of England* 88 (3), 82–3.

Bain, C. (2003) *Treatment Planning in General Dental Practice*, London: Churchill Livingstone.

Bakewell, J. (2006) *View from Here: Life at Seventy*, London: Atlantic Books.

Bruce, M. (2005) Assessment within a values-based curriculum pilot in dental vocational training, *VT Newsletter* October, 2.

COPDEND (2006) *Child Protection and the Dental Team*, http://www.cpdt.org.uk.

Cottingham, J. and Toy, A. (2009) The industrialisation of the dental profession, *British Dental Journal* 206, 347–50.

Darzi, Professor the Lord Darzi of Denham KBE (2008) *High Quality Care For All. NHS Next Stage Review Final Report*, London: The Stationery Office.

Dental Vocational Training Authority (2003) *Curriculum, Quality, Assessment: A Consultation Paper on Dental Vocational Training in the NHS GDS*, Eastbourne: DVTA.

Department of Health (2001) Medicines for older people, in *National Service for Older People*, London: Department of Health.

Department of Health (2002) *NHS Dentistry: Options for Change*, London: Department of Health.

de Ronde (2008) *The Last Amateurs: To Hell and Back with the Cambridge Boat Race Crew*, Thriplow, Cambs: Icon Books (as reported during Radio 4 discussion).

General Dental Council (2005) *Standards Guidance: Standards for Dental Professionals*, London: General Dental Council.

General Dental Council (2006) *Standards Guidance: Principles of Dental Team Working*, London: General Dental Council.

General Dental Council (2009) *Scope of Practice*, London: General Dental Council.

Grace, M. (2004) Cost-effective teamwork, *British Dental Journal* 197, 447.

Gratton, L. (2007) *Hot Spots: Why Some Companies Buzz with Energy and Innovation and – Others Don't*, Harlow: Pearson Education.

Hancocks, S. (2009) Does the team think? *British Dental Journal* 207, 301.

Hocken, C. (2009) Lead! Don't manage, *BDA News* 22 (12), 11–12.

Holt, R. D. (2004) Cost-effectiveness study of therapists in general practice (comment on Harris and Burnside), *British Dental Journal* 197, 477.

Lambert-Humble, S. (2003) Teamwork, in P. Rothwell (ed.) *Pathways in Practice, volume 2*, London: Faculty of General Dental Practitioners (UK).

Lewin, K., LIippit, R. and White, R. K. (1939) Patterns of aggressive behaviour in experimentally created social climates, *Journal of Social Psychology* 10, 271–301.

Mathewson, H. and Rudkin, D. (2008) The GDC – lifting the lid. Part One: professionalism and standards, *British Dental Journal* 204, 571–4.

McHarg, J. and Kay, E. (2008) The anatomy of a new dental curriculum, *British Dental Journal* 204, 635–8.

McHarg, J. and Kay, E. (2009) Designing a dental curriculum for the 21st century, *British Dental Journal* 207, 493–7.

Mossy, P. (2004) The changing face of dental education, *British Dental Journal Education and Training Supplement* 3–4.

Nettleton, S. (1992) *Power, Pain and Dentistry*, Buckingham: Open University Press.

Parsloe, P. (1981) *Social Services Area Teams*, London: Allen and Unwin.

Payne, M. (2005) *Skills for Collaborative Working: Proposal to the Learning Partnership, Leicester/Leicestershire*, Leicester: School of Applied Social Sciences, De Montfort University.

Pirrie, A., Wilson, V., Harden, R. M. and Elsegood, J. (1998) AMEE Guide No. 12: multiprofessional education: part 2 – promoting cohesive practice in health care, *Medical Teacher* 20: 409–16.

Preston, T. (2010) The considerations in the management of the elderly patient in restorative dentistry, *Dental Practice* April, 14.

Sennett, R. (2008) *The Craftsman*, London: Allen Lane.

Steele, J. (2009) *NHS Dental Services in England: An Independent Review led by Professor Jimmy Steele*, London: Department of Health.

Tate, P. (2002) *The Doctor's Communication Handbook*, 4th edn, Oxford: Radcliffe Medical Press.

Townsend, A. (2005) Dental nurse to dentist in one easy move? *Vital* Spring, 18–19.

Ward, P. (2006) The changing skill-mix – experiences on the introduction of the dental therapist into general dental practice, *British Dental Journal* 200, 93–197.

Wenger, E. (1999) *Communities of Practice: Learning, Meaning and Identity*, Cambridge: Cambridge University Press.

Index